CRASH COURSE
Endocrine and Reproductive Systems

Endocrine and Reproductive Systems

J. Gary Meszaros, PhD

Department of Physiology and Pharmacology
Northeastern Ohio Universities College of Medicine
Rootstown, Ohio

Student authors
Erik R. Olson and Jennifer E. Naugle

UK edition authors
Stephan Sanders and Madeleine Debuse

UK series editor
Daniel Horton-Szar

ELSEVIER
MOSBY

ELSEVIER
MOSBY

1600 John F. Kennedy Blvd.
Ste 1800
Philadelphia, PA 19103-2899

CRASH COURSE: ENDOCRINE AND REPRODUCTIVE SYSTEMS   ISBN-13: 978-1-4160-2961-8
Copyright 2006, Elsevier, Inc. All rights reserved.   ISBN-10: 1-4160-2961-3

Notice

Knowledge and best practice in this field are constantly changing. As new research and experience broaden our knowledge, changes in practice, treatment and drug therapy may become necessary or appropriate. Readers are advised to check the most current information provided (i) on procedures featured or (ii) by the manufacturer of each product to be administered, to verify the recommended dose or formula, the method and duration of administration, and contraindications. It is the responsibility of the practitioner, relying on their own experience and knowledge of the patient, to make diagnoses, to determine dosages and the best treatment for each individual patient, and to take all appropriate safety precautions. To the fullest extent of the law, neither the Publisher nor the Author assumes any liability for any injury and/or damage to persons or property arising out or related to any use of the material contained in this book.

The Publisher

Adapted from Crash Course Endocrine and Reproductive Systems 2e by Stephan Sanders, ISBN: 0-7234-3245-7. © 2003, Elsevier Science Limited. All rights reserved.

The rights of Stephan Sanders to be identified as the author of this work have been asserted by him in accordance with the Copyright, Designs and Patents Act, 1988.

Library of Congress Cataloging-in-Publication Data
Meszaros, J. Gary.
    Endocrine and reproductive systems / J. Gary Meszaros, Erik R. Olson, Jennifer E. Naugle.—1st ed.
        p. ; cm.—(Crash course)
    Includes index.
    ISBN 1-4160-2961-3
    1. Endocrinology. 2. Endocrine glands. 3. Human reproduction—Endocrine aspects. I. Olson, Erik R. II. Naugle, Jennifer E. III. Title. IV. Series
    [DNLM: 1. Endocrine System. 2. Genitalia. WK 100 M586e 2006]
    QP187.M47 2006
    612.4—dc22   2005052213

Commissioning Editor: *Alex Stibbe*
Project Development Manager: *Stan Ward*
Project Manager: *David Saltzberg*
Designer: *Andy Chapman*
Cover Design: *Antbits Illustration*
Illustration Manager: *Mick Ruddy*

Printed in China

Last digit is the print number:
9 8 7 6 5 4 3 2 1

Preface

The endocrine system controls a multitude of complex physiological functions in a highly directed and coordinated manner. To this end, the endocrine system can be viewed as "the ultimate" in integrative physiology, and a sound base of knowledge in the anatomy and physiology of nearly all systems throughout the body is needed to fully understand the endocrine system. In addition to this knowledge base, there are several hormones, mechanisms, and functions within the study of endocrinology that must be committed to memory; at the same time, they must be applied to the overall goal of maintaining homeostasis throughout the body.

Crash Course: Endocrine and Reproductive Systems is designed to provide a clear and concise outline of endocrine and reproductive physiology and should be a valuable study guide for medical school courses as well as board examinations. Basic principles are covered along with topics in clinical medicine, and relevant review items and study questions are included to provide important and immediate feedback to facilitate preparation for examinations. Ample figures, diagrams, and charts are supplied as additional streams of information and visualization.

We wish all of our readers the best luck in their future careers!

J. Gary Meszaros, PhD
Erik R. Olson
Jennifer E. Naugle

Acknowledgments

We should like to thank Alex Stibbe and Stan Ward for this opportunity and for their feedback and assistance with this project. Thanks also to the authors and editors of the UK editions: Stephan Sanders, Susan Whiten, Daniel Horton-Szar, and Madeleine Debuse.

Contents

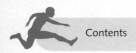

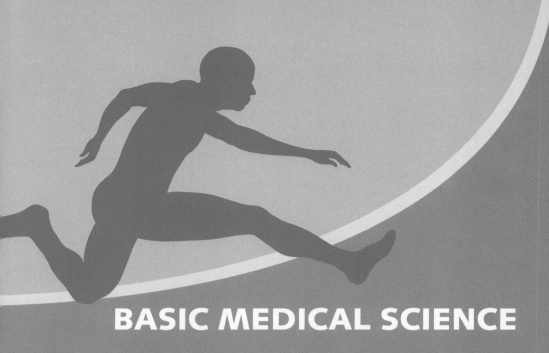

BASIC MEDICAL SCIENCE

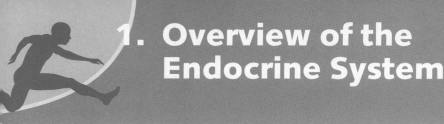

1. Overview of the Endocrine System

The role of the endocrine system

The endocrine system allows cells to communicate using chemical messengers called hormones. This communication is essential for the maintenance of homeostasis (Greek for "staying the same"). Homeostasis is an ongoing process that minimizes change from the ideal physiological conditions, creating a suitable environment for life. As a result, hormones are important components of all major body systems; you cannot escape them.

The endocrine system also regulates long-term changes in the body, including:
- Growth.
- Sexual development.
- Pregnancy.

After reading this chapter you should be able to:
- Explain what is meant by the term "hormone."
- Picture the general organization of the endocrine system.
- Understand how hormone secretion is controlled.
- Describe the synthesis of the main types of hormones.
- Understand how these hormones act through their cellular receptors.
- Discuss the integration and role of the endocrine and nervous systems.

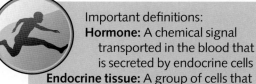

Important definitions:
Hormone: A chemical signal transported in the blood that is secreted by endocrine cells
Endocrine tissue: A group of cells that secrete hormones
Target cell: A cell that responds to a specific hormone
Receptor: A protein in target cells that recognizes and binds hormones
Second messenger: A chemical that transmits the hormone message from the receptor to the effector
Effector: A protein regulated by a hormone that mediates the cellular effects

Hormones and endocrine secretion

Hormones
Classical definition
Classically a hormone is described as a chemical substance that is secreted by specialized endocrine cells directly into the blood to exert an effect on distant target cells.

The word "endocrine" means "internal secretion," while "hormone" is derived from the Greek verb *hormao*, meaning "I excite."

Modern definition
Recent research has revealed many locally acting chemical substances that have challenged the

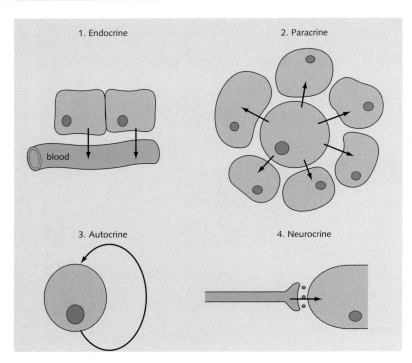

1. Endocrine   2. Paracrine

blood

3. Autocrine   4. Neurocrine

Fig. 1.1 The routes by which chemical signals are delivered to cells.

classical definition of hormones. Four modes of delivery are recognized (Fig. 1.1). They are:
- Endocrine—chemicals that act on distant cells via the blood stream (e.g., thyroxine).
- Paracrine—chemicals that act on the surrounding cells without entering the blood (e.g., gut hormones).
- Autocrine—chemicals that act on the cell from which they are secreted (e.g., nitric oxide).
- Neurocrine—signals between neurons (e.g., neurotransmitters).

Different textbooks suggest different explanations of the term "hormone," ranging from the classical definition to a definition that encompasses all chemical signals external to cells. In a clinical setting, the term "hormone" generally refers to a chemical signal that passes through the blood (endocrine delivery).

Types of hormones
Three classes of hormones are secreted into the blood; the characteristics of these are explained later in the chapter:
- Polypeptides (also called proteins).
- Steroids.
- Modified amino acids.

Endocrine tissues
Definition
An endocrine tissue is one that produces and secretes a hormone. These tissues respond to signals that either stimulate or inhibit the release of the specific hormone.

Arrangement of endocrine tissues
Endocrine tissues contain cells that secrete hormones; these cells can be arranged in three patterns:
- As an endocrine organ devoted to hormone synthesis (e.g., the thyroid gland).
- As clusters of cells within an organ (e.g., the islets of Langerhans in the pancreas).
- Individual cells scattered diffusely throughout an organ (e.g., the gastrointestinal [GI] tract).

Endocrine organs
The term "endocrine organ" originally referred to organs in which specialized endocrine cells formed a significant component. These "traditional" endocrine organs are shown in Fig. 1.2 along with the hormone they secrete.

However, we now know that almost all organs contain some endocrine tissue. For example:

Fig. 1.2 The location of major endocrine organs and the hormones secreted by them.

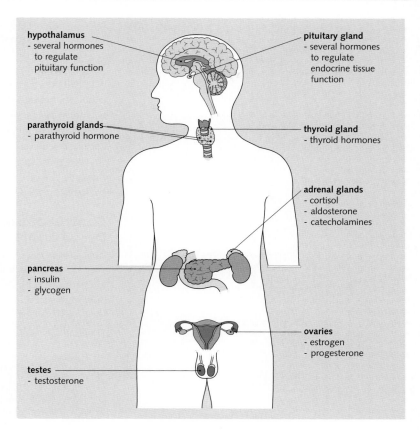

hypothalamus
- several hormones to regulate pituitary function

pituitary gland
- several hormones to regulate endocrine tissue function

parathyroid glands
- parathyroid hormone

thyroid gland
- thyroid hormones

adrenal glands
- cortisol
- aldosterone
- catecholamines

pancreas
- insulin
- glycogen

ovaries
- estrogen
- progesterone

testes
- testosterone

- Adipose tissue secretes leptin.
- Lungs secrete 5-hydroxytryptamine (5-HT; serotonin).
- Heart secretes atrial natriuretic factor (ANF).

Endocrinology is a relatively new medical science. The first hormone was demonstrated in 1902, and the connection between the endocrine and nervous systems through the hypothalamus was not found until halfway through the 20th century.

Organization of the endocrine system

The regulation and control of many major hormones follows a similar pattern that starts in the brain and ends with a hormone being secreted. Understanding this pattern is the key to understanding how the endocrine system works. There are three steps, each of which involves the secretion of a hormone that stimulates the next step (Fig. 1.3). The control of hormones released by the thyroid gland will be used to illustrate this pathway throughout.

The main components
Hypothalamus

The endocrine system is coordinated by the hypothalamus. This is a part of the brain that acts as a bridge between the nervous system and endocrine system, translating neural messages into chemical (hormonal) signals. It initiates the secretion of hormones by controlling the function of the pituitary gland via "releasing hormones." These hormones do not act directly on peripheral endocrine tissues. Hormones secreted from the hypothalamus are released in pulsatile manner, often with a circadian rhythm (regular changes through a 24-hour cycle). Thyrotropin-releasing hormone (TRH) is secreted

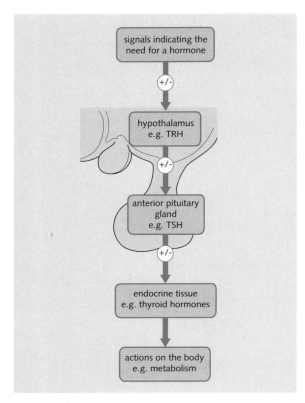

signals indicating the
need for a hormone

+/-

hypothalamus
e.g. TRH

+/-

anterior pituitary
gland
e.g. TSH

+/-

endocrine tissue
e.g. thyroid hormones

actions on the body
e.g. metabolism

Fig. 1.3 The organization of the endocrine system.

into the blood by the hypothalamus; this initiates the hormone cascade resulting in the release of thyroid hormones.

Pituitary gland

The pituitary gland is found at the base of the brain beneath the hypothalamus. It releases hormones into the blood in response to signals from the hypothalamus. The hormones from the pituitary gland regulate the function of peripheral endocrine tissues throughout the body. TRH from the hypothalamus acts on the pituitary gland to cause the release of thyroid-stimulating hormone (TSH) into the blood stream.

Peripheral endocrine tissues

The hormones secreted by the pituitary gland act on peripheral endocrine tissues. These tissues respond by increasing or decreasing secretion of specific hormones into the blood. It is the hormones secreted by these peripheral tissues that affect the state of the body by acting on target cells. TSH from the

pituitary gland stimulates the thyroid gland to release thyroid hormones into the blood.

Target cells

The cells that respond to a specific hormone are called its target cells; they can be found anywhere in the body. All target cells have receptors to detect the specific hormone, but the effect of the hormone can vary between cells. Thyroid hormones from the thyroid gland act on almost every cell in the body to increase the rate of metabolism through receptors on the cell surface.

Control of hormone secretion
Overall control

Endocrine tissues are regulated by signals from a variety of neural and systemic sources. These signals are processed by cells to determine the rate of hormone secretion. The strength and importance of the signals varies so that hormone secretion fits the needs of the body.

Hormone secretion rates can vary by the minute, hour, day, month, and stage of life.

Neural control

Higher neural centers can influence the activity of the endocrine system by acting on the hypothalamus. They can increase or decrease the secretion of hypothalamic releasing hormones, which regulate the secretion of pituitary gland hormones. For example, stress or fear will inhibit reproductive hormone secretion, and cold external temperatures will stimulate TRH.

Feedback regulation

An almost universal feature of endocrine system regulation is feedback from the hormones that are released. Feedback regulation occurs by two means:
- Direct—the hormone itself acts on the hypothalamus and pituitary to affect its subsequent release.
- Indirect—the physiological change induced by the hormone affects its further production.

Feedback is usually inhibitory; thus a hormone can inhibit its own production. This process is called

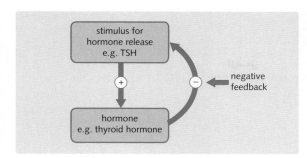

Fig. 1.4 Negative feedback.

negative feedback. It is an essential mechanism that prevents excess secretion of many hormones. The level at which the feedback acts varies between hormones; however, many hormones act at the level of the hypothalamus and pituitary gland. For example, thyroid hormones feed back to the anterior pituitary, where they inhibit the release of TSH (Fig. 1.4).

Why is it so complex?
At first glance the endocrine system seems incredibly complex for no obvious reason. Many students wish that the system had fewer hormones and organs, but there are a number of advantages.

Amplification
As described, endocrine signals begin in the hypothalamus and result in a cascade of hormones from different endocrine glands. There is only a small population of cells in the hypothalamus that secrete each hormone; for example, about 2000 neurons secrete gonadotropin-releasing hormone (GnRH). Because of the small number of cells involved, they are able to respond to important but small neural signals, but they cannot secrete large amounts of hormone.

The very small quantities of hormone secreted directly into the blood stream by the hypothalamus can be detected by the closely related pituitary gland. This gland is able to secrete a greater quantity of hormone than the hypothalamus, but it is still too small to secrete enough for the whole body.

In response to hormones from the pituitary gland the peripheral endocrine tissues secrete hormones in large quantities that can act throughout the body. In this manner the signal of a small number of neurons in the hypothalamus is amplified in three stages to affect the entire body.

Control
The endocrine system regulates all major body processes that are essential for life, including:
- Metabolic rate.
- Nutrient levels.
- Cardiac output and blood pressure.
- Reproduction.

Since they are so important, these processes must be controlled very tightly. The complex interactions of the endocrine system allow for many sites of regulation in order to prevent excessive or deficient hormone release and to maintain homeostasis.

Hormone types and secretion

This section describes the properties and synthesis of the three classes of hormone (Fig. 1.5).

Polypeptide hormones
As their name suggests, polypeptide hormones are proteins that act as hormones. The size of the polypeptide varies widely from 3 to 200 amino acid residues; they cannot pass through cell membranes owing to their size and water-soluble nature. Protein hormones are the most numerous type (often a safe bet in an exam). Accordingly, they are secreted by many glands, including:
- Hypothalamus—TRH, GnRH, growth hormone-releasing hormone (GHRH), etc.
- Pituitary—TSH, follicle-stimulating hormone (FSH), luteinizing hormone (LH), oxytocin, etc.
- Pancreas and GI tract—insulin, glucagon, cholecystokinin (CCK), etc.

Synthesis
Polypeptide hormones are synthesized in the same manner as any other protein. DNA in the nucleus is transcribed to mRNA, which is translated into the protein by ribosomes. The protein is then processed by the Golgi apparatus and stored in secretory granules. Many hormones undergo modification in the Golgi apparatus or secretory granules, including:
- Cleavage reactions to free a smaller polypeptide hormone from the larger prohormone.
- Addition of carbohydrate groups to form glycoproteins.

Fig. 1.5 Comparison of the different types of hormones.

Comparison of different types of hormone			
	Polypeptides	Modified amino acids	Steroids
Size	Medium–large	Very small	Small
Ability to cross cell membrane	×	✓	✓
Receptor type	Cell-surface	Cell-surface or intracellular	Intracellular
Soluble in:	Water	Water	Fat
Action	Protein activation	Protein activation or synthesis	Protein synthesis
Transport in the blood	Dissolved in the plasma	Dissolved in the plasma or bound to plasma proteins	Bound to plasma proteins

Secretion

The secretory granules are released by exocytosis, in which the membrane of the granule fuses with the membrane of the cell, causing the contents to be released. This process is triggered by calcium entering the cell. Polypeptide hormone release is controlled mainly by regulating secretion rather than synthesis.

Polypeptide-secreting cells

Polypeptide-secreting cells all have a similar histological appearance (Fig. 1.6):

- Large, prominent nuclei.
- Small amount of cytoplasm.
- Prominent Golgi apparatus.
- Abundant rough endoplasmic reticulum (RER).
- Large numbers of secretory granules.
- Surrounded by fenestrated blood sinusoids.

Steroid hormones

Steroids are small, fat-soluble molecules that can pass through cell membranes but must circulate bound to plasma proteins since they are insoluble in the blood. They are secreted by:

- Adrenal cortex—cortisol and aldosterone.
- Ovaries—estrogen and progesterone.
- Placenta—estrogen and progesterone.
- Testes—testosterone.

Synthesis

Steroids are derived from cholesterol by a series of reactions in the mitochondria and smooth

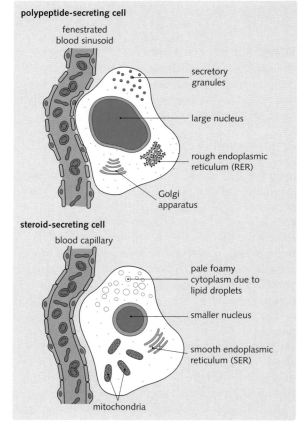

Fig. 1.6 Appearance of a polypeptide-secreting cell and steroid-secreting cell.

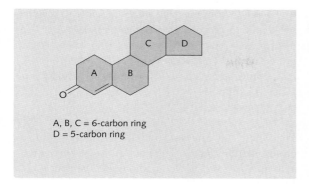

A, B, C = 6-carbon ring
D = 5-carbon ring

Fig. 1.7 Basic structure of a steroid hormone.

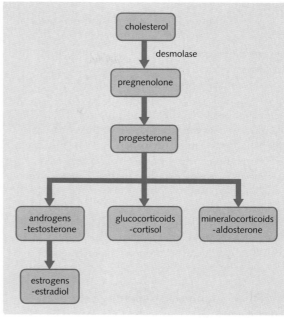

Fig. 1.8 Steroid synthesis. The initial stages are the same for all steroid hormones.

endoplasmic reticulum (SER). Cholesterol is acquired from the diet or synthesized within the cells; it is stored within lipid droplets seen in the cytoplasm of steroid cells. All steroids have the same basic structure formed by four rings of carbon (Fig. 1.7), but individual hormones differ in the following ways:

- Side chains attached to these rings.
- Bonds within the rings (double or single).

The exact sequence of reactions to synthesize each hormone varies, since there are many different enzyme pathways. However, the vast majority of steroid hormones share two common steps.

Step 1

Cholesterol is converted into pregnenolone by desmolase, an enzyme found within the mitochondria of steroid-producing cells. Desmolase removes six carbon atoms from the cholesterol side chain of ring D. This reaction is the rate-limiting step in steroid synthesis.

Step 2

Pregnenolone is converted to progesterone by enzymes found in the mitochondria and cytoplasm. This reaction involves:

- Isomerization—the double bond moves from ring B to ring A.
- Oxidation—the hydroxyl group (—OH) of ring A becomes a keto group ($=O$).

Further steps are highly variable, but the general pattern is shown in Fig. 1.8.

Secretion

The steroid hormone is released immediately so that the rate of release is determined by the rate of synthesis, especially the synthesis of pregnenolone.

Steroid-secreting cells

Steroid-secreting cells also have a similar histological appearance to each other (see Fig. 1.6):

- Small, rounded nuclei.
- Large amount of cytoplasm.
- Large numbers of lipid droplets (foamy appearance).
- Abundant smooth ER.
- Many mitochondria.
- Highly vascularized.

Modified amino acids

Several hormones are formed by altering the structure of amino acids, producing small, water-soluble hormones that can cross cell membranes. They are secreted by the:

- Thyroid gland—T_3 and T_4.
- Adrenal medulla—catecholamines (norepinephrine and epinephrine).
- Hypothalamus—dopamine.
- Pineal gland—melatonin.

Synthesis

These hormones are synthesized from two amino acids:

- Tyrosine—precursor of thyroid hormones, dopamine, and catecholamines.
- Tryptophan—precursor of melatonin and 5-HT.

The reactions to modify these amino acids vary significantly between hormones so the synthesis is described in the individual chapters. The hormones are stored in secretory granules except thyroid hormones, which are unique in that they are stored in follicles.

Secretion

The granules are released by exocytosis in the same way as polypeptide hormones. The rate of release is regulated by negative feedback.

Modified amino acid-secreting cells

The cells that secrete modified amino acid hormones vary more than the cells secreting polypeptide or steroid hormones. However, the following features are often found:

- Large nuclei.
- Many mitochondria.
- Abundant rough ER.
- Prominent Golgi apparatus.
- Large numbers of secretory granules.
- Highly vascularized.

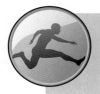

A single hormone may have multiple actions, and multiple hormones may have the same action.

Paracrine hormones

Eicosanoids

Eicosanoids are not always considered as hormones, and they do not fit into any of the main classes of hormones. However, they are important in many physiological processes. They are therefore included in most endocrine courses. They are small, lipid-soluble molecules that act in a paracrine (local) manner. They are derived from a phospholipid found in the cell membrane called arachidonic acid which is broken down by the enzyme phospholipase A_2. There are two pathways, which synthesize different groups of eicosanoids:

- Cyclooxygenase pathway—forms prostaglandins and thromboxanes.
- Lipoxygenase pathway—forms leukotrienes.

Eicosanoids are released immediately and readily cross cell membranes. Their action varies between cells and the specific eicosanoid molecule that is formed.

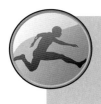

Aspirin and NSAIDs produce their anti-inflammatory action by blocking the cyclooxygenase pathway to prevent prostaglandin synthesis.

Hormone receptors

Target cells possess unique receptors that bind specific hormones; without these receptors the hormones can have no effect. The number of receptors per cell can be increased or decreased to alter the sensitivity of the hormone's effect. Receptors are found in two locations:

- Cell-surface receptors—for polypeptides and catecholamines; they activate or inhibit enzymes, which may affect protein synthesis.
- Intracellular receptors—for steroids and thyroid hormones; they stimulate or inhibit protein synthesis directly by regulating gene transcription.

The response to a hormone varies between target cells so that the same hormone can have different actions on different tissues. This variation is partly due to different receptor types but also the response to receptor stimulation.

Hormones that act via cell-surface receptors can respond faster than those stimulating intracellular receptors because the activation of preexisting enzymes takes less time than synthesizing new proteins. This explains why catecholamines released for the "fight or flight" response use cell-surface receptors, even though they can cross cell membranes.

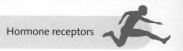

Cell-surface receptors

Cell-surface receptors are necessary for polypeptide hormones, which cannot cross the cell membrane, and catecholamines. The receptor must transmit the external signal into the cell where it can have an effect; therefore, cell-surface receptors are glycoproteins that span the cell membrane to create extracellular and intracellular domains. When the hormone binds to the receptor it triggers a cascade of changes within the cell that alter protein activity. There are two types of cell-surface receptors involved in the endocrine system:

- G-protein coupled receptors.
- Tyrosine kinase receptors.

G-protein coupled receptors

G-protein coupled receptors are extremely common throughout the endocrine system. They consist of two main elements:

- Receptor with seven transmembrane spanning domains.
- Heterotrimeric G-protein.

The receptor is a glycoprotein with a hormone-binding site on the extracellular surface and a G-protein-binding site on the intracellular surface. When the hormone binds, the receptor changes conformation, affecting the attached G-protein.

The G-protein is an enzyme that can break down guanosine triphosphate (GTP); hence the name. It is made of two functional subunits:

- α-subunit—bound to guanosine diphosphate (GDP) in the resting state.
- βγ-complex—bound to the α-subunit if GDP is present.

Binding of a specific ligand induces a conformational change of the receptor, which facilitates exchange of GDP for GTP by the α-subunit of the G-protein. The βγ-complex dissociates from the α-subunit, and both move away from the receptor and bind to intracellular effector proteins.

One critical effector protein of the α-subunit is the enzyme adenylyl cyclase, which synthesizes cyclic AMP (cAMP) from ATP. Cyclic AMP acts as a second messenger, an intracellular chemical signal that activates or inhibits target proteins to mediate the effects of the hormone. The target proteins are often kinases (e.g., protein kinase A), which phosphorylate other downstream proteins to affect their activities.

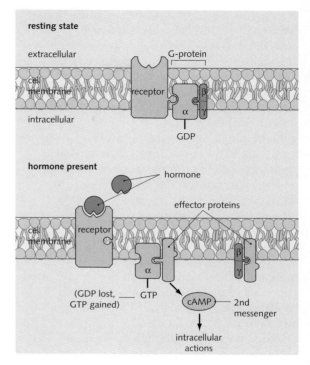

Fig. 1.9 Mechanism of action of a G-protein receptor.

The α-subunit has intrinsic GTPase activity, and a short time after activation it will cleave one phosphate group from the bound GTP, converting it to GDP. The GDP-bound α-subunit then associates with the βγ-complex and the G-protein returns to its inactive resting state. Figure 1.9 shows the action of a Gs (stimulatory of adenylyl cyclase)-coupled protein receptor.

Other G-protein coupled receptors can use different effectors or second messengers, including:

- Inhibition of adenylyl cyclase via Gi.
- Stimulation of inositol triphosphate production and subsequent calcium release via Gq.
- Facilitation of the ion channel opening.

Tyrosine kinase receptors

Insulin and insulin-like growth factors act through tyrosine kinase receptors. These receptors are glycoproteins with kinase activity (ability to add phosphate groups) that is triggered by the binding of the hormone. The receptors phosphorylate each other by adding phosphate to tyrosine residues within their structure. This phosphorylation promotes the association of multiple docking proteins and initiates activation of serine–threonine

11

signaling cascades, including the mitogen-activated protein kinase (MAPK) cascade and the phosphatidylinositol-3-kinase/protein kinase B (P13-K/PKB) cascade. Activation of the MAPK cascade results in gene transcription and DNA replication, while the P13-K/PKB pathway stimulates protein translation and progression through the cell cycle.

One example of the importance of tyrosine kinase receptors and the downstream serine–threonine cascades involves the insulin receptor. Insulin is released in response to elevated blood glucose. Activation of the insulin receptor results in an increase in cellular glucose uptake by stimulating GUTI (a glucose transporter) expression directly via MAPK activation and translocation of GLUT4 from the cytoplasm to the cell in a PK-dependent manner. Activation of the insulin receptor also reduces blood glucose by stimulating glycogen synthesis and inhibiting glycogenolysis by a P13-K/PKB-dependent mechanism.

The activation mechanism is shown in Fig. 1.10.

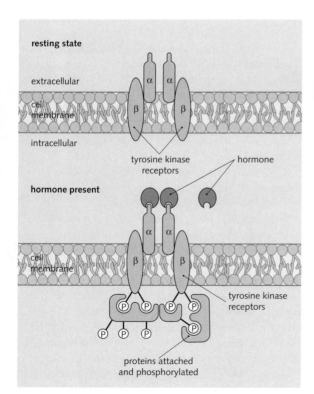

Fig. 1.10 Mechanism of activation of a tyrosine kinase receptor.

Intracellular receptors

Hormones that readily cross the cell membrane, especially steroids, use intracellular receptors. The receptors stimulate gene transcription and protein synthesis directly.

The hormone binds to the receptor in the cytoplasm, and this complex enters the nucleus, where it binds to specific sections of DNA called hormone response elements. This binding stimulates or inhibits the transcription of specific genes, causing changes in protein synthesis. It is this change that brings about the effects of the hormone. This action is shown in Fig. 1.11.

Receptor-mediated control

Hormone receptors are an important site of endocrine regulation. The number of active receptors can be increased or decreased to alter the strength of an endocrine signal. This allows the cell to respond to the deficiency or excess of a hormone. This control can be very subtle, for example, GnRH receptors in the pituitary gland are downregulated if GnRH secretion is not pulsatile. This effect is used clinically to suppress the reproductive hormones.

Relationship of the nervous and endocrine systems

Integration

The nervous and endocrine systems have a very close relationship, since they both use chemical signals to communicate between cells, and they may share a common evolutionary origin. The overlap between some hormones and neurotransmitters also supports this idea (e.g., somatostatin is found in both systems). The close relationship allows the two systems to coordinate responses to maintain homeostasis.

Neural control of hormones

The nervous system can control the endocrine system through two routes:
- Hypothalamus.
- Autonomic nervous system (sympathetic and parasympathetic).

The endocrine system often acts as a long-term output from the brain to complement the action of

Fig. 1.11 Mechanism of action of an intracellular receptor.

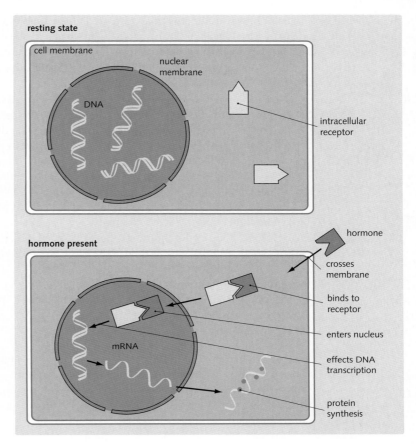

short-term neural responses. This is demonstrated by the three responses to stress listed in the order in which they take effect:

- Norepinephrine is released from sympathetic nerves.
- Preformed epinephrine is released from the adrenal medulla.
- Cortisol is synthesized by the adrenal cortex.

Hormonal control of neurons

To complete this circuit, the hormones of the endocrine system also affect the nervous system. Negative feedback to the hypothalamus has already been described. However, many hormones affect other areas of the brain. For example:

- Thyroid hormone deficiency causes depression.
- Leptin and insulin regulate feelings of hunger.
- Epinephrine increases mental activity.
- Melatonin regulates the feeling of tiredness.

Comparison between the nervous and endocrine systems

While the two systems function closely, they have different modes of action. The hypothalamus combines these actions since it is an endocrine tissue composed of nerve cells called neurosecretory cells.

Nervous system

The nervous system uses very localized chemical signals at synapses to transmit membrane depolarization between neurons. The effects of the nervous system are very rapid but of short duration and expensive metabolically (i.e., the neurotransmitters and depolarization require a lot of energy). The specific target cell is determined mostly by the location of chemical release rather than the receptors.

Endocrine system

The endocrine system uses very generalized chemical signals, though a few endocrine tissues can

13

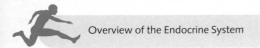

depolarize. These signals require less energy than neural signals. The signals travel throughout the body in the blood stream, and the target cell is determined mainly by the presence and specificity of receptors. The signals of the endocrine system tend to be slower but with a longer duration.

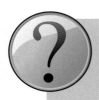

- Define the terms hormone, endocrine, target cell, and paracrine.
- Name five hormones along with the gland that secretes them.
- Outline the role of the hypothalamus in the endocrine system.
- Where do hormones from the hypothalamus act?
- Outline the role of the anterior pituitary gland in the endocrine system.
- Where do hormones from the anterior pituitary gland act?
- Describe the control of thyroid hormones starting in the hypothalamus.
- What is an eicosanoid? Is it a hormone?
- Define negative feedback, and give an example of this process.
- Describe the role of amplification in the endocrine system.
- State the three types of hormone along with an example of each.
- Describe the synthesis and properties of polypeptide hormones.
- Describe the mode of action of a G-protein receptor along with three examples of hormones that act through these receptors.
- Describe the mode of action of a tyrosine kinase receptor along with the hormones that act through these receptors.
- Describe the synthesis and properties of steroid hormones.
- Describe the receptors on which steroid hormones act.
- Describe the properties of modified amino acid hormones.
- Where can neurons affect the endocrine system?
- List examples of hormones that act on neurons.
- Compare the action of hormones and neurons.

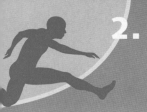

2. The Hypothalamus and the Pituitary Gland

The hypothalamus and pituitary gland control the endocrine system. To understand how the other endocrine organs function it is essential to know how they relate to these controllers.

The hypothalamus is a part of the brain that controls the secretion of many hormones. It can release small quantities of hormones in response to neuronal signals and thus acts as an interface between the nervous and endocrine systems, converting neural signals into chemical signals.

Hypothalamic hormones are carried locally in the blood stream. They are detected by cells in the anterior part of the pituitary gland, which is found just below the hypothalamus. In response, the pituitary gland secretes distinct effector hormones that regulate other endocrine organs (e.g., thyroid-stimulating hormone) or exert direct effects on the body (e.g., prolactin).

The posterior part of the pituitary gland functions in a slightly different way because it is a direct extension of the hypothalamus. Neurosecretory cells in the hypothalamus synthesize hormones that are transported along their axons. These hormones are released into capillaries within the posterior pituitary gland to affect body parts directly.

The secretory activity of the hypothalamus and pituitary gland can also be affected by hormones released from other endocrine organs (e.g., thyroxine from the thyroid gland). This feedback helps to control hormone levels and is a key component of endocrine function.

At first glance the hypothalamus and pituitary gland seem needlessly complicated to perform a simple task. There are two main reasons for this arrangement:
- It allows intricate regulation of hormone levels.
- It amplifies the initial signal so that a few neurons can affect cells throughout the body.

After reading this chapter you should be able to:
- Describe the structure and development of the hypothalamus and pituitary gland.
- List the hormones released by these structures and state their effects.
- Explain the major disorders associated with these structures.

Important terms:
Hypothalamus: a part of the brain that controls the endocrine system
Pituitary gland: an endocrine gland beneath the hypothalamus that controls other endocrine glands
Adenohypophysis: the anterior pituitary gland
Neurohypophysis: the posterior pituitary gland
Adenoma: a benign tumor

Anatomy

Hypothalamus

The hypothalamus is located at the base of the forebrain beneath the thalamus, and together they form the lateral walls of the third ventricle. The optic chiasma is anterior to the hypothalamus, and the mammillary bodies are found posteriorly. The inferior part of the hypothalamus—called the median eminence—gives rise to the pituitary stalk, which is continuous with the posterior pituitary gland. This arrangement is shown in Figs. 2.1 and 2.2.

The hypothalamus receives multiple inputs about the homeostatic state of the body. These signals arrive by two means:
- Circulatory (e.g., temperature, blood glucose, hormone levels).
- Neuronal (e.g., autonomic function, emotional).

It responds to these inputs by the secretion of hormones that either regulate the release of hormones from the anterior pituitary or are released directly from the posterior pituitary (e.g., antidiuretic hormone [ADH]). It also responds by neuronal signals to other areas of the central nervous system (CNS).

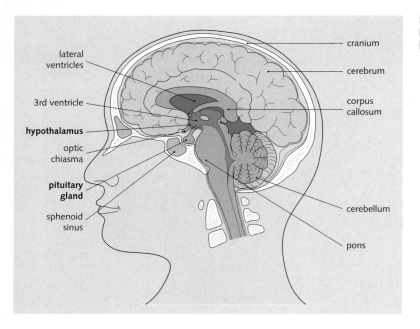

Fig. 2.1 Medial sagittal section of head showing the location of the hypothalamus and pituitary gland.

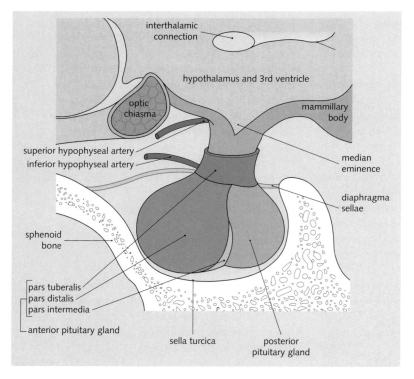

Fig. 2.2 Anatomical relationship of the pituitary gland and the hypothalamus to surrounding structures.

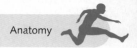

 The hypothalamus is V-shaped because it surrounds the third ventricle.

Pituitary gland

The pituitary gland is divided into two lobes with distinct embryological origins, structure, and function:

- Anterior pituitary or adenohypophysis.
- Posterior pituitary or neurohypophysis.

The pituitary gland gets its name from the incorrect belief that it secreted nasal mucus. This belief was put forward by the Greek physician Galen (129–216 A.D.). "Pituitary" means "mucus."

The pituitary gland lies in a deep bony hollow in the sphenoid bone (the sella turcica), and it is covered by the fibrous diaphragma sellae. The optic chiasma lies above this diaphragm directly superior to the anterior lobe. The posterior lobe is connected to the median eminence of the hypothalamus by the pituitary stalk (infundibulum). The cavernous sinuses including the cranial nerves III–VI lie laterally (see Figs. 2.1 and 2.2).

Tumors of the pituitary gland are surrounded by the bone of the sella turcica. Thus they can expand only upward into the optic chiasma, causing visual field defects. Further expansion compresses cranial nerves III, IV, V, and VI in the wall of the cavernous sinus.

Blood supply

The blood supply to the anterior pituitary gland first passes through the median eminence, creating a vascular communication. The median eminence of the hypothalamus is supplied by the superior hypophyseal artery, which forms a plexus within it. The blood then drains into portal veins, which supply the anterior pituitary gland. Hormones secreted from the median eminence pass directly to the anterior pituitary in the blood stream, as shown in Fig. 2.3.

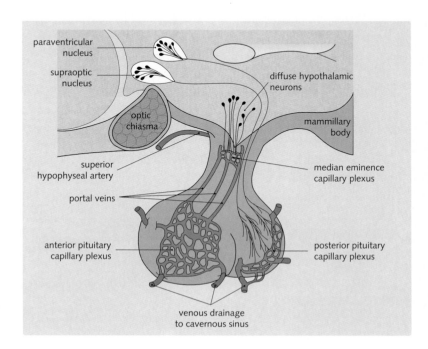

Fig. 2.3 Communication between the hypothalamus and pituitary gland. Note the difference between the anterior and posterior pituitary gland.

The posterior pituitary gland is supplied by the inferior hypophyseal arteries. These vessels do not communicate with the median eminence.

The veins exiting the pituitary gland drain to the cavernous sinuses.

Development

Hypothalamus

The hypothalamus develops from the embryological forebrain; it can be identified at week six of gestation.

Anterior pituitary

The anterior pituitary develops as an outgrowth of the ectoderm of the primitive mouth called Rathke's pouch. It grows upward until it fuses with the infundibulum of the hypothalamus. The anterior pituitary is composed of nonneural secretory epithelial tissue; it is not directly connected to the hypothalamus.

The connection to the roof of the primitive mouth is gradually lost along with its blood supply. The portal veins from the hypothalamus grow downward to replace this blood supply, and these are the only communication between the hypothalamus and the anterior pituitary.

As the connection to the primitive mouth is lost, nests of epithelial cells may be left behind. These can give rise to cysts or tumors, which may secrete ectopic hormones (e.g., craniopharyngiomas—see the disorders section, p. 22).

The embryology of the pituitary gland is shown in Fig. 2.4.

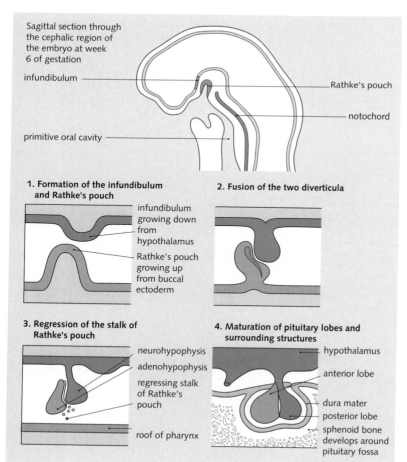

Fig. 2.4 Embryological development of the anterior and posterior lobes of the pituitary gland.

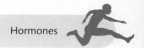

Posterior pituitary

The posterior pituitary is derived from the neuroectoderm of the primitive brain tissue. It develops as an outgrowth from the hypothalamus called the infundibulum. Axons from neurosecretory cells in the hypothalamus pass downward in the stalk of the pituitary gland and terminate in the posterior pituitary. A direct neuronal connection between the hypothalamus and posterior pituitary is formed, and this is the only means of communication between these structures.

Microstructure

Hypothalamus

There are a number of different secretory neurons in the hypothalamus, each specialized to secrete specific hormones. Neurons that secrete the same chemical may be arranged in clusters called nuclei, or they may be scattered diffusely. Some neurons can secrete more than one hormone.

Anterior pituitary

The anterior pituitary is composed of cords of secretory cells in a rich network of capillaries. Six types of secretory cells can be distinguished using immunohistochemical staining. These are listed with the hormones that they synthesize:

- Somatotrophs—growth hormone (GH).
- Gonadotrophs—luteinizing hormone (LH) and follicle-stimulating hormone (FSH).
- Corticotrophs—adrenocorticotropic hormone (ACTH) and melanocyte-stimulating hormone (MSH).
- Thyrotrophs—thyroid-stimulating hormone (TSH).
- Lactotrophs—prolactin.
- Chromophobes—inactive secretory cells.

In the past, cells were differentiated by their pH; the terms acidophil and basophil in older textbooks refer to this distinction.

The anterior pituitary is divided into three distinct areas (see Fig. 2.2):

- Pars distalis—the majority of the gland.
- Pars tuberalis—a layer of mostly gonadotroph cells around the pituitary stalk.
- Pars intermedia—a thin layer of corticotroph cells between the anterior and posterior pituitary. It is very small in humans.

Posterior pituitary

The posterior pituitary is composed of two cell types, but it contains no secretory cells:

- Nonmyelinated axons, originating from the hypothalamus.
- Pituicytes, which are stellate (star-shaped) glial support cells.

Within the axons there are microtubules and mitochondria that are involved in the transport of neurosecretory granules. These granules travel from the hypothalamus to the axon terminals in the posterior pituitary, where they are stored before release. The axon terminals lie close to blood sinusoids, where the neurosecretory granules are released into the systemic circulation (Fig. 2.5).

Hormones

Hormones of the hypothalamus

The hypothalamus secretes very small quantities of hormones into the portal veins to exert control over the anterior pituitary. The quantity is so small that the hormones can rarely be detected in systemic blood, but by traveling in the portal veins directly to the anterior pituitary, their concentration is high enough to produce an effect. This system allows for a rapid response and amplification of the signal. The hypothalamic hormones are often released in a pulsatile manner. The pulses vary in amplitude and rate, often with a circadian rhythm (see Chapter 6).

Hormones that regulate anterior pituitary function

The hormones secreted by the hypothalamus are small peptides (between 3 and 44 amino acid residues), except for dopamine, which is derived from the amino acid tyrosine. These hormones are shown in Fig. 2.6 along with their effects.

The factors that regulate the secretion of these hormones are discussed independently in the subsequent chapters. They act on the secretory cells in an excitatory (e.g., thyrotropin-releasing hormone [TRH]) or inhibitory (e.g., growth hormone-inhibiting hormone [GHIH]) manner. There is some promiscuity or overlap in function between these peptides; for example, TRH can stimulate prolactin release.

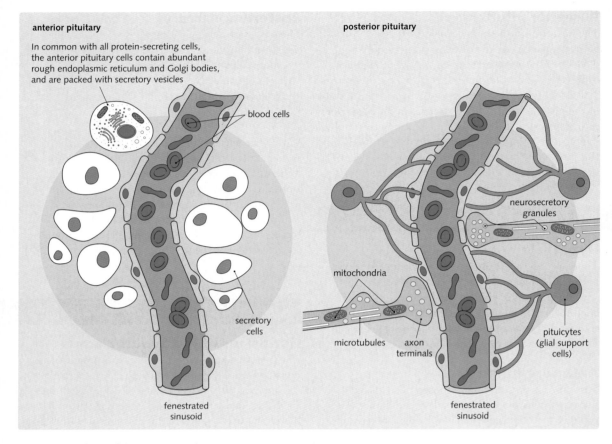

Fig. 2.5 Histology of the anterior and posterior pituitary gland.

Hormones of the hypothalamus		
Hormone	**Target cells in the anterior pituitary gland**	**Effect on the anterior pituitary gland**
Growth hormone-releasing hormone (GHRH)	Somatotrophs	↑ GH release
Growth hormone-inhibiting hormone (GHIH, also called somatostatin)	Somatotrophs and thyrotrophs	↓ GH and TSH release
Corticotropin-releasing hormone (CRH)	Corticotrophs	↑ ACTH release
Gonadotropin-releasing hormone (GnRH)	Gonadotrophs	↑ LH and FSH release
Thyrotropin-releasing hormone (TRH)	Thyrotrophs and lactotrophs	↑ TSH and prolactin release
Prolactin-releasing factors (PRF)	Lactotrophs	↑ Prolactin release
Dopamine (prolactin-inhibiting hormone)	Lactotrophs	↓ Prolactin release

Fig. 2.6 Hormones secreted by the hypothalamus and their effects on the secretion of the anterior pituitary hormones. (ACTH, adrenocorticotropic hormone; FSH, follicle-stimulating hormone; GH, growth hormone; LH, luteinizing hormone; TSH, thyroid-stimulating hormone.)

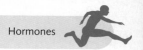

Hormones released from the posterior pituitary

The small peptides ADH and oxytocin are synthesized in the cell bodies of magnocellular neurons arranged into two nuclei in the hypothalamus:
- Supraoptic nucleus.
- Paraventricular nucleus.

While both nuclei secrete both hormones, the supraoptic tends to secrete more ADH, whereas the paraventricular produces oxytocin. The hormones pass along the axons bound to glycoproteins. They pass through the median eminence to the posterior pituitary where they are stored before release. Their actions are described below in the section "Hormones of the posterior pituitary."

Hormones of the anterior pituitary

The hormones secreted by the anterior pituitary are large peptides (about 200 amino acid residues) or glycopeptides. The six main hormones are:
- Growth hormone (GH).
- Thyroid-stimulating hormone (TSH; also called thyrotropin).
- Adrenocorticotropic hormone (ACTH).
- Luteinizing hormone (LH).
- Follicle-stimulating hormone (FSH).
- Prolactin (PRL).

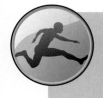

The hormones of the anterior pituitary can be remembered using the mnemonic: **F**resh **P**ituitary **T**astes **A**lmost **L**ike **G**uinness.

The hormones synthesized by the anterior pituitary are released into the systemic circulation. They act in two ways:
- Regulation of other endocrine organs—TSH, ACTH, GH, LH, and FSH.
- Direct effects on distant organs—prolactin.

GH and prolactin are large peptides whereas the others are glycopeptides. The individual hormones are discussed in more detail in later chapters (see also Figs. 2.7 and 2.8). The secretion and release of these hormones often follows the pulsatile pattern of the releasing hormones from the hypothalamus.

The pars intermedia of the anterior pituitary gland also secretes a number of less important hormones including:
- Melanocyte-stimulating hormone (MSH), which stimulates melanocytes in the skin.
- Beta-endorphin, an endogenous morphine, which may have a role in the control of pain.

Hormonal feedback

In response to the small quantities of releasing hormones secreted by the hypothalamus, the anterior pituitary is stimulated to secrete hormones in quantities large enough to act on endocrine organs throughout the body. The release of pituitary hormones is also regulated by hormones from other endocrine glands mainly through negative feedback mechanisms (e.g., thyroxine from the thyroid inhibits the release of TSH from the anterior pituitary).

Hypothalamic regulation of prolactin release is unique because the main control is inhibitory: dopamine secreted from the hypothalamus inhibits release of prolactin from the pituitary. This is important if a tumor stops the hypothalamic releasing hormones from reaching the anterior pituitary. The levels of most pituitary hormones will fall, while the levels of prolactin will increase.

Hormones of the posterior pituitary

Two major hormones are synthesized in the hypothalamus and released into the systemic circulation from the posterior pituitary:
- Antidiuretic hormone (ADH), also called arginine vasopressin (AVP).
- Oxytocin.

Both hormones are peptides consisting of nine amino acid residues that vary by a single residue. The main actions of these hormones are shown in Figs. 2.9 and 2.10.

Antidiuretic hormone

ADH acts mainly on the collecting duct of the kidney to prevent water excretion. It also has a vasoconstricting action at high doses, hence the name vasopressin. Low blood volume detected by peripheral baroreceptors stimulates very high ADH release to increase blood pressure.

A small proportion of ADH is released into the portal veins, where it stimulates corticotrophs in the anterior pituitary gland to secrete ACTH.

Hormones of the anterior pituitary gland						
Hormone	Synthesized by	Stimulated by	Inhibited by	Target organ	Effect	Chapter
GH	Somatotrophs	GHRH	GHIH and IGF-1	Liver	Stimulates IGF-1 production and opposes insulin	9
TSH	Thyrotrophs	TRH	T_3	Thyroid gland	Stimulates thyroxine release	3
ACTH	Corticotrophs	CRH	Glucocorti-coids	Adrenal cortex	Stimulates glucocorticoid and androgen release	4
LH + FSH	Gonadotrophs	GnRH, sex steroids	Prolactin, sex steroids	Reproductive organs	Release of sex steroids	11
Prolactin	Lactotrophs	PRF and TRH	Dopamine	Mammary glands and reproductive organs	Promotes growth of these organs and initiates lactation	11
MSH	Corticotrophs	—	—	Melanocytes in skin	Stimulates melanin synthesis	—
Beta-endorphin	Corticotrophs	—	—	Unknown	May be involved in pain control	—

Fig. 2.7 Hormones synthesized and secreted by the anterior pituitary and their effects. (ACTH, adrenocorticotropic hormone; CRH, corticotropin-releasing hormone; FSH, follicle-stimulating hormone; GH, growth hormone; GHRH, growth hormone-releasing hormone; GnRH, gonadotropin-releasing hormone; GHIH, growth hormone-inhibiting hormone; LH, luteinizing hormone; MSH, melanocyte-stimulating hormone; TRH, thyrotropin-releasing hormone; TSH, thyroid-stimulating hormone.)

Oxytocin

When a baby suckles the mother's breast, stretch receptors in the nipple send signals to the brain via sensory nerves. These signals reach the paraventricular neurons causing depolarization and oxytocin release from the posterior pituitary. The oxytocin reaches the myoepithelial cells of the breast, which contract pushing milk out of the breast. This reflex is illustrated in Fig. 14.19 (p. 194).

Disorders of the hypothalamus

Primary diseases of the hypothalamus are very rare, but they tend to cause deficiency of hypothalamic hormones and the corresponding pituitary hormones. Dopamine deficiency has the opposite effect, resulting in excessive prolactin secretion from the anterior pituitary. The main causes of hypothalamic hormone deficiency are:

- Trauma/surgery.
- Radiotherapy.
- Congenital gonadotropin-releasing hormone (GnRH) deficiency (Kallmann's syndrome), causing infertility.
- Congenital GHRH deficiency, causing dwarfism.
- Primary glial cell tumors of the hypothalamus.

Lesions in the hypothalamus can cause many other abnormalities, including disorders of consciousness, behavior, thirst, satiety, and temperature regulation. These disorders usually occur together with hypopituitarism and diabetes insipidus.

Disorders of the anterior pituitary

Etiology

The nine I's of pituitary pathology are:
- Iatrogenic (e.g., surgery or radiotherapy).
- Invasion (i.e., tumors).

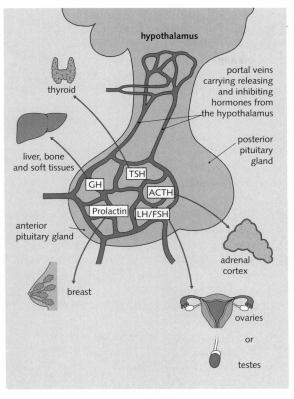

Fig. 2.8 Hormones of the anterior pituitary gland and their respective target organs.

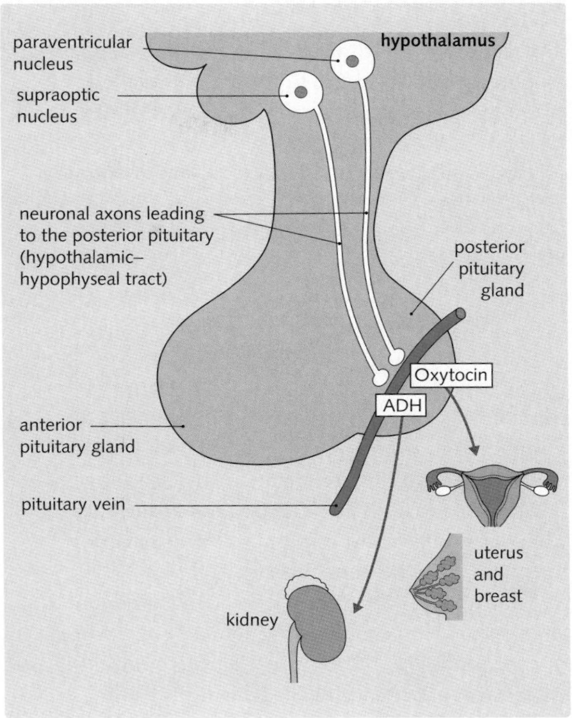

Fig. 2.10 Hormones of the posterior pituitary gland and their respective target organs.

Hormones secreted by the posterior pituitary gland						
Hormone	Synthesized by	Stimulated by	Inhibited by	Target organ	Effect	Chapter
Antidiuretic hormone (ADH)	Supraoptic vasopressinergic neurons	Raised osmolarity; low blood volume	Lowered osmolarity	Kidney	Increases the permeability of the collecting duct to reabsorb water	7
Oxytocin	Paraventricular oxytocinergic neurons	Stretch receptors in the nipple and cervix; estrogen	Stress	Uterus and mammary glands	Smooth muscle contraction leading to birth or milk ejection	14

Fig. 2.9 Hormones secreted by the posterior pituitary and their effects.

- Infarction (e.g., Sheehan's syndrome).
- Idiopathic (i.e., no underlying cause known).
- Injury (e.g., severe head trauma).
- Infection (e.g., tuberculosis; very rare).

- Infiltration (e.g., sarcoidosis; very rare).
- Immunological (e.g., lymphocytic hypophysitis; very rare).
- Inherited (e.g., congenital hormone deficiency; very rare).

Tumors

The majority of pituitary gland disorders are caused by benign tumors of the secretory cells called adenomas. Disease occurs as a result of three processes:

- Hyperpituitarism—excess pituitary hormone secretion.
- Hypopituitarism—insufficient pituitary hormone secretion.
- Compression of surrounding structures—caused by space-occupying lesions.

These tumors are classified into two groups: functioning and nonfunctioning adenomas. Functioning adenomas present early while still very small. These microadenomas cause disease by excess hormone release, which can be fatal if untreated. They also cause compression, so other pituitary hormones may be deficient (Fig. 2.11).

Nonfunctioning adenomas usually present at a later stage as larger macroadenomas. They cause disease indirectly by compressing surrounding structures, often causing insufficient pituitary hormone release by compressing the portal vessels or secretory cells.

Hyperpituitarism
Prolactinomas

All of the anterior pituitary secretory cells can form tumors; however, the vast majority are prolactinomas (i.e., tumors of the prolactin-secreting cells) (Fig. 2.12). They are more common in women and tend to present earlier, before visual disturbance occurs. Excess prolactin secretion—hyperprolactinemia—causes galactorrhea and hypogonadism, the symptoms of which are shown in Fig. 2.13.

Investigations

A number of symptoms and investigations are assessed to achieve a diagnosis:

- Are there symptoms of a specific endocrine abnormality?
- Visual field assessment is carried out to detect compression of the optic chiasma.
- Are there abnormal hormone levels in the blood? If an excess is suspected, all pituitary hormones should be tested as an adenoma can cause related deficiencies.
- Suppression tests are carried out—these assess pituitary response to hormone analogs or inhibiting factors to locate the lesion on the endocrine axis. Adenomas generally display reduced negative feedback.
- Magnetic resonance imaging (MRI) or computed tomography (CT) scans are used to detect abnormal anatomy.

Anterior pituitary hormones and the disorders caused by their deficiency and excess		
Hormone	Deficiency	Excess
GH	Dwarfism in children or adults GH deficiency syndrome	Gigantism in children, acromegaly in adults
LH and FSH	Gonadal insufficiency (decreased sex steroids)	Extremely rare but causes infertility
ACTH	Adrenocortical insufficiency (decreased cortisol and adrenal androgens)	Cushing's disease (increased cortisol and adrenal androgens)
TSH	Hypothyroidism (decreased thyroid hormones)	Extremely rare but causes hyperthyroidism (increased thyroid hormones)
Prolactin	Hypoprolactinemia (failure in postpartum lactation)	Hyperprolactinemia (impotence in males, amenorrhea in females, and decreased libido)

Fig. 2.11 Disorders caused by the deficiency or excess of anterior pituitary hormones. (ACTH, adrenocorticotropic hormone; FSH, follicle-stimulating hormone; GH, growth hormone; LH, luteinizing hormone; TSH, thyroid-stimulating hormone.)

Fig. 2.12 Adenomas of the anterior pituitary gland and their effects. (ACTH, adrenocorticotropic hormone; FSH, follicle-stimulating hormone; GH, growth hormone; LH, luteinizing hormone; TSH, thyroid-stimulating hormone.)

Adenomas of the anterior pituitary gland and their effects				
Tumor	Hormone excess	Percentage of all pituitary tumors	Disease	Chapter
Prolactinoma	Prolactin	50%	Hyperprolactinemia	2
Nonsecretory prolactinoma	None	20%	Hypopituitarism	2
Somatotropic cell adenoma	GH	20%	In children: gigantism In adults: acromegaly	9
Corticotropic cell adenoma	ACTH	5%	Cushing's disease	4
Gonadotropic cell adenoma	LH and FSH	Very rare	Infertility	—
Thyrotropic cell adenoma	TSH	Very rare	Hyperthyroidism	3

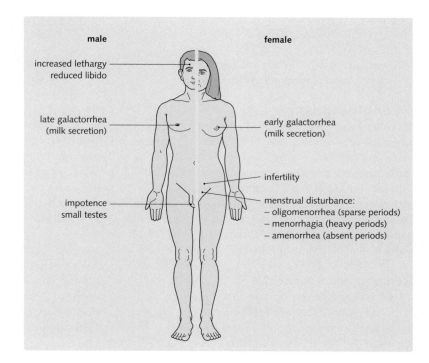

Fig. 2.13 Symptoms and signs of hyperprolactinemia.

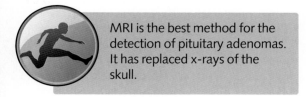

MRI is the best method for the detection of pituitary adenomas. It has replaced x-rays of the skull.

The main suppression tests for anterior pituitary levels are to measure:
- GH in response to an oral glucose tolerance challenge, which normally suppresses GH levels.
- ACTH in response to dexamethasone, a steroid that normally suppresses CRH and ACTH release.

Hypogonadism caused by hyperprolactinemia is a very common feature of pituitary adenomas. Prolactin-secreting adenomas are the most common type of functioning adenoma and secrete excess prolactin by definition. Nonfunctioning adenomas prevent hypothalamic dopamine inhibition of prolactin release by compression so that excess prolactin is released.

Treatment

There are three methods of treating excess hormone production, but they all carry the risk of causing hypopituitarism:

- Bromocriptine (dopamine agonist) to reduce prolactin secretion.
- Octreotide (synthetic somatostatin) to reduce GH secretion.
- Surgical removal of pituitary adenoma.
- Irradiation to prevent adenoma recurrence.

Hypopituitarism

Pituitary insufficiency (hypopituitarism) often presents with insidious onset depression, tiredness, and hypogonadism as most hormone levels fall and prolactin levels rise. A deficiency of more than one pituitary hormone is called panhypopituitarism. The causes of pituitary insufficiency are more varied than those of hyperpituitarism. However, the common causes include head or neck injuries (e.g., whiplash) or treatment of hyperpituitarism.

Nonfunctioning adenomas

About 20% of pituitary tumors do not produce hormones so they are called nonfunctioning adenomas (sometimes called chromophobe adenomas). They are almost always nonactive prolactinomas. Since there is no excess hormone production, they present late with symptoms caused by compression of surrounding structures, which become progressively severe:

- Headaches.
- Pituitary hormone deficiencies.
- Hypogonadism due to hyperprolactinemia.
- Loss of peripheral vision due to compression of the optic nerve (bitemporal hemianopia).

- Cranial nerve palsies (starting with nerve IV).
- Raised intracranial pressure.

The tumor can cause hormone deficiencies by direct compression of the secretory cells or by compressing the portal veins that bring the hypothalamic releasing factors. Secretion of anterior pituitary hormones is inhibited in a characteristic order: GH, LH and FSH, ACTH, TSH (see Fig. 2.11 for symptoms). Unless the compression is very severe, prolactin secretion often increases initially since dopamine inhibition is lost. This excess prolactin secretion is not from the cells of the adenoma, but it causes the symptoms shown in Fig. 2.13.

The Bible according to endocrinology: Goliath was a giant due to excessive GH secretion from a somatotroph tumor. This grew to compress his optic nerve, causing a bilateral hemianopia so that he failed to see David's stone coming from the side.

Other tumors

Tumors in surrounding tissues can also compress the pituitary gland, causing panhypopituitarism. The most common are:

- Craniopharyngiomas.
- Gliomas (especially in the optic chiasma).

Craniopharyngiomas are rare tumors formed in the remnants of Rathke's pouch and left behind when the connection with the pharynx regresses. They can form above, below, or within the sella turcica.

Gliomas are primary tumors of the glial support cells found throughout the brain.

Infarction of the pituitary gland

Infarction of the pituitary gland causes necrosis of all secretory cells and results in complete panhypopituitarism, including loss of prolactin secretion. Sheehan's syndrome is a rare condition that can cause this disorder. It may develop if a woman suffers a severe hemorrhage during childbirth, resulting in a blood pressure drop due to volume loss. Since the pituitary gland is enlarged

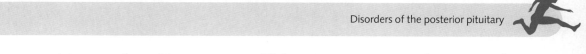

during pregnancy, it is extremely sensitive to hypotension and the resulting hypoxia. The ensuing panhypopituitarism causes a failure to lactate, amenorrhea, and eventually death if untreated.

A more catastrophic infarction can occur through spontaneous hemorrhage of the pituitary itself. This is called pituitary apoplexy; it is a neurosurgical emergency.

Compression of the pituitary gland

Empty sella syndrome is a condition in which the sella turcica partially fills with cerebrospinal fluid, causing the pituitary gland to be compressed. It is not always pathological (some cerebrospinal fluid is found within the sella in at least 50% of normal individuals). Causes include congenital incompetence of the diaphragma sellae, pituitary surgery or irradiation, postpartum pituitary infarction (Sheehan's syndrome), and coexisting pituitary tumor.

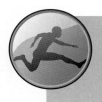

The pituitary has a great secretory reserve—more than 75% must be affected before clinical manifestations are evident.

Diagnosis of hypopituitarism

Diagnosis of hypopituitarism involves the same steps as for hyperpituitarism; however, stimulation is used instead of suppression:

- Visual field assessment.
- Basal hormone levels in the blood.
- Stimulation tests.
- MRI or CT scan.

The main stimulation tests for anterior pituitary levels are to measure:

- GH in response to an insulin tolerance test, which normally increases GH levels.
- Cortisol in response to hypoglycemia or the ACTH analog Synacthen®.
- LH and FSH in response to GnRH or the antiestrogen clomiphene.

Treatment of hypopituitarism

The main treatment of hypopituitarism is hormone replacement, which requires frequent monitoring.

All the major anterior pituitary hormones can be replaced, although prolactin is not readily available since it is rarely needed:

- Subcutaneous GH replacement using human recombinant GH.
- Oral cortisol replacement.
- Oral thyroxine once cortisol replacement has begun.
- Oral or intramuscular testosterone in males.
- Oral estrogen and progesterone cyclically in females.
- Intramuscular human chorionic gonadotropin, LH, and FSH are given if male or female fertility is required.

Surgery may be required to remove adenomas, gliomas, or craniopharyngiomas.

Disorders of the posterior pituitary

Diabetes insipidus

A deficiency of ADH (vasopressin) secretion prevents osmotic control of the kidney so that very dilute polyuria occurs. Up to 20 liters of urine can be passed in a day, causing a potentially fatal dehydration and constant thirst. It is rare and usually idiopathic, but it can be caused by trauma, surgery, or tumors (Fig. 2.14).

An ADH stimulation test is used to distinguish between deficient ADH and unresponsive kidneys. The condition is treated with desmopressin, a long-acting vasopressin analog, to control fluid loss.

Posterior pituitary hormones and the disorders caused by their deficiency and excess		
Hormone	Deficiency	Excess
ADH	Diabetes insipidus (polyuria, hypotension)	Syndrome of inappropriate ADH secretion (SIADH)
Oxytocin	Failure to progress in labor and difficulty with breastfeeding	No effect

Fig. 2.14 Disorders caused by the deficiency or excess of posterior pituitary hormones. (ADH, antidiuretic hormone.)

Excessive antidiuretic hormone secretion

The syndrome of inappropriate secretion of ADH (SIADH) can be caused by neurological, endocrine, malignant, or infective diseases, but it can also be idiopathic, postoperative, or caused by medications (see Fig. 2.14). Excess ADH causes water retention resulting in hypoosmotic hyponatremia (low sodium). The symptoms progress from malaise and weakness to confusion and coma. If untreated it can be fatal.

- Describe the anatomical location of the hypothalamus.
- Explain how the hypothalamus regulates the anterior pituitary gland including relevant vasculature.
- List the hormones secreted by the hypothalamus along with their effects.
- Describe the role of the hypothalamus in the release of posterior pituitary hormones.
- Describe the anatomical relationships of the pituitary gland.
- Explain the embryological development of the pituitary gland and how it affects hypothalamic control.
- List the hormones of the anterior pituitary gland along with their effects.
- List the hormones of the posterior pituitary gland along with their effects.
- Name the most common types of pituitary adenoma.
- List the effects of compression by a pituitary tumor. In what order do they occur?
- List the anterior pituitary hormones in the order that they are affected by compression.
- List the symptoms of hyperprolactinemia in males and females. Which sex presents to the doctor earliest?
- List three treatment options for adenomas.
- Describe the investigations of pituitary hormone excess and deficiency.
- Describe the difference between a suppression and stimulation test along with an example of each.
- The deficiency of which pituitary hormone is life-threatening?
- Perform a musical interpretation of a pituitary gland undergoing infarction.
- Describe the treatment of panhypopituitarism.
- Name and describe the disorders of excess and deficient ADH secretion.
- Draw a diagram to illustrate the reflex that initiates lactation.

3. The Thyroid Gland

Diseases of the thyroid gland are the second most common endocrine disorder, after diabetes. The main diseases are caused by excess or deficiency of thyroid hormones, and they tend to affect middle-aged or elderly women.

The thyroid gland regulates the body's metabolism (Fig. 3.1). It is the largest endocrine organ in the body, and it is found anterior to the trachea in the lower neck. The gland is composed of two lobes that are joined by a narrow isthmus in the center.

Within the gland the cells are arranged in spherical follicles that surround a thyroid hormone store. The thyroid is the only endocrine gland to store large quantities of preformed hormones. These thyroid hormones are released in response to thyroid-stimulating hormone (TSH) from the anterior pituitary gland. The follicles release two hormones:

- T_4—a prohormone that acts as a plasma reservoir.
- T_3—the active hormone.

These hormones increase the rate of metabolism in almost every cell in the body.

Excessive release is called hyperthyroidism, which causes abnormally fast metabolism. The patients feel hot and sweaty; they often lose weight.

Deficient release is called hypothyroidism. Metabolism is slow, making the patients feel lethargic; they frequently gain weight.

After reading this chapter you should be able to:
- Explain the structure and development of the thyroid gland.
- Describe the synthesis of thyroid hormones.
- Understand the regulation and physiological effects of thyroid hormones.
- Discuss the major disorders associated with thyroid function.

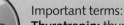

Important terms:
Thyrotropin: thyroid-stimulating hormone (TSH)
Thyroglobulin: the store of thyroid hormones found in the thyroid follicles
Parathyroid glands: endocrine organs found behind the thyroid gland that regulate calcium metabolism and are essential to life
Deiodination: removal of an iodine molecule
Goiter: an enlarged thyroid gland

Anatomy

Thyroid gland

The thyroid gland is palpable in about 50% of women and 25% of men. It is located in the neck, inferior to the larynx and cricoid cartilage. It has two lobes, each about 5 cm long and joined by a narrow isthmus. The lobes lie on either side of the trachea and esophagus, and the isthmus crosses the trachea anteriorly, usually over the second and third tracheal cartilages (Fig. 3.2).

The thyroid gland is bound to the trachea by the pretracheal fascia so that it moves with the trachea and larynx on swallowing, but not when the tongue is protruded. The gland is surrounded by a fibrous capsule within the pretracheal fascia (Fig. 3.3).

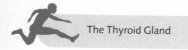

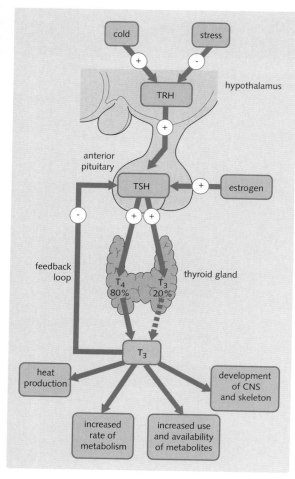

Fig. 3.1 Hormonal regulation of the thyroid hormones. (T_3, triiodothyronine; T_4, thyroxine; TRH, thyrotropin-releasing hormone; TSH, thyroid-stimulating hormone.)

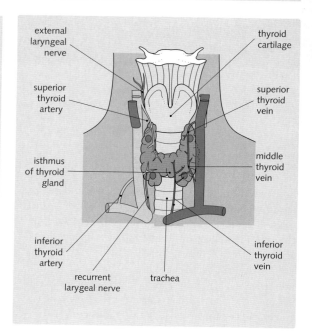

Fig. 3.2 Anterior view of the neck, showing the location and blood supply of the thyroid gland.

The thyroid gland derives its name from the Greek word *thyreos*, meaning "shield," and the suffix *-oid*, meaning "like." It is unclear whether the Greeks had shields with slits in the middle or whether anatomists knew nothing about shields.

Blood supply, nerves, and lymphatics

The thyroid gland is highly vascular; in fact, the blood flow per gram is greater than that of the kidneys. It is supplied by two arteries that anastomose (join) within the gland: the inferior and superior thyroid arteries.

The inferior thyroid artery is a branch of the thyrocervical trunk that arises from the subclavian arteries. It ascends behind the carotid sheath to enter the thyroid posteriorly. The right recurrent laryngeal nerve is intimately related to this artery near the inferior pole of the thyroid gland. Surgery to the thyroid gland can bruise this nerve, causing temporary difficulty with speaking. To minimize the risk to this nerve, the artery is ligated far away from the thyroid gland during thyroidectomy.

The superior thyroid artery is the first branch of the external carotid artery. The external laryngeal nerve is related to this artery, but it is at less risk than the recurrent laryngeal nerve during thyroid surgery. The superior thyroid artery is ligated close to the thyroid gland to reduce this risk (see Fig. 3.2).

A third artery, called the thyroid ima artery, is present in 10% of people. It supplies the isthmus and arises near the aortic arch, although the exact origin varies.

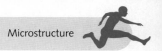

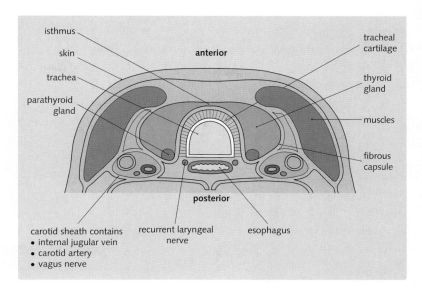

Fig. 3.3 Horizontal section of the anterior neck at the level of the sixth cervical vertebra, showing the location of the thyroid and parathyroid glands and their surrounding structures.

isthmus

skin

trachea

parathyroid gland

anterior

tracheal cartilage

thyroid gland

muscles

fibrous capsule

posterior

carotid sheath contains
• internal jugular vein
• carotid artery
• vagus nerve

recurrent laryngeal nerve

esophagus

The thyroid gland is drained by three veins:
• Superior thyroid vein.
• Middle thyroid vein.
• Inferior thyroid vein.

The first two veins drain into the internal jugular, whereas the inferior vein drains into the brachiocephalic veins.

Thyroid lymphatics drain into four groups of nodes:
• Prelaryngeal lymph nodes.
• Pretracheal lymph nodes.
• Paratracheal lymph nodes.
• Deep cervical lymph nodes.

Parathyroid glands

The parathyroid glands are four oval-shaped structures about 5 mm across; they are embedded in the thyroid capsule behind both lateral lobes. These glands are described as superior and inferior pairs. The number of parathyroid glands often varies between two and six, and the location of the inferior pair differs widely. They are supplied by branches of the inferior thyroid artery. Their function is described in Chapter 8.

Microstructure

Thyroid gland

The thyroid is composed of about one million spherical follicles or acini. Each follicle is lined by a single layer of secretory epithelial cells (follicular cells) around a colloid-filled space. These cells secrete thyroglobin—a storage form of thyroid hormone—into the colloid. When the thyroid gland is not actively secreting hormones, the size of the colloid store and the follicle itself increase in diameter.

When the follicular cells enter an active secretory phase, microvilli form on their inner surface and thyroglobin is absorbed. The colloid store shrinks as a result. The absorbed thyroglobin is broken down to release thyroid hormone. The histology of the thyroid gland is shown in Fig. 3.4.

Another type of secretory cell is found between the follicles. These parafollicular cells (C cells) synthesize and secrete calcitonin.

The thyroid gland is the only endocrine gland to store its hormone in an extracellular compartment: 2–3 months of thyroid hormone are stored within the follicles. This reservoir delays the onset of symptoms in deficiency diseases.

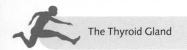
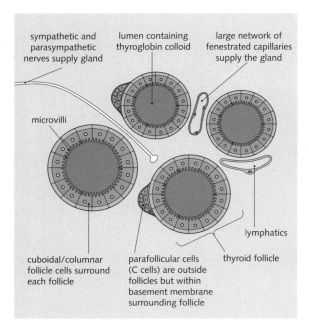

sympathetic and parasympathetic nerves supply gland

lumen containing thyroglobin colloid

large network of fenestrated capillaries supply the gland

microvilli

cuboidal/columnar follicle cells surround each follicle

parafollicular cells (C cells) are outside follicles but within basement membrane surrounding follicle

thyroid follicle

lymphatics

Fig. 3.4 Histology of the thyroid gland.

Parathyroid glands

There are three cell types in the parathyroid glands:

- Chief cells—synthesize parathyroid hormone (PTH).
- Oxyphil cells—exhausted chief cells; their numbers increase with age.
- Adipocytes—contain fat; their numbers also increase with age.

Development

Thyroid gland

The thyroid gland is an endodermal structure that develops as an outpouching in the floor of the pharynx behind the tongue. It descends in the neck but remains attached to the tongue by the thyroglossal duct until it reaches its final position.

In 50% of people a remnant of this duct forms a small pyramidal lobe extending superiorly from the isthmus. Thyroglossal cysts can form anywhere along the course taken by the thyroid. They present as neck lumps that rise when the tongue is protruded.

Parathyroid glands

The parathyroid glands are endodermal structures that develop from the pharyngeal pouches. The

inferior parathyroid glands are formed by the dorsal portion of the third pouch while the dorsal portion of the fourth pouch forms the superior parathyroid glands.

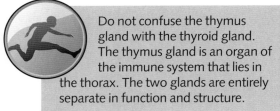

Do not confuse the thymus gland with the thyroid gland. The thymus gland is an organ of the immune system that lies in the thorax. The two glands are entirely separate in function and structure.

Hormones

The thyroid gland synthesizes and secretes three hormones:

- Thyroxine (T_4).
- Triiodothyronine (T_3).
- Calcitonin.

Calcitonin is involved with calcium homeostasis (discussed in Chapter 8).

Synthesis

T_3 and T_4 are derived from two molecules of the amino acid tyrosine and iodine. T_3 contains three iodine atoms, and T_4 contains four. Their structures are shown in Fig. 3.5.

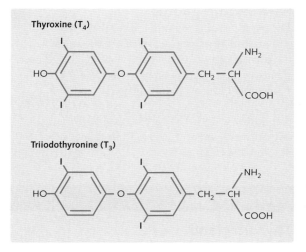

Fig. 3.5 Structures of T_3 and T_4.

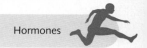

Thyroid hormones are formed in the follicle lumen, not in the cells. The process of T_3 and T_4 synthesis involves the processing of tyrosine and iodine followed by a reaction to bind them together. These steps (Fig. 3.6) are as follows:

1. Thyroglobulin synthesis   Tyrosine is converted into the glycoprotein thyroglobulin, which contains approximately 110 tyrosine residues.

2. Processing of iodine   This involves two stages since plasma iodine concentrations are very low:
- In *iodine trapping*, plasma iodide ions (I^-) are actively transported from the plasma into the follicular cells against a steep concentration gradient. This is a rate-limiting step.
- In *iodide oxidation*, I^- is rapidly oxidized into iodine (I_2) by a peroxidase enzyme near the luminal membrane. This increases reactivity.

3. Iodination of thyroglobulin   The two components are then combined in the extracellular follicle lumen. Reactive iodine rapidly attaches to the tyrosine molecules within the extracellular thyroglobulin. The reaction requires thyroperoxidase, an enzyme on the luminal membrane of the follicle cells. Monoiodotyrosine

(MIT or T_1) and diiodotyrosine (DIT or T_2) are formed.

4. Coupling   Tyrosine molecules within thyroglobulin are coupled together. Combinations of T_1 and T_2 can form thyroid hormones:
- T_3 is made from $T_1 + T_2$.
- T_4 is made from $T_2 + T_2$.

5. Secretion   The iodinated thyroglobulin is taken into the follicular cells by pinocytosis and broken down by lysosomal enzymes. Coupled tyrosine molecules are released, including some T_3 and T_4, which diffuse into the blood. T_1 and T_2 are also released, but they are broken down to rescue iodine molecules.

Iodine metabolism

Iodine is acquired from the diet mainly from iodized salt, meat, and vegetables. About 150 mg of iodine is needed per day, although only a fraction of this is absorbed. The thyroid gland cells are the only cells that can actively absorb and utilize plasma iodine; a considerable quantity of iodine is stored in the thyroid as preformed thyroid hormones. Iodine is returned to the plasma by the breakdown of these

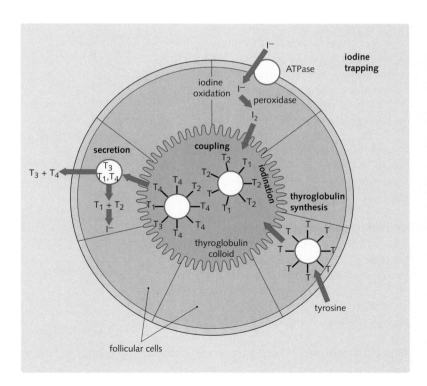

Fig. 3.6 Steps in the synthesis and secretion of T_3 and T_4.

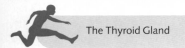

thyroid hormones. Iodine is excreted mainly via the kidneys.

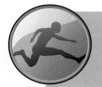

Thyroid hormones are the only molecules in humans that contain organically bound iodine.

Regulation

Hypothalamic thyrotropin-releasing hormone (TRH) stimulates the release of thyroid-stimulating hormone (TSH or thyrotropin) from the anterior pituitary gland. TSH acts on extracellular receptors on the surface of thyroid follicle cells. Cyclic AMP (cAMP) is formed and stimulates five of the stages of synthesis and secretion:

- Iodine uptake.
- Thyroglobin synthesis.
- Iodination.
- Coupling.
- Pinocytosis for secretion.

As a result T_3 and T_4 are synthesized and secreted more rapidly (see Fig. 3.1). TSH also has long-term actions on the thyroid gland by increasing its size and vascularity to improve hormone synthesis.

A number of factors affect thyroid hormone release. Three main factors stimulate secretion:

- Long-term exposure to cold temperatures acting on the anterior pituitary.
- Estrogens acting on the anterior pituitary.
- Epinephrine acting directly on the thyroid gland.

Thyroid hormone release is inhibited by excess thyroid hormones and glucocorticoids (e.g., cortisol) by acting on the anterior pituitary to suppress TSH release.

Transport of thyroid hormones

The thyroid hormones circulate bound to plasma proteins produced in the liver, which protect the hormones from enzymic attack:

- 70% are bound to thyroid-binding globulin (TBG).
- 30% are bound to albumin.

Only 0.1% of T_4 and 1% of T_3 are carried unbound—this free (unbound) fraction is responsible for their hormonal activities. Both T_3 and T_4 can cross cell membranes.

The concentration of circulating T_4 is much higher than that of T_3 (50:1). There are two reasons:

- The thyroid secretes more T_4 than T_3.
- T_4 has a longer half-life (7 days vs. 1 day).

Actions

Figure 3.7 describes some of the differences between T_4 and T_3. T_4 is a relatively inactive, stable molecule that can be thought of as a prohormone. T_3 is the active hormone, since it is readily available and has more effect on receptors. The benefit of producing both hormones is that T_4 can maintain a background level of activity while T_3 levels can adapt rapidly to changing environments.

Peripheral tissues can regulate local T_3 levels by increasing or decreasing T_3 synthesis. T_4 is converted to T_3 by deiodination, i.e., removal of one iodine atom catalyzed by deiodinase enzymes (5'-monodeiodinase [MIT]). Two main forms of this enzyme have been found:

- Type 1—found on the cell surface in most tissues. It raises local T_3.
- Type 2—intracellular enzymes that raise cellular T_3 in the central nervous system (CNS) and pituitary gland.

A further deiodinase enzyme can remove a different iodine molecule from T_4 to form reverse T_3 (rT_3). This is an inactive molecule that is rapidly cleared from the circulation by the kidney and liver. Production of rT_3 is favored by low energy stores and illness, so that energy is conserved.

Comparison of T_3 and T_4		
	T_3	T_4
Proportion of secreted thyroid hormone	10%	90%
Percentage free in plasma	1%	0.1%
Relative activity	10	1
Half-life (days)	1	7

Fig. 3.7 Comparison of T_3 and T_4.

The majority of plasma T_3 is formed by the deiodination of T_4—*not* from the thyroid gland. This is important in the treatment of hypothyroidism since only T_4 is given.

Free plasma T_3 enters cells and binds to intracellular T_3 receptors located in the membrane, mitochondria, and nucleus of the target cells. The intracellular actions are described in Fig. 3.8 and related to physiological effects.

In general, T_3 promotes energy production in every cell in the body. This causes heat production and maintains metabolism.

Feedback

T_3 receptors are also found in the pituitary gland, where they inhibit the release of TSH to create a negative feedback loop. Excess T_3 concentrations inhibit TSH release while deficient T_3 concentrations stimulate TSH release. This mechanism helps to maintain T_3 levels and therefore stabilizes metabolic rate.

Disorders of the thyroid gland

The thyroid gland is prone to a number of diseases that can alter its function and structure. These diseases frequently have wide-ranging systemic effects because thyroid hormones regulate the metabolism of almost every cell in the body. The main categories of disease are:

- Hyperthyroidism—excess of thyroid hormone production.
- Hypothyroidism—deficiency of thyroid hormone production.
- Goiter formation.
- Adenoma (benign growths) of the thyroid.
- Carcinoma of the thyroid.

Hyperthyroidism

Hyperthyroidism is defined as an overactive thyroid gland leading to excess thyroid hormones (T_4 and T_3). When this becomes symptomatic, it is called thyrotoxicosis. It is a common disorder affecting 1/50 females and 1/250 males. The symptoms and signs of thyrotoxicosis are illustrated in Fig. 3.9. Presentation is usually slow with a history lasting over 6 months.

The major symptoms of hyperthyroidism can be remembered by the mnemonic, "**D**on't **e**vade **f**eeling **h**ot **a**nd **s**weaty **p**atients." The symptoms are **d**iarrhea, **e**motional lability, **f**atigue, **h**eat intolerance, increased **a**ppetite, **s**weating, and **p**alpitations.

Actions of T_3		
Site of action	**Intracellular effects**	**Physiological results**
Cell membrane	Stimulates the Na^+/K^+ ATPase pump	Increased demand for metabolites, e.g., glucose
Mitochondria	Stimulates growth, replication, and activity; basal metabolic rate is raised	Increased heat production, oxygen demand, heart rate, and stroke volume
Nucleus	Increases expression of enzymes necessary for energy production	Lipolysis, glycolysis, and gluconeogenesis increased to raise blood metabolite levels and cellular metabolite use
Neonatal cells	Essential for cell division and maturation	Essential for normal development of CNS and skeleton

Fig. 3.8 Intracellular and physiological actions of T_3.

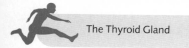

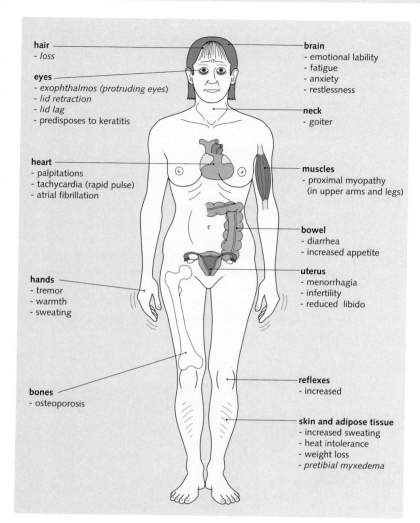

Fig. 3.9 Symptoms and signs of thyrotoxicosis (hyperthyroidism). The features in italics are found only in Graves' disease.

hair
- *loss*

eyes
- *exophthalmos (protruding eyes)*
- *lid retraction*
- *lid lag*
- *predisposes to keratitis*

heart
- palpitations
- tachycardia (rapid pulse)
- atrial fibrillation

hands
- tremor
- warmth
- sweating

bones
- osteoporosis

brain
- emotional lability
- fatigue
- anxiety
- restlessness

neck
- goiter

muscles
- proximal myopathy
  (in upper arms and legs)

bowel
- diarrhea
- increased appetite

uterus
- menorrhagia
- infertility
- reduced libido

reflexes
- increased

skin and adipose tissue
- increased sweating
- heat intolerance
- weight loss
- *pretibial myxedema*

An acute exacerbation of symptoms is called a thyrotoxic crisis; it is usually brought on by infection in previously undiagnosed patients. Surgery or radioactive ablation of the thyroid gland can also be responsible as the damaged thyroid follicles release their contents.

The main causes of hyperthyroidism are:
- Graves' disease—an autoimmune disease.
- Multinodular goiter—nodular enlargement of the thyroid in the elderly.
- Toxic adenoma—a benign thyroid hormone-producing tumor.

Diagnosis
Thyroid function tests are the main component of diagnosis. Serum TSH, free T_3, and free T_4 are measured by radioimmunoassay (RIA). Elevated T_3 and T_4 indicate that hyperthyroidism is present. Raised TSH suggests the fault lies in or above the pituitary gland, whereas low TSH points to a thyroid organ lesion.

Other tests include:
- Autoantibody detection (e.g., Graves' disease).
- Radioisotope scanning to show the size of the thyroid gland and any abnormal "hot" areas such as a toxic adenoma.
- ECG for sinus tachycardia or atrial fibrillation.

Treatment
There are three methods of treatment:
- Pharamacological intervention. Oral medications may be used to inhibit peroxidase activity

(propylthiouracil, carbimazole) or iodine trapping and transport (thiocyanate, perchloride). Most of these drugs take 3–4 weeks to have an effect.

- Radioactive iodine therapy. ^{131}I is taken up only by thyroid tissue; it kills the cells, leading to reduced T_3 and T_4 synthesis. The response is slow, and other pharmacological agents may be required.
- Partial thyroidectomy. The thyroid gland is surgically removed, leaving some tissue and the parathyroid glands.

Both radioactive iodine and partial thyroidectomy carry a high risk of long-term hypothyroidism. The remaining thyroid tissue may be insufficient to meet the body's needs, especially as the patient ages. Their treatment is described under hypothyroidism.

Graves' disease

Graves' disease is an autoimmune disease in which autoantibodies against the TSH receptors stimulate the receptors so that thyroid hormones are produced in excess. Graves' disease is the most common cause of hyperthyroidism; it is especially common in middle-aged women and has a genetic component.

The disease follows either a relapsing-remitting course or one with fluctuating severity. In rare cases, Graves' disease can progress to hypothyroidism with time.

Graves' disease can cause the classic picture of hyperthyroidism with bulging eyes (exophthalmos), goiter (with bruit), and swollen legs (pretibial myxedema). It is diagnosed by detection of autoantibodies along with low TSH and raised T_3. The treatment is consistent with other causes of hyperthyroidism, but radioactive iodine and surgery are especially likely to cause hypothyroidism.

Eye disease is an important symptom of Graves' disease. Inflammation of the orbit causes the eye to protrude, which can lead to discomfort and double vision. This symptom may occur before thyroid hormone levels rise. It does not always respond to treatment, and it may develop in patients with well-controlled disease.

In Graves' disease, the vasculature of the thyroid gland can increase to such an extent that a bruit can be heard over the goiter using a stethoscope.

Hypothyroidism

Hypothyroidism is defined as an underactive thyroid gland leading to deficient thyroid hormones (T_4 and T_3). When this becomes symptomatic, it is called myxedema. It is slightly less common than hyperthyroidism, affecting 1/100 females and 1/500 males. The symptoms and signs of myxedema are illustrated in Fig. 3.10. Presentation is even more gradual than in hyperthyroidism with many symptoms frequently being ignored.

Thyroid hormones are essential between birth and puberty for the normal development of the CNS. Deficiency can cause irreversible mental retardation called cretinism. TSH levels are checked in all newborns for this relatively common abnormality; the levels will be raised if the thyroid gland is not functioning correctly.

Undertreated hypothyroidism can progress to a life-threatening myxedemic coma. This rare condition is characterized by bradycardia and hypotension. Plasma levels of glucose and sodium can also drop, and type II respiratory failure may develop.

Diagnosis

Hypothyroidism is not investigated as thoroughly as hyperthyroidism, since treatment does not vary. Free T_3 and T_4 levels are low, whereas TSH levels are usually raised. If TSH is low, a lesion of the hypothalamus or pituitary is likely. Autoantibodies can be detected in Hashimoto's thyroiditis, which gradually destroys the thyroid gland.

Treatment

All hypothyroidism is treated with thyroxine (T_4) administered as an oral tablet in varying doses. The dose is increased over several months with regular monitoring of TSH levels until TSH levels are within the normal boundaries. This process is slow since it takes 4 weeks for TSH levels to reflect an increased dose owing to the long half-life of thyroxine. Thyroxine therapy is usually maintained for life.

Overtreatment of hyperthyroidism

Radioactive ablation and surgical removal of the thyroid gland initially cure hyperthyroidism but, with time, the remaining thyroid tissue is often insufficient. Hypothyroidism can develop, and lifelong thyroxine treatment is required.

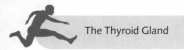

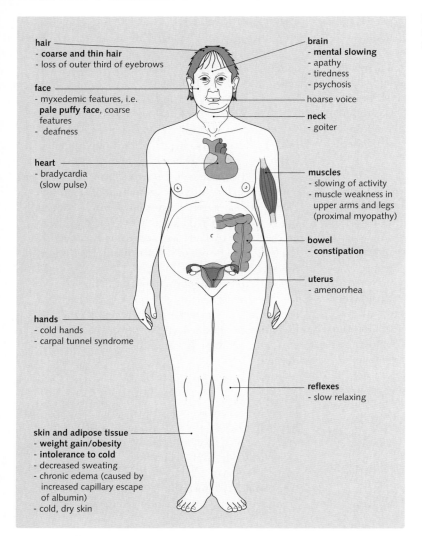

Fig. 3.10 Symptoms and signs of myxedema (hypothyroidism). The main features are shown in bold.

Many drugs can also cause reversible hypothyroidism, including lithium, amiodarone, and excess iodine.

Hashimoto's thyroiditis
When the thyroid gland is inflamed, the disease is called thyroiditis. This can be caused by autoimmune or viral processes. Hashimoto's thyroiditis is a destructive autoimmune disease that is especially common in middle-aged women. It is mediated by autoantibodies against rough endoplasmic reticulum (microsomal antibodies) or thyroglobulin. The presence of these antibodies can be tested to confirm the diagnosis. The thyroid gland is infiltrated by lymphocytes that cause the gland to enlarge, forming a goiter.

The initial destruction of the thyroid gland can release the thyroglobulin colloid, causing temporary hyperthyroidism. The patients usually progress to a euthyroid (normal) state and finally develop progressive hypothyroidism.

De Quervain's thyroiditis
De Quervain's thyroiditis is inflammation of the thyroid gland caused by a virus. It is common in young or middle-aged women, in whom it causes a tender, swollen gland along with a febrile illness. The inflammation destroys the follicles, which causes

hypothyroidism and leakage of the thyroglobulin colloid. An immune reaction against this colloid causes the formation of granulomas so this disease is also called granulomatous thyroiditis.

Primary atrophic hypothyroidism

Spontaneous or primary atrophic hypothyroidism is a disease resulting in hypothyroidism in the elderly. The thyroid gland becomes shrunken and fibrosed so that there is no goiter. It is suspected that this disease is the end-stage of many thyroid diseases, including Hashimoto's and de Quervain's thyroiditis.

Goiters

A goiter is a swelling in the neck caused by an enlarged thyroid gland. It is a common finding that is usually asymptomatic; however, large goiters can compress the esophagus and trachea. If a goiter is associated with hyperthyroidism, it is described as "toxic." Nontoxic goiters secrete normal or reduced levels of thyroid hormones. Goiters are treated by correcting the underlying pathology or by surgical removal for cosmetic reasons or to prevent compression of surrounding structures.

An enlarged thyroid gland can be distinguished from a thyroglossal cyst by asking the patient to swallow and stick out the tongue. The thyroid gland will move with the trachea on swallowing, whereas a thyroglossal cyst rises when the tongue is protruded.

Iodine deficiency

Iodine deficiency was once a common cause of goiter in regions where the soil lacked iodine (e.g., the Great Lakes), but nowadays iodine is added to salt to prevent this. Deficient iodine means that thyroid hormones cannot be synthesized so TSH levels rise owing to a lack of negative feedback. TSH stimulates follicle and blood vessel growth and development of new blood vessels; as a result, the thyroid gland enlarges. Because this does not cure the iodine deficiency, the goiter continues to grow.

The goiter formed by this process is diffusely enlarged and smooth. It is sometimes called an endemic goiter because it occurred in certain geographical regions.

Graves' disease

The constant stimulation of TSH receptors in Graves' disease causes a goiter in a similar manner to iodine deficiency with similar characteristics. The gland becomes highly vascular, to the extent that a bruit can be heard using a stethoscope.

Puberty and pregnancy

Because higher levels of thyroid hormones are required in puberty and pregnancy, the thyroid gland often enlarges to meet the increased demand. This enlargement is a physiological response, not a pathological process. The goiter regresses once the demand lessens.

During pregnancy the secretion of T_4 increases. However, blood levels remain constant owing to the increase in thyroid-binding globulin controlled by estrogen.

Multinodular goiter

Many elderly people have an enlarged thyroid that contains many nodules of varying sizes. These nodules are formed from hyperplasia (increased number) of thyroid cells. The excess cells sometimes cause excess thyroid hormone production (i.e., hyperthyroidism). The disease is then called toxic multinodular goiter.

Thyroiditis

Inflammation of the thyroid gland can cause swelling, and infiltration by lymphocytes can also cause enlargement. The goiter formed is usually slightly nodular, but it may be tender if the inflammation is acute.

Thyroid gland neoplasia

Thyroid lumps are common and usually benign, but they must be investigated. Solitary thyroid lumps are found in 5% of women, and it is difficult to distinguish between benign (80%) and malignant (20%) on clinical grounds. A fine-needle aspiration should be performed along with thyroid function

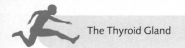

Characteristics of primary thyroid gland malignancies

Type	Cell type	Age group	Route of metastasis	Prognosis
Papillary	Follicle cells	All	Cervical lymphatics	Excellent
Follicular	Follicle cells	Middle-aged	Blood to bone, lung, and brain	Good
Medullary	Parafollicular cells	Middle-aged and elderly	Cervical lymphatics	Variable but usually good
Malignant lymphoma	Lymphatics	Elderly	Local invasion	Poor
Anaplastic	Follicle cells	Elderly	Local invasion	Very poor

Fig. 3.11 The characteristics of the five primary thyroid gland malignancies.

tests. Aspiration alone will not distinguish a follicular adenoma from a follicular carcinoma, but low TSH suggests the former. Ultrasound can be performed to detect cysts.

Causes of solitary thyroid lumps include:
• Thyroid cysts.
• Nodule of multinodular goiter.
• Follicular adenoma.
• Malignancy.

Five separate forms of cancer can arise in the thyroid gland, but three of these are derived from the follicle cells. These tumors are summarized in Fig. 3.11.

Medullary carcinomas of the parafollicular cells often secrete ectopic hormones, including:
• Calcitonin—usually asymptomatic.
• Adrenocorticotropic hormone (ACTH)—Cushing's syndrome.
• 5-Hydroxytryptamine (5-HT; serotonin)—carcinoid syndrome.

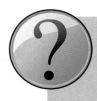

• Describe the anatomical shape and location of the thyroid and parathyroid glands. Why does the thyroid gland move during swallowing?
• Describe the blood supply to the thyroid gland, and describe the nerves that are related to these vessels.
• Describe how the cells of the thyroid gland are arranged.
• How do the thyroid and parathyroid glands develop in the embryo?
• List the hormones secreted by the thyroid gland, and describe their actions.
• Describe the five steps in thyroid hormone synthesis.
• Explain the endocrine control of the thyroid gland.
• State the main symptoms and signs of thyrotoxicosis. What is the most common cause?
• State the main symptoms and signs of myxedema. What is the main cause?
• Describe the treatment of hyperthyroidism and hypothyroidism.

4. The Adrenal Glands

The two adrenal glands allow the body to deal with both the emotional and physical stresses of life. They secrete four groups of hormones that have a wide range of effects.

The adrenal glands are located above each kidney. They are composed of two different types of endocrine tissue, which have different embryological origins.

The adrenal cortex is derived from embryonic mesoderm. It is regulated by adrenocorticotropic hormone (ACTH) from the pituitary gland, and it responds by secreting three types of steroid hormone:

- Glucocorticoids to deal with stress.
- Mineralocorticoids to regulate blood volume.
- Androgens for sexual development.

The adrenal medulla is derived from ectodermal tissue and consists of sympathetic nerve cells. It is under the direct control of the sympathetic nervous system, and it responds by secreting two modified amino acid hormones:

- Epinephrine.
- Norepinephrine.

The most important hormones produced by the adrenal glands are glucocorticoids, such as cortisol. They are regulated by hypothalamic and anterior pituitary hormones to form the hypothalamic–pituitary–adrenal (HPA) axis (Fig. 4.1). Synthetic versions of these hormones are commonly used to treat inflammatory illness, and they are referred to as "steroids" or "corticosteroids."

An excess of glucocorticoids causes Cushing's syndrome, and a deficiency causes Addison's disease.

Important terms:
Catecholamine: hormone secreted from the adrenal medulla
Cushing's syndrome: an excess of glucocorticoids
Cushing's disease: Cushing's syndrome caused by an ACTH-secreting tumor of the anterior pituitary gland
Conn's syndrome: an excess of aldosterone caused by a tumor of the adrenal cortex
Addison's disease: deficiency of cortisol and aldosterone caused by progressive destruction of the adrenal gland

After reading this chapter you should be able to:
- Picture the structure and development of adrenal glands.
- Explain the regulation and physiological effects of steroid hormones secreted by the adrenal cortex.
- Describe the major disorders of the adrenal cortex.
- Discuss the physiological effects of hormones secreted by the adrenal medulla.
- Discuss the major disorders of the adrenal medulla.

Anatomy

There are two adrenal glands, superior to each kidney, which differ significantly in their relations and shape. Both glands are retroperitoneal and are embedded in adipose tissue. Each gland is composed of an internal medulla and external cortex.

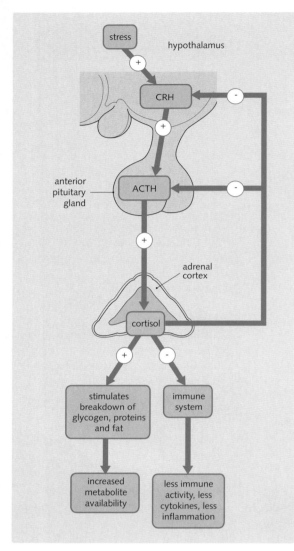

Fig. 4.1 Hormonal regulation of cortisol. (ACTH, adrenocorticotropic hormone; CRH, corticotropin-releasing hormone.)

Right adrenal gland

The right adrenal gland is pyramidal in shape, lying between the inferior vena cava and the right crus (a large tendon) of the diaphragm. The liver is located superiorly.

Left adrenal gland

The left adrenal gland is crescent-shaped; it lies medially to the left crus of the diaphragm. Anteriorly, the body of the pancreas and the splenic artery are adjacent. The stomach is situated

superiorly, separated by the peritoneum. The location of both glands is shown in Fig. 4.2.

Blood supply, nerves, and lymphatics

The outer cortex receives no significant innervation; instead it is regulated primarily by ACTH from the pituitary gland.

The adrenal gland's name comes from the Latin meaning "toward the kidney."

The medulla is innervated directly by the splanchnic nerves, which arise from the thoracic spinal cord and do not synapse before reaching the adrenal medulla. The nerves are therefore preganglionic sympathetic nerves that release acetylcholine, while all other tissues receive only postganglionic sympathetic innervation. The cause of this relationship is apparent from their development (see below).

The glands receive a rich blood supply from the adrenal arteries, which are branches of the inferior phrenic arteries and renal arteries. They are drained by the adrenal veins into the inferior vena cava and renal vein. Lymphatic drainage passes to the paraaortic nodes.

Development

Adrenal cortex

The adrenal cortex is formed from an area of mesoderm that surrounds the adrenal medulla; this is close to the origin of the gonads. The cortical layer thickens to form the fetal cortex, which stimulates the differentiation of the adrenal medulla.

Later, more mesodermal cells surround the fetal cortex to form the permanent cortex found in adults. At birth, the permanent cortex has two layers while a third (the zona reticularis) develops by the third year. During this time the fetal cortex regresses until only the developed medulla and permanent cortex are left.

Adrenal medulla

The adrenal medulla is derived from ectodermal neural crest cells of the embryo. These cells

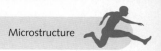

Fig. 4.2 Location and blood supply of the adrenal glands.

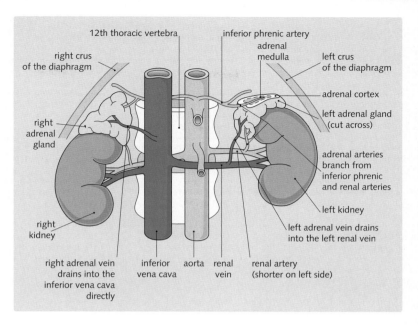

Fig. 4.3 Comparison between the adrenal medulla and the sympathetic nervous system. (ACh, acetylcholine; CNS, central nervous system; NE, norepinephrine.)

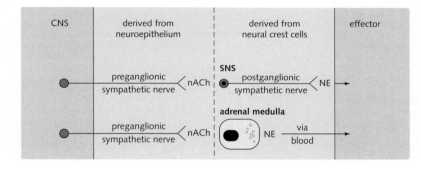

contribute to many diverse structures, including all the norepinephrine-secreting postganglionic neurons in the sympathetic nervous system. The secretory cells in the adrenal medulla secrete either epinephrine or norepinephrine, and they are essentially highly specialized neurons (Fig. 4.3).

Microstructure

Adrenal cortex
The adult adrenal cortex makes up about 90% of the adrenal gland by weight. It is divided into three layers, which secrete the following groups of steroid hormones (Figs. 4.4 and 4.5):
- Outer zona glomerulosa secretes mineralocorticoids.
- Middle zona fasciculata secretes glucocorticoids.
- Inner zona reticularis secretes androgens and glucocorticoids.

These hormone groups will be explained later in the chapter.

The cells of the zona fasciculata and zona reticularis are arranged in columns around blood sinusoids. The blood in these sinusoids passes directly into the adrenal medulla.

To remember the order of the layers in the adrenal cortex, think of GFR which stands for glomerular filtration rate in the nearby kidney.

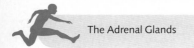

Microstructure of the adrenal gland and the major hormones secreted in each region			
Region	**Name**	**Cell structure**	**Hormones synthesized**
Outer cortex	Zona glomerulosa	Cells arranged in clumps (Latin, *glomerulus*: little ball)	Mineralocorticoids (mainly aldosterone)
Middle cortex	Zona fasciculata	Cells arranged in cords alongside blood sinusoids; (Latin, *fasciculus*: bundle)	Glucocorticoids (mainly cortisol)
Inner cortex	Zona reticularis	Network of smaller cells (Latin, *reticularis*: network)	Glucocorticoids and androgens (DHEA)
Center of gland	Adrenal medulla	Loose network of neurosecretory cells surrounded by blood sinusoids	Catecholamines (epinephrine and norepinephrine)

Fig. 4.4 Microstructure of the adrenal gland and the major hormones secreted in each region.

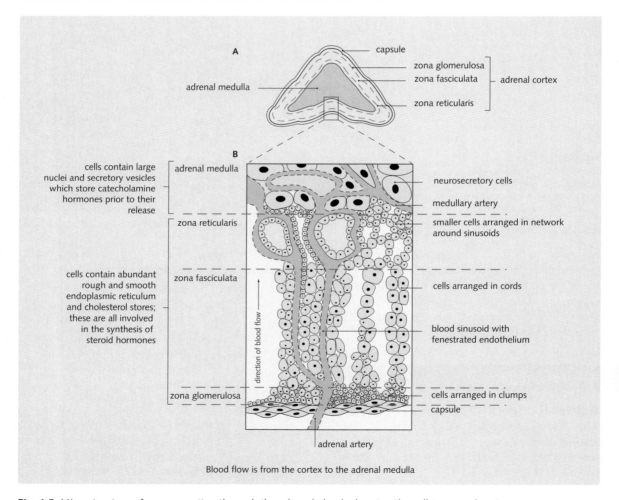

Fig. 4.5 Microstructure of a cross-section through the adrenal glands showing the cell types and regions.

Adrenal medulla

The adrenal medulla is composed of two types of neuroendocrine cell:

- Norepinephrine-secreting cells (20%).
- Epinephrine-secreting cells (80%).

Both types contain neuroendocrine granules that store the hormone. In older textbooks these cells are called chromaffin cells because they turn a dark-brown color if exposed to oxygen after fixation in chrome salts. The cells are arranged around blood sinusoids.

Medullary cells require the steroid cortisol to convert norepinephrine to epinephrine. Cortisol is produced in the cortex and travels in the cortical capillaries to the medulla. Separate medullary arteries supply oxygenated blood directly.

Hormones of the adrenal cortex

The adrenal cortex secretes three groups of steroid hormones:

- Mineralocorticoids (e.g., aldosterone).
- Glucocorticoids (e.g., cortisol)
- Androgens (e.g., DHEA).

Steroid hormones are synthesized from cholesterol. They are small lipid-soluble molecules that cross membranes readily. Inside cells they act on intracellular receptors to regulate gene expression. The synthesis and mechanism of action of steroid hormones are discussed in more detail in Chapter 1.

Mineralocorticoids and aldosterone
Regulation of aldosterone

Mineralocorticoids help to regulate the electrolyte balance of plasma; their name is derived from this action on the body's minerals. Aldosterone is the main mineralocorticoid secreted by the outer layer of the cortex, called the zona glomerulosa. Its release is stimulated by three main factors:

- Angiotensin II.
- High plasma potassium.
- ACTH.

Angiotensin II is released in response to low blood volume as part of the renin–angiotensin system (see Chapter 7 and Fig. 4.6). ACTH from the anterior pituitary gland is less important as a regulator; therefore, pituitary failure does not severely impair aldosterone secretion. An excess of aldosterone due to an adrenal adenoma is called Conn's disease.

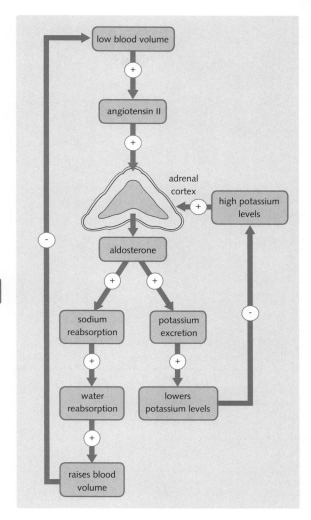

Fig. 4.6 Control of aldosterone secretion.

Actions of aldosterone

Aldosterone acts mainly on the distal convoluted tubule (DCT) and the collecting duct of the kidney. It causes reabsorption of sodium ions in exchange for potassium and hydrogen ions. Water is also reabsorbed and blood volume is increased. Other hormones involved in this mechanism are discussed in more detail in Chapter 7 on fluid balance.

Intracellular actions of aldosterone

To cause these physiological effects, aldosterone acts on the nucleus via an intracellular receptor known as the mineralocorticoid receptor. Only cells that express this receptor can respond to aldosterone. The expression of four genes encoding the Na^+/K^+ ATPase, Na^+ channel, K^+ channel, and

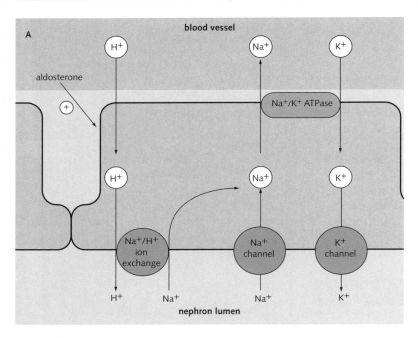

Fig. 4.7 Intracellular and physiological actions of aldosterone in the nephron. Aldosterone acts to increase the levels of the four proteins shown (A), causing the physiological responses (B).

B	Effects of proteins induced by aldosterone in the nephron		
Protein	Location	Action	Physiological response
Na⁺/K⁺ ATPase	Cell membrane on the side of the blood supply	Active pump that increases cell potassium and lowers cell sodium levels	Creates an ion gradient that drives the other proteins
Na⁺ channel	Cell membrane on the side of the nephron	Reabsorbs sodium from the nephron lumen	Increases plasma sodium and water to increase blood volume
K⁺ channel	Cell membrane on the side of the nephron	Excretes potassium into the nephron lumen	Decreases plasma potassium
Na⁺/H⁺ ion exchanger	Cell membrane on the side of the nephron	Reabsorbs sodium in exchange for hydrogen ions	Makes the plasma more alkaline

Na^+/H^+ ion exchanger is increased in the cells of the DCT and collecting duct, the actions of which are described in Fig. 4.7.

Aldosterone circulates in the plasma with 60% bound to albumin and 40% free and, therefore, active. The high proportion of free hormone causes aldosterone to be rapidly degraded by the liver, giving a short half-life of about 15 minutes.

Glucocorticoids and cortisol

Glucocorticoids act on the metabolism of carbohydrate, protein, and to a lesser extent fat. It is the action on glucose (a carbohydrate) that is responsible for their name. Glucocorticoids also depress the immune system, and it is for this effect that "steroids" are most often used as medication. Cortisol is the main glucocorticoid. Cushing's syndrome is a result of elevated systemic levels of glucocorticoids due to either treatment or pathology.

Regulation of cortisol

Corticotropin-releasing hormone (CRH) is secreted by the hypothalamus and stimulates the anterior pituitary to release ACTH. This hormone acts on the zona fasciculata and zona reticularis of the adrenal cortex, which secrete cortisol. Cortisol has a negative feedback effect on the hypothalamus and anterior pituitary gland to inhibit CRH and ACTH release.

Cortisol release displays a circadian rhythm, i.e., the rate of secretion changes through a 24-hour period (Fig. 4.8). The highest levels of cortisol release are in the early morning, peaking at about 6 a.m., then falling through the day. This circadian variation is initiated in the hypothalamus by changes in sensitivity to cortisol levels. Cortisol exerts a weaker negative feedback effect in the morning so CRH release rises.

> The inhibitory action of cortisol on ACTH release is important clinically. Patients treated with long-term "steroids" cannot simply stop because ACTH release and, therefore, cortisol production would also stop. Instead the dose must be lowered over a number of months.

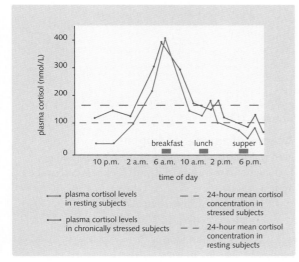

Fig. 4.8 Circadian variation in plasma cortisol in resting and chronically stressed subjects.

Actions of cortisol

Like epinephrine, cortisol allows the body to deal with "stress" such as trauma, hemorrhage, and fever. This effect is very important, and cortisol deficiency can rapidly become life-threatening. The response to stress is called the general adaptation syndrome (GAS) and is divided into three phases:

1. *Alarm reaction* (Also called the "fight or flight" response.) A stressful stimulus causes:
- Norepinephrine release from sympathetic nerves.
- Epinephrine and norepinephrine release from adrenal medulla.
- Cortisol release from adrenal cortex.

2. *Resistance* Cortisol has a slower and longer-lasting action than epinephrine and norepinephrine; it allows the resistance to stress to be maintained. It also counteracts the effects of other hormones (e.g., insulin) to maintain substrates required to combat stress.

3. *Exhaustion* Prolonged stress causes continued cortisol secretion, which results in muscle wastage, immune system suppression, and hyperglycemia.

Cortisol affects almost every cell in the body. The physiological effects are described in Fig. 4.9. The main actions of cortisol are:
- Increase of energy metabolite levels in the blood.
- Suppression of the immune system and inhibition of allergic and inflammatory processes.

There is some overlap between the actions of mineralocorticoids and glucocorticoids. Cortisol can have mineralocorticoid actions, whereas aldosterone can act as a glucocorticoid.

Intracellular actions of cortisol

Like all steroid hormones, cortisol acts via intracellular receptors to regulate gene expression. The receptor and genes vary between cells, and this accounts for the wide range of actions. The anti-inflammatory actions are produced by inhibiting phospholipase A_2, an enzyme that is essential for the production of prostaglandins from arachidonic acid.

Most cortisol (95%) is transported through the circulation bound to plasma proteins:
- 80% bound to cortisol-binding protein.
- 15% bound to albumin.
- 5% free and active.

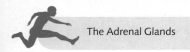

Physiological effects of cortisol and the symptoms of Cushing's syndrome		
Process/system affected	Effect of cortisol	Related pathology in Cushing's syndrome
Carbohydrate metabolism	Raises blood glucose by stimulating gluconeogenesis and preventing glucose uptake	Hyperglycemia and diabetes
Protein metabolism	Increases breakdown of proteins in skeletal muscle, skin, and bone to release amino acids	Muscle weakness and wasting; thin, easily bruising skin
Fat metabolism	Stimulates lipolysis and increases fatty acid levels in the blood	Fat redistributed to the face and trunk causing a moon face, buffalo hump, and abdominal stretch marks
Immune system	Suppresses the action and production of immune cells; inhibits the production of cytokines and antibodies	Infections, poor healing, peptic ulceration
Endocrine system	Suppresses the secretion of anterior pituitary hormones: ACTH, LH, FSH, TSH, and GH	Suppression of growth in children
Nervous system	Influences fetal and neonatal neuron development; influences behavior and cognitive function; augments the actions of the sympathetic system	Depression, insomnia, psychosis, and confusion
Water metabolism	Has weak mineralocorticoid actions: raises sodium and water retention	Hypertension and heart failure
Calcium metabolism	Decreases calcium absorption from the gut; increases calcium excretion in the kidneys; increases calcium resorption from bones	Osteoporosis

Fig. 4.9 Physiological effects of cortisol related to the symptoms of Cushing's syndrome. (ACTH, adrenocorticotropic hormone; FSH, follicle-stimulating hormone; GH, growth hormone; LH, luteinizing hormone; TSH, thyroid-stimulating hormone.)

It is inactivated in the liver by conjugation and then excreted from the kidney. About 1% of cortisol is excreted into the urine without metabolism. This can be detected by 24-hour urine collection to estimate blood cortisol levels.

Androgens

Androgens are male sex steroids, i.e., hormones involved in the growth and function of the male genital tract. They also stimulate muscle growth (anabolism), hence their use as an illicit drug in sports. They are secreted by the adrenal glands in both males and females; in males, however, testicular androgen secretion accounts for a much greater proportion of total production.

Actions of adrenal androgens

Adrenal androgens are synthesized in the zona reticularis of the adrenal gland; the main adrenal androgens are:
- Dehydroepiandrosterone (DHEA).
- Androstenedione.

Androgens secreted by the adrenal glands have weak biological activity, but they are converted to more active androgens, such as testosterone, by enzymes in peripheral tissues.

Adrenarche

The initiation of androgen secretion from the adrenal glands is called adrenarche. It occurs a few years before puberty (about 7–9 years of age) and is marked by maturation of the zona reticularis.

In males, the early development of the male sex organs may result from adrenal androgens released after adrenarche. In male adult life adrenal androgens account for only 5% of total activity and are physiologically negligible. Androgens are discussed in greater detail in Chapter 13.

In females, adrenal androgens are responsible for about 50% of total androgen activity from adrenarche to the end of life. These hormones help to promote the growth of female pubic and axillary hair.

Disorders of the adrenal cortex

The main diseases of the adrenal cortex are caused by an excess or deficiency of mineralocorticoids or glucocorticoids. There are four named diseases affecting the adrenal cortex hormones that are a common cause of pre-exam tremor; however, they are rare diseases:

- Cushing's syndrome—excessive cortisol production.
- Cushing's disease—ACTH-secreting tumor.
- Conn's syndrome—aldosterone-secreting tumor.
- Addison's disease—deficiency of cortisol and aldosterone.

Hyperaldosteronism

Excess aldosterone production causes sodium ion and water retention with increased excretion of potassium and hydrogen ions. The main symptoms and signs (Fig. 4.10) are:

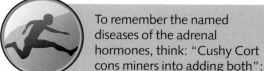

To remember the named diseases of the adrenal hormones, think: "Cushy Cort cons miners into adding both":
Cushing's—cortisol (excess)
Conn's—mineralocorticoids (excess)
Addison's—both (deficiency)

- Hypertension (high blood pressure).
- Hypokalemia (low potassium).
- Alkalosis (raised blood pH).
- Polyuria and polydipsia (thirst).
- Muscle weakness and spasm.

A number of blood tests are used for diagnosis:
- Urea and electrolytes (U + Es) for hypokalemia.
- Aldosterone levels (raised).
- Renin levels (variable).

Aldosterone increases blood volume, which inhibits renin secretion. If renin levels are low, the disorder is primary hyperaldosteronism (i.e., the disease originates in the adrenal glands). The adrenal glands can then be imaged by CT/MRI scanning.

Renin stimulates aldosterone release via angiotensin II; thus, high renin levels suggest secondary hyperaldosteronism. This disorder is external to the adrenal glands; it is a common response to heart failure and renal disease.

Primary hyperaldosteronism and Conn's syndrome

Primary hyperaldosteronism is a rare disease that is responsible for about 1% of patients with hypertension. The vast majority of primary

Clinical symptoms of hyperaldosteronism and hypoaldosteronism		
Action of aldosterone	Hyperaldosteronism	Hypoaldosteronism
Increases plasma Na$^+$	Hypernatremia rarely occurs because of other mechanisms regulating fluid volume	Loss of Na$^+$ is accompanied by loss of water, so plasma Na$^+$ concentration does not change
Decreases plasma K$^+$	Hypokalemia	Hyperkalemia
Decreases plasma H$^+$	Metabolic alkalosis	Mild metabolic acidosis
Maintains extracellular fluid volume	Hypertension	Volume depletion and postural hypotension

Fig. 4.10 Clinical symptoms caused by hyperaldosteronism (e.g., Conn's syndrome) and hypoaldosteronism (e.g., Addison's disease).

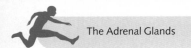

hyperaldosteronism is caused by Conn's syndrome, in which the patients have an adenoma of the zona glomerulosa. This is discussed later in the chapter.

Secondary hyperaldosteronism

Secondary hyperaldosteronism is a very common problem caused by activation of the renin–angiotensin system. The most common cause is excessive diuretic therapy, but it is also a feature of:

- Congestive heart failure.
- Renal artery stenosis.
- Nephritic syndrome.
- Cirrhosis with ascites.

All these conditions result in decreased renal perfusion, which stimulates renin release.

Excess cortisol
Cushing's syndrome

Cushing's syndrome is a rare condition caused by a chronic excess of glucocorticoids. The disorder can be in the anterior pituitary gland or the adrenal cortex, or it may result from excess medication. It has a 5-year mortality rate of about 50% if it is not treated. The symptoms and signs of Cushing's syndrome are shown in Figs. 4.9 and 4.11; it is most common in adult women.

Diagnosing excess cortisol is complicated by the circadian variation in cortisol secretion. Two main tests are employed to overcome this problem:

- 24-hour urinary free cortisol: 1% of free cortisol is excreted unmetabolized, and this can be measured to give an accurate reflection of plasma cortisol.

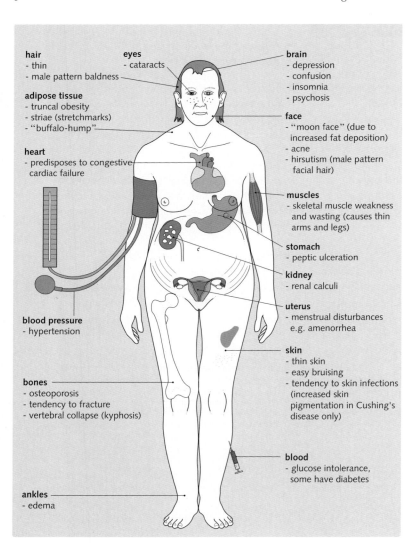

Fig. 4.11 Symptoms and signs of Cushing's syndrome.

- Dexamethasone suppression test: plasma cortisol is measured before an oral dexamethasone (a synthetic glucocorticoid) dose and then at 8 a.m. the next morning. In a normal person, plasma cortisol will be suppressed; in a patient with Cushing's syndrome, cortisol levels will remain high.

Once cortisol excess has been confirmed, further tests using higher doses of dexamethasone and measuring ACTH levels can distinguish between adrenal hyperplasia and other causes. CT scans are used once a source has been identified.

Treatment with glucocorticoids

Glucocorticoids (often simply called "steroids") are used to treat a wide range of medical conditions, usually to reduce immune reactions. These conditions include asthma, inflammatory bowel disease, rheumatoid arthritis, and post-transplantation. Patients are treated with the lowest dose that will control their condition because prolonged use can cause the features of Cushing's syndrome. Inhaled steroids are used in asthma to reduce the systemic dose, especially in children, in whom growth retardation may occur.

Cushing's disease

Adenomas of the corticotroph cells in the anterior pituitary can release excess ACTH. This stimulates the adrenal cortex to secrete excess cortisol, leading to bilateral enlargement of the cortex or adrenal hyperplasia. The negative feedback that normally prevents excess ACTH release is absent in the tumor.

This type of tumor causes Cushing's syndrome with the additional sign of pigmented skin. The prohormone proopiomelanocortin is cleaved to form several smaller peptide hormones, including ACTH and melanocyte-stimulating hormone (α-MSH), which stimulates the activity of melanocytes in the skin. Cushing's disease occurs most frequently in young adult women.

Cushing's disease is treated by surgical removal of the pituitary adenoma. This may result in panhypopituitarism (see Chapter 2 for more details).

Ectopic adrenocorticotropic hormone production

Ectopic ACTH can be secreted by the rare, but highly malignant, small-cell anaplastic carcinoma of the lung (also called oat-cell carcinoma). This carcinoma displays the characteristics of a neuroendocrine cell despite developing from bronchial epithelium. Even more rarely, tumors of the thymus, ovary, or pancreas and carcinoid tumors can secrete ACTH or CRH. The excess production is so dramatic that patients rarely exhibit features of Cushing's syndrome before death. Ectopic hormones are discussed in Chapter 10.

> Cushing's disease and syndrome are named after the American neurosurgeon Harvey Cushing (1869–1939), who clarified the function of the anterior pituitary gland and described the effects of excess cortisol. In his spare time he also developed the first surgical technique for removing pituitary tumors.

Neoplasia of the adrenal cortex

Benign adenoma of the adrenal cortex is relatively common, but only a small proportion secrete hormones. If cortisol is secreted, Cushing's syndrome develops; aldosterone-secreting adenomas cause Conn's syndrome.

Adrenal adenomas are the most common cause of Cushing's syndrome in children, but they account for only 10% of adult disease. In Conn's syndrome, adenomas of the adrenal cortex are the most common cause of primary hyperaldosteronism in all age groups. Adenomas associated with either syndrome are removed surgically, but cortisol replacement is necessary due to long-term ACTH inhibition.

Carcinoma of the adrenal cortex is a very rare condition. These tumors secrete vast excesses of glucocorticoids and androgens. The patient usually dies before the physical features of Cushing's syndrome develop.

Deficiency of cortisol and aldosterone
Congenital adrenal hyperplasia

This is an autosomal recessive condition causing deficiency of 21-hydroxylase, an enzyme normally found in the adrenal cortex. Since this enzyme is required for the synthesis of aldosterone and cortisol, both hormones are deficient. Low cortisol triggers ACTH release, resulting in hyperplasia of the adrenal cortex. Low aldosterone results in salt loss and neonatal shock in some babies. Full-blown congenital adrenal hyperplasia is rare (1 in 10,000 births); however, 1 in 100 births partially express this condition.

The enlarged adrenal cortex secretes excess androgens, causing adrenogenital syndrome. This presents differently in each sex. In males, it causes early (precocious) pseudopuberty. Signs of secondary sexual development can be found by 6 months of age, but the child is not fertile. Early bone maturation causes short adult height.

In females, androgen excess causes masculinization (also called virilization). The symptoms are similar to those found in polycystic ovarian syndrome, as described in Chapter 12. They include:

- Masculine body shape.
- Balding of temporal skull.
- Increased muscle bulk.
- Deepening of the voice.
- Enlargement of the clitoris.

Adrenal cortex insufficiency

Adrenal cortex insufficiency tends to affect the whole adrenal cortex rather than specific layers. Accordingly, deficiencies of glucocorticoids, mineralocorticoids, and androgens occur together, although clinical effects are due to cortisol and aldosterone deficiency. These effects are shown in Fig. 4.12. Hydrocortisone (cortisol) and

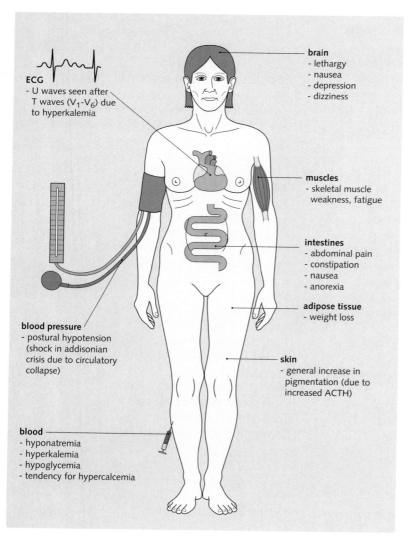

ECG
- U waves seen after T waves (V_1-V_6) due to hyperkalemia

brain
- lethargy
- nausea
- depression
- dizziness

muscles
- skeletal muscle weakness, fatigue

intestines
- abdominal pain
- constipation
- nausea
- anorexia

adipose tissue
- weight loss

blood pressure
- postural hypotension (shock in addisonian crisis due to circulatory collapse)

skin
- general increase in pigmentation (due to increased ACTH)

blood
- hyponatremia
- hyperkalemia
- hypoglycemia
- tendency for hypercalcemia

Fig. 4.12 Symptoms and signs of Addison's disease.

fludrocortisone (a mineralocorticoid) therapy must be initiated before the underlying disease process is treated.

Suspected adrenal cortex insufficiency is investigated using the ACTH stimulation test. A synthetic ACTH analog is injected, and plasma cortisol levels are measured every 30 minutes. If the cortisol levels do not rise sufficiently, the disease is of the adrenal cortex (i.e., Addison's disease).

Addison's disease
Primary insufficiency of the adrenal cortex is called Addison's disease; it is characterized by deficient secretion of glucocorticoids and mineralocorticoids. It is a rare chronic condition caused by progressive destruction of the adrenal cortex. This destruction can result from autoimmune adrenalitis, infection (e.g., tuberculosis, fungi), or tumor. Addison's disease presents with adrenal cortex insufficiency, but the high levels of circulating ACTH can cause skin pigmentation too.

An acute exacerbation of Addison's disease is called an adrenal crisis. It is a life-threatening emergency caused by stressful events such as infection. Its presentation is the same as acute adrenal cortical failure.

Acute adrenal cortical failure
Acute adrenal cortex failure is a life-threatening condition characterized by:
- Hypotensive shock.
- Hypovolemic shock.
- Hypoglycemia.

The adrenal cortex can be destroyed acutely by bilateral hemorrhagic necrosis following disseminated intravascular coagulation. Essentially blood clots block the venous drainage of the adrenal cortex causing cell death. These clots can form following severe septicemia. Meningococcal septicemia is the most common cause; it is called Waterhouse–Friderichsen syndrome.

A similar situation can occur if long-term high-dose steroid treatment is stopped abruptly. The prolonged treatment chronically suppresses ACTH release from the anterior pituitary gland so that no cortisol is secreted from the adrenal cortex for a number of weeks.

Secondary adrenocortical insufficiency
Disorders of the hypothalamus and anterior pituitary gland can also cause deficiency of adrenal cortex steroid hormones. Any condition that causes a reduction in CRH or ACTH release will prevent the synthesis of glucocorticoids especially. These conditions are described in more detail in Chapter 2.

Hormones of the adrenal medulla

The adrenal medulla secretes two hormones, norepinephrine and epinephrine. Both of these hormones are catecholamines, a term that is derived from their chemical structure (Fig. 4.13). Eighty per cent of catecholamine released from the adrenal glands is epinephrine.

Regulation
Catecholamines are released in response to stress (e.g., exercise, pain, shock, hypoglycemia, and imminent exams). Stress stimulates an area of the hypothalamus that activates the sympathetic system, including the adrenal medulla. It receives no direct regulation from the pituitary gland.

Actions
Catecholamines from the adrenal medulla perform similar functions to direct sympathetic neuronal connections in that they prepare the body for fight or flight. Their effects last longer than the neuronal signals; thus they help to minimize the harm caused

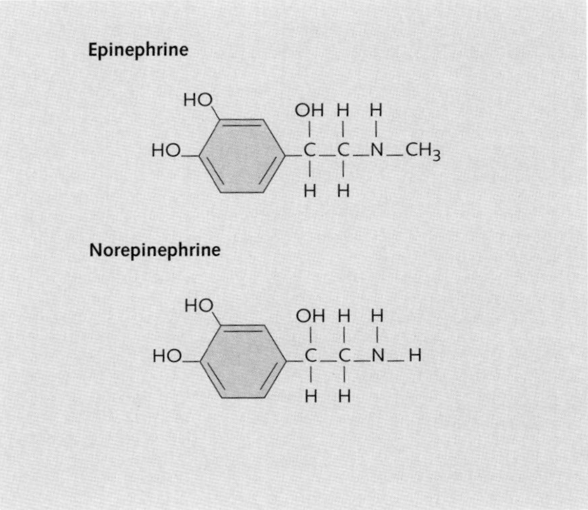

Fig. 4.13 Structure of epinephrine and norepinephrine.

53

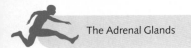
by repeated stress. Epinephrine and norepinephrine have similar effects to each other.

Their main actions are described in Fig. 4.14. Generally they improve mental and physical abilities to overcome the stressor; for more detail about the sympathetic nervous system see *Crash Course: Nervous System*.

Intracellular actions

Catecholamines bind to adrenergic receptors. These transmembrane receptors are linked to intracellular G-proteins that initiate a signal cascade. The effect of the signal depends on the subtype of receptor present and the cell type.

Synthesis

Norepinephrine is synthesized from the amino acid tyrosine, which is then converted to epinephrine in response to cortisol from the adrenal cortex.

The medullary cells store catecholamines in cytoplasmic granules. They are released into blood sinusoids by exocytosis in response to acetylcholine from preganglionic sympathetic neurons.

Metabolism

Catecholamines circulate bound to albumin. They are degraded by two enzymes in the liver:
- Monoamine oxidase (MAO).
- Catechol-O-methyl transferase (COMT).

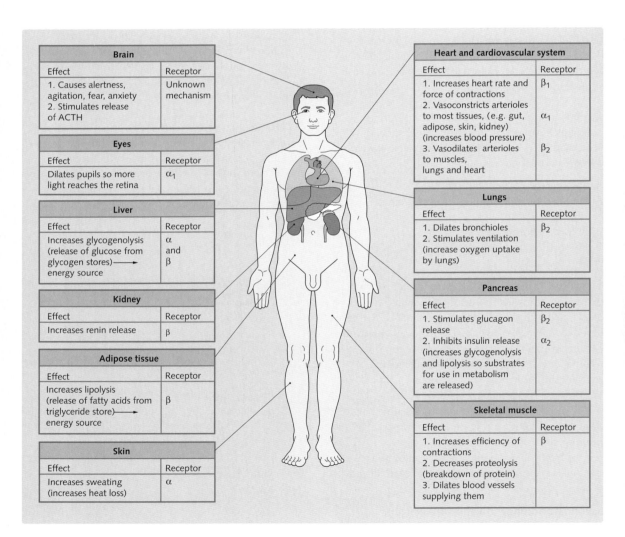

Fig. 4.14 Physiological effects of epinephrine and norepinephrine and the receptors present in each tissue/organ.

Epinephrine and norepinephrine are converted to vanillyl mandelic acid (VMA or HMMA), which is released into the urine. Urinary VMA levels are measured to detect pheochromocytomas, a rare tumor of the adrenal medulla that is discussed below.

> Monoamine oxidase (MAO)—the enzyme that degrades catecholamines in the liver—is also present in the brain. Inhibitors of this enzyme are used as antidepressants.

Disorders of the adrenal medulla

Pheochromocytomas

Pheochromocytomas are very rare tumors of the catecholamine-producing cells in the adrenal medulla. They are usually benign and present in only one gland (unilateral). Epinephrine and norepinephrine are secreted in large quantities, causing severe, sporadic (paroxysmal) hypertension that can produce headaches. With time the hypertension can become constant, leading to heart failure.

The tumor is detected by the high levels of catecholamine breakdown products in the urine (e.g., VMA). It is treated by surgical excision. The surgery has a high perioperative mortality rate due to the unstable blood pressure.

Catecholamine-producing tumors can also develop in sympathetic ganglia. These usually occur beside the abdominal aorta near the bifurcation.

> It is an essential component of your medical education to diagnose at least one pheochromocytoma in yourself or a friend. Thankfully these usually resolve spontaneously with practice at taking blood pressures!

Multiple endocrine neoplasia syndromes

A very rare autosomal dominant mutation causes inheritable pheochromocytoma. These tumors can also develop in both glands (bilaterally) as a component of multiple endocrine neoplasia syndromes (MEN type II), described in Chapter 10.

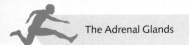

- List the five major hormones secreted by the adrenal gland.
- Describe the shape and location of each adrenal gland.
- Describe the innervation of the adrenal medulla and the developmental origins of this relationship.
- State the functions of the adrenal cortex.
- Name the blood vessels that supply and drain the adrenal gland.
- List the three layers of the adrenal cortex and state which group of hormones each layer secretes. Bonus point: which layer develops last?
- Describe the regulation and actions of mineralocorticoids.
- State the main target tissues and intracellular actions of mineralocorticoids.
- Describe the regulation of glucocorticoid release, including variation through the day.
- List the physiological actions of glucocorticoids.
- Describe the actions of adrenal androgens in males and females. How important are these effects in each sex?
- List the symptoms of Conn's syndrome.
- List the main causes of hyperaldosteronism. Which are most common?
- Describe the diagnosis of excess glucocorticoids. What makes this more complicated?
- State the difference between Cushing's disease and Cushing's syndrome. List the symptoms of these conditions.
- What is the most common cause of Cushing's syndrome? Bonus point: what is the rarest and most obscure cause that you can think of?
- Describe congenital adrenal hyperplasia including the symptoms in males and females.
- List the symptoms of Addison's disease. Which hormones are deficient?
- Describe the regulation and action of catecholamine hormones from the adrenal medulla.
- What is a pheochromocytoma? What symptoms does it cause?

5. The Pancreas

The pancreas is an important exocrine gland that secretes digestive enzymes; it also has a significant endocrine function. This chapter focuses on cells within the pancreas that secrete insulin. Insulin is an important hormone essential for the regulation of blood glucose levels. Its secretion is not controlled by the hypothalamus and pituitary gland in the same manner as many other important hormones.

The pancreas is a retroperitoneal organ found between the duodenum and the spleen. The endocrine cells are arranged within the pancreas in clusters called the islets of Langerhans. These clusters contain four types of cells, the most important and numerous of which are the insulin-producing β-cells. After a meal, glucose enters the blood from the gastrointestinal (GI) tract. Insulin is released from the pancreas to promote the uptake and use of glucose by cells and to keep blood glucose within tightly controlled limits. When blood glucose levels drop, insulin secretion is inhibited in favor of another pancreatic hormone called glucagon. This hormone opposes many of the actions of insulin; for example, it causes cells to release glucose into the blood. Figure 5.1 shows how these hormones regulate blood glucose.

> **Important terms:**
> **Metabolite:** a molecule that can be broken down to release energy (ATP)
> **Glucose:** an important metabolite that is a type of simple sugar or monosaccharide (i.e., carbon atoms)
> **Anabolism:** processes that build large molecules
> **Catabolism:** processes that break down large molecules
> **Glycosuria:** glucose in the urine
> **Polyuria:** large volume of urine

Insulin deficiency or insulin resistance causes diabetes mellitus. It is the most common endocrine disorder, affecting at least 2% of people. Blood glucose rises, causing hyperglycemia, and glucose is excreted in the urine (glycosuria). Water follows the movement of glucose; thus the patient produces excess urine and becomes dehydrated.

There are two types of diabetes mellitus. Type 1 (insulin-dependent diabetes mellitus [IDDM]) is more common in the young and always requires insulin injections. Type 2 (non-insulin-dependent diabetes mellitus [NIDDM]) is very common in the elderly and can sometimes be controlled through diet alone. Poor control of diabetes causes a number of serious and potentially life-threatening complications.

After reading this chapter you should be able to:
- Visualize the structure and development of the pancreas and its ducts.
- Understand the regulation and physiological effects of insulin and glucagon.
- Describe the control of glucose homeostasis.
- Explain the etiology, symptoms, complications, and treatment of diabetes mellitus.
- Briefly discuss neoplasia of the endocrine pancreas.

Location and anatomy

The pancreas is a long, flat organ that lies on the posterior of the abdominal wall, anterior to the vertebral bodies, aorta, and inferior vena cava. It is a retroperitoneal structure situated between the duodenum and spleen. For descriptive purposes it is divided into four sections (Fig. 5.2):
- Head.
- Uncinate process.
- Body.
- Tail.

> The word "pancreas" is derived from the Greek words *pan*, meaning "all," and *kreas*, meaning "flesh." Uncinate is the Latin word for "hooked."

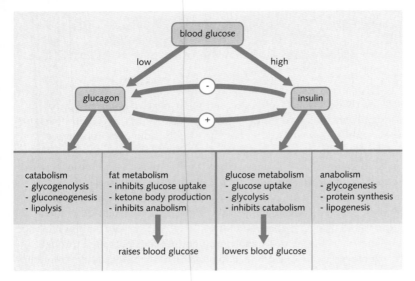

Fig. 5.1 Hormonal regulation of blood glucose and metabolism by insulin and glucagon.

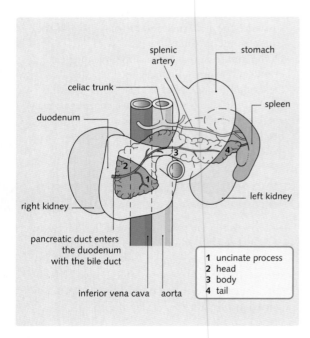

Fig. 5.2 Location of the pancreas in the retroperitoneal abdomen.

Head and uncinate process

The head lies within the curve of the duodenum with the uncinate process located posteriorly and inferiorly. The uncinate process is a "hook" of pancreatic tissue that lies left and posteriorly to the head of the pancreas; it is separated from the head by the superior mesenteric vessels. The inferior vena cava and bile duct lie posteriorly; a clinical consequence of this is that the bile duct can be obstructed by masses in the head of the pancreas.

The shape of the uncinate process joining the pancreas is similar to the shape of a thumb (uncinate process) and a flat hand (head). The superior mesenteric vessels would lie between the thumb and index finger.

Body and tail

The body of the pancreas passes over the aorta and the left kidney, while the stomach lies in front. The body slopes upward as it passes from right to left. The celiac trunk (a large branch of the aorta) is a superior relation, giving rise to the splenic artery that runs along the upper pancreatic border. The tail crosses the left kidney to touch the hilum of the spleen.

Pancreatic duct

The exocrine secretions of the pancreas, which are rich in digestive enzymes, are carried in the pancreatic duct to the duodenum. The main duct runs from the tail to the head with numerous small branches joining on the way. It joins the bile duct, and they open into the duodenum at the major

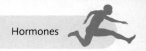

duodenal papilla (ampulla of Vater). In some people a smaller accessory duct drains the superior part of the head of the pancreas. It opens into the duodenum separately, at the minor duodenal papilla, about 2 cm proximal to the main papilla.

Blood, lymphatics, and nerves

The pancreas is supplied with blood from branches of the splenic artery. Blood drains into the splenic vein and the portal vein to the liver. Both splenic vessels lie along the upper border of the body and tail. Lymph drains to preaortic lymph nodes via a number of routes.

The main control of the endocrine pancreas is hormonal; however, a few autonomic nerves reach the pancreas via the celiac plexus and splanchnic nerves.

Microstructure

The pancreas contains exocrine (enzyme-secreting) and endocrine (hormone-secreting) tissue. The endocrine cells are arranged in spherical clusters called islets of Langerhans within the exocrine tissue (see Fig. 5.3). Each islet has a rich network of fenestrated capillaries; however, only 10% of endocrine cells are innervated by the autonomic nervous system.

The islets are made up of endocrine cells containing dense secretory granules. These cells are APUD (amine precursor uptake and decarboxylation) cells (see Chapter 6). There are four types of endocrine cell:
- Glucagon-secreting α-cells (20%).
- Insulin-secreting β-cells (70%).
- Somatostatin-secreting δ-cells (8%).
- Pancreatic polypeptide-secreting F-cells (2%).

Insulin and glucagon help regulate blood glucose levels. Somatostatin inhibits the release of insulin and glucagon. Pancreatic polypeptide inhibits the exocrine (i.e., nonendocrine) functions of the pancreas.

Development

The pancreas is an endodermal structure that develops from two buds derived from the foregut:

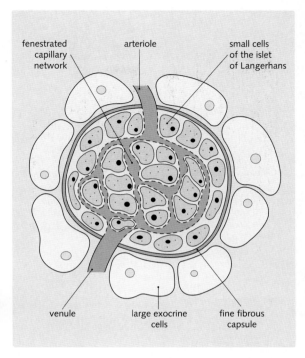

Fig. 5.3 Microstructure of the pancreas showing an islet of Langerhans surrounded by exocrine tissue.

- Dorsal bud—the larger bud that forms the majority of the gland.
- Ventral bud—the smaller bud from the right side near the bile duct.

The ventral bud rotates behind the duodenum, along with the bile duct, to lie posterior to the dorsal bud. This smaller ventral bud forms the uncinate process as it fuses with the larger dorsal bud. The ducts usually fuse so that the end of the pancreatic duct is formed from the smaller ventral bud. The duct of the dorsal bud may persist as the accessory pancreatic duct. This sequence of events is shown in Fig. 5.4.

Hormones

Insulin

Insulin is a hormone that promotes the uptake, storage, and use of glucose. The pancreas secretes insulin when glucose levels are high—for example, after a meal.

As glucose levels fall a few hours after a meal, insulin secretion is reduced. The stored glucose can

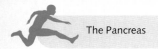

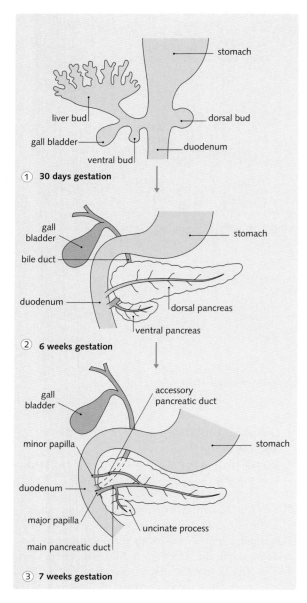

① **30 days gestation**

② **6 weeks gestation**

③ **7 weeks gestation**

Fig. 5.4 Embryological development of the pancreas.

then be released to maintain blood levels. Insulin secretion never ceases completely; there is always a basal level of insulin in the blood.

Synthesis

Insulin is a polypeptide hormone consisting of two short chains (A and B) linked by disulfide bonds. A single gene controls the production of pre-proinsulin, which is broken down to form proinsulin. Further cleavage occurs within intracellular secretory vesicles, resulting in two molecules, insulin and C peptide.

Since equal quantities of insulin and C peptide are produced, C peptide acts as a useful marker for β-cell activity in diabetics who receive insulin treatment.

Control of insulin secretion

Insulin secretion is increased by high blood glucose levels. The pancreatic cells detect this stimulus directly because it raises ATP production. Other metabolites (energy molecules such as amino acids and triglycerides—i.e., fat) have a similar but weaker effect. The raised intracellular ATP levels inhibit membrane-bound potassium channels, causing the β-cell to depolarize. The depolarization opens voltage-sensitive calcium channels raising intracellular calcium, which promotes the secretion of preformed insulin secretory granules by exocytosis. This pathway is shown in Fig. 5.5.

Although metabolite concentrations are the main regulators of insulin release, a number of stimuli can also affect this pathway. These stimuli can have an inhibitory or stimulatory effect, but insulin secretion cannot be totally inhibited. The hormone glucagon, which is released when metabolite levels fall, acts as an important inhibitor of insulin's action; however, it stimulates insulin secretion. Figure 5.6 shows the main factors that control secretion.

Insulin receptors

Insulin causes a cascade of activity by acting through a tyrosine kinase receptor located on the cell membrane. It must act via cell-surface receptors because it is a polypeptide hormone and cannot readily cross the cell membrane. Insulin receptors are present in most cells, and they can be withdrawn into the cell to inactivate them.

When insulin binds to the tyrosine kinase receptor, it causes phosphorylation of tyrosine side chains within the receptor (autophosphorylation). The phosphorylated receptor attracts and phosphorylates insulin receptor substrate 1 (IRS-1). This activated molecule then initiates a cascade of phosphorylation and aggregation of other proteins to bring about intracellular effects of insulin.

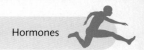

Fig. 5.5 Intracellular stimulation of insulin secretion by glucose.

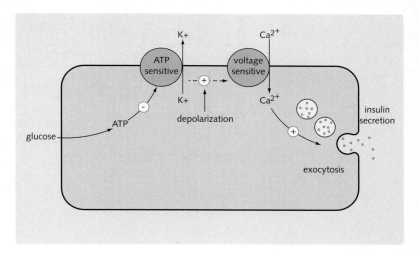

Factors controlling insulin and glucagon secretion				
	Insulin		**Glucagon**	
	Stimulants	**Inhibitors**	**Stimulants**	**Inhibitors**
Blood glucose	High	Low	Low	High
Metabolites	Amino acids, fatty acids, and ketones	—	Amino acids	Fatty acids and ketones
Hormones	Glucagon Some gastrointestinal tract peptides Growth hormone Adrenocorticotropic hormone (ACTH), thyroid-stimulating hormone (TSH)	Epinephrine Somatostatin	Epinephrine Some gastrointestinal tract peptides	Insulin Somatostatin
Innervation	Parasympathetic	Sympathetic	Parasympathetic and sympathetic	—
Other	—	Hypocalcemia	—	—

Fig. 5.6 Factors that control insulin and glucagon secretion.

Insulin receptors are unusual because they phosphorylate the tyrosine side chains of proteins using tyrosine kinase. Most receptors phosphorylate serine and threonine side chains.

Actions of insulin

Insulin has an anabolic effect; it promotes the synthesis of larger molecules. The stimulation of insulin receptors regulates many enzymes associated with metabolism. The specific enzymes vary among cells (Fig. 5.7), but the overall effects are:

- Increased uptake of metabolites.
- Conversion of metabolites to stored forms (this is an anabolic effect).

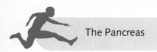
Fig. 5.7 Metabolic effects of insulin on target cells.

Metabolic effects of insulin on target cells	
Target cells	**Action of insulin**
Muscle cells and many other cells	Stimulates glucose uptake
	Stimulates glycogenesis (glucose → glycogen)
	Stimulates glycolysis (glucose → energy)
	Stimulates amino acid uptake and protein synthesis
	Inhibits glycogenolysis (glycogen → glucose)
	Inhibits proteolysis (protein → amino acids)
Adipose cells	Stimulates glucose uptake
	Stimulates lipogenesis (glucose → fatty acids)
	Inhibits lipolysis (fatty acids → energy)
Liver cells	Stimulates glycogenesis (glucose → glycogen)
	Inhibits glycogenolysis (glycogen → glucose)
	Inhibits gluconeogenesis (amino acids → glucose)
Hypothalamus	May stimulate satiety (fullness)

- Decreased breakdown of stored metabolites.
- Use of glucose for energy over other metabolites.

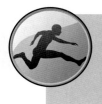

Insulin is the only hormone that lowers blood glucose levels, but a number of hormones, including glucagon and epinephrine, can raise them.

Glucagon

Glucagon is released when blood levels of metabolites are low, causing the release of stored metabolites. In many respects glucagon has the opposite effect of insulin. Its secretion from α-cells is stimulated by a number of factors, of which falling blood glucose is the most important. The main factors are shown in Fig. 5.6.

Synthesis and actions

Glucagon is a single chain polypeptide hormone formed from a larger precursor in a similar manner to insulin. The precursor is pre-proglucagon, which is cleaved in the storage vesicles to yield proglucagon and, finally, glucagon.

Glucagon is a catabolic hormone; it promotes the breakdown of large molecules. Glucagon binds to a G-protein-coupled receptor on the cell membrane, and cAMP acts as a second messenger to initiate a cascade effect. Its effects vary between tissues (Fig. 5.8), but broadly its actions are:
- Inhibition of glucose and amino acid uptake.
- Breakdown of stored metabolites into usable metabolites (catabolism).
- Use of fatty acids for energy over other metabolites.

Endocrine control of glucose homeostasis

All cells in the body are capable of using glucose as an energy source by the process of glycolysis. Most cells can also use fatty acids with two important exceptions:
- Neurons (particularly in the CNS), although they can adapt to use ketone bodies.
- Blood cells.

If blood glucose levels drop too low (hypoglycemia), the brain is starved of energy. If levels rise too high (hyperglycemia), glucose can become toxic. Blood glucose is tightly controlled within narrow limits to

Fig. 5.8 Metabolic effects of glucagon on target cells.

Metabolic effects of glucagon on target cells	
Target cells	**Action of glucagon**
Muscle cells and many other cells	Stimulates glycogenolysis (glycogen → glucose)
	Inhibits glucose uptake
	Inhibits glycolysis (glucose → energy)
	Inhibits amino acid uptake and protein synthesis
Adipose cells	Stimulates lipolysis (fatty acids → energy)
Liver cells	Stimulates glycogenolysis (glycogen → glucose)
	Stimulates gluconeogenesis (amino acids → glucose)
	Stimulates ketogenesis (fatty acids → ketone bodies)

Responses that alter blood glucose levels	
Responses that raise blood glucose	**Responses that lower blood glucose**
Ingestion of glucose in the diet	Increased uptake in cells
Gluconeogenesis—the irreversible conversion of amino acids to glucose (liver)	Metabolism to produce energy
Glycogenolysis—the reversible breakdown of glycogen to release glucose (liver)	Glycogenesis—the reversible conversion of glucose to glycogen
	Lipogenesis, the irreversible conversion of glucose to fatty acids

Fig. 5.9 Responses that alter blood glucose levels.

prevent either scenario. Fasting glucose levels are normally 3.5–5.5 mmol/L.

For glucose levels to be maintained (glucose homeostasis), the body must be able to increase or decrease these levels in response to changes. There are a number of ways that the body can respond (Fig. 5.9). The liver is especially important in raising blood glucose.

Insulin and glucagon

Glucose homeostasis is maintained by the interplay between insulin and glucagon. These two hormones act as antagonists of each other. Their blood concentrations mirror each other because they are secreted in opposite conditions (Fig. 5.10).

- Insulin lowers blood glucose by stimulating uptake, metabolism, and anabolism. It also inhibits the actions of glucagon.

- Glucagon raises blood glucose by simulating gluconeogenesis (synthesis of glucose from amino acids) and glycogenolysis (breakdown of glycogen to release glucose). It also inhibits the actions of insulin but stimulates insulin secretion.

Other hormones

Three nonpancreatic hormones also significantly increase blood glucose:

- Epinephrine—released in response to stress and the sympathetic nervous system; it inhibits insulin.
- Cortisol—released in response to stress; it reduces sensitivity to insulin.
- Growth hormone—released at night; it reduces sensitivity to insulin.

All three hormones can stimulate glycogenolysis and gluconeogenesis to raise blood glucose levels directly.

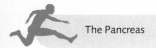
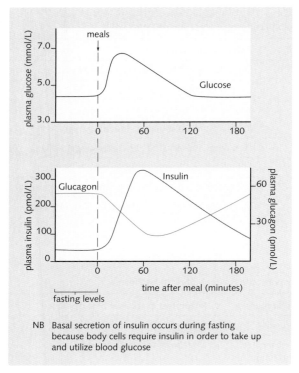

NB Basal secretion of insulin occurs during fasting because body cells require insulin in order to take up and utilize blood glucose

Fig. 5.10 Changes in blood levels of glucose, insulin, and glucagon after a carbohydrate-rich meal.

Neural signals and other hormones can cause less significant rises in blood glucose.

Hyperglycemia

Hyperglycemia is an excess of glucose in the blood; it is defined as a fasting concentration >7.8 mmol/L. This can occur in:

- Diabetes mellitus—a common disease caused by insulin deficiency or insulin resistance (reduced sensitivity).
- Glucagonoma—a very rare tumor of the α-cells that secrete glucagon.

Hypoglycemia

Hypoglycemia is a deficiency of blood glucose; it is defined as a concentration <2.5 mmol/L. It can be caused by:

- Overtreatment of diabetes mellitus, either excess insulin or β-cell-stimulating drugs.
- Nondiabetic disorder causing fasting hypoglycemia.
- Idiopathic excessive insulin secretion causing hypoglycemia after glucose ingestion.

Diabetes mellitus
Types of diabetes mellitus
Diabetes mellitus (DM) is caused by insulin deficiency or insulin resistance (reduced sensitivity). These abnormalities result in chronic hyperglycemia (excess blood glucose) and metabolic chaos. It is a very common disease affecting about 2% of the population. There are two types:

- Type 1—insulin-dependent DM (IDDM) caused by insulin deficiency.
- Type 2—non-insulin-dependent DM (NIDDM) caused by insulin deficiency and/or resistance.

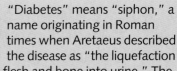

"Diabetes" means "siphon," a name originating in Roman times when Aretaeus described the disease as "the liquefaction of the flesh and bone into urine." The term "mellitus," referring to "honey or sweet-tasting" urine, was added in the 17th century by Thomas Willis (of the circle), who also observed that diabetics "piss a great deal." Next time you meet a diabetic why not try a sample?

Type 1 diabetes (IDDM)
IDDM is an autoimmune disease resulting in destruction of the islet β-cells, which causes insulin deficiency. Autoimmune antibodies can be detected in the blood. It is most common in the young, but it can occur at any age. There is a genetic component of about 30% mostly due to HLA genes.

Type 2 diabetes (NIDDM)
NIDDM is usually a disease of the elderly, especially those who are obese; it is about twice as common as IDDM. It can be caused by insulin deficiency, insulin resistance, or a combination of both. Family history is very important since there is almost 100% concordance in identical twins. NIDDM often occurs alongside obesity, hypertension, and hyperlipidemia (excess fatty acids in the blood); together these features are called syndrome X.

NIDDM can develop in young people in whom it is called maturity-onset diabetes in the young

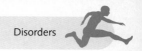

(MODY). This is becoming more common with rising juvenile obesity.

Other causes of diabetes mellitus

Diabetes can also develop secondary to a number of diseases. These include pancreatitis, prolonged corticosteroid use (Cushing's syndrome), acromegaly, and thyrotoxicosis.

> Do not confuse diabetes insipidus with diabetes mellitus. They both cause polyuria (hence the similar name). But diabetes insipidus is a disorder of antidiuretic hormone (ADH) causing excess, pale (insipid) urine, whereas patients with DM have glucose in the urine.

Symptoms

Insulin has many important effects on the regulation of glucose and metabolism. Accordingly, the effects of diabetes can appear quite complicated. The effects make more sense if they are thought of in four categories:

- Symptoms of **hyperglycemia** in both IDDM and NIDDM.
- Symptoms of **starvation**, particularly in IDDM.
- Symptoms of **ketoacidosis** in IDDM.
- Symptoms of **chronic complications** in NIDDM and IDDM.

Symptoms of hyperglycemia

Hyperglycemia causes dehydration because glucose is an osmotically active substance, i.e., it draws water toward it. In hyperglycemia, glucose concentration is high in the blood and low in the cells so the cells become dehydrated. The excess glucose is also excreted in the kidney and again water follows this movement. Excess water is lost from the body along with electrolytes. The resulting symptoms are shown in Fig. 5.11.

Symptoms of starvation

In IDDM the body enters a state of starvation because cells cannot use the excess glucose; this is caused by the high levels of glucagon. The lack of insulin prevents glucose entering cells and being metabolized. Muscle protein and adipose tissue are broken down to release metabolites, and this causes the symptoms shown in Fig. 5.11.

Symptoms of ketoacidosis

Ketoacidosis develops only in IDDM. In IDDM, lipolysis (fat breakdown) is a major component, resulting in raised blood fatty acid levels. These fatty acids are converted to acetyl coenzyme A (acetyl

Symptoms of diabetes mellitus			
Symptoms due to hyperglycemia	Symptoms due to starvation	Symptoms due to ketoacidosis	Symptoms due to chronic complications
Polyuria (increased urine volume)	Weight loss	Vomiting	Decreased visual acuity
Glycosuria (glucose in the urine)	Wasting	Acetone smell on the breath	Reduced sensation in the limbs
Polydipsia (thirst)	Weakness	Ketonuria, polyuria, and dehydration	Proteinuria
Tiredness		Hyperventilation	Edema
Tendency to infections		Reduced consciousness	Intermittent claudication
Dehydration (loose skin, hypotension, and tachycardia)		Convulsions	Ischemic heart disease
Coma		Coma	Hypertension

Fig. 5.11 Symptoms of diabetes mellitus.

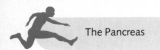

CoA). The excess acetyl CoA can overload the tricarboxylic acid (TCA) or Krebs cycle so that the liver uses the excess to synthesize ketone bodies. The ketone bodies are synthesized more quickly than they are metabolized by peripheral tissues; hence they build up in the blood.

Because the excess ketone bodies are osmotically active, they compound the dehydration caused by

glucose. Because they are acidic, they can cause a metabolic acidosis (ketoacidosis), which causes severe symptoms (see Fig. 5.11).

Presentation of IDDM

IDDM presents with a short history of polyuria, tiredness, and weight loss followed by dehydration and ketoacidosis (Fig. 5.12). The onset is relatively

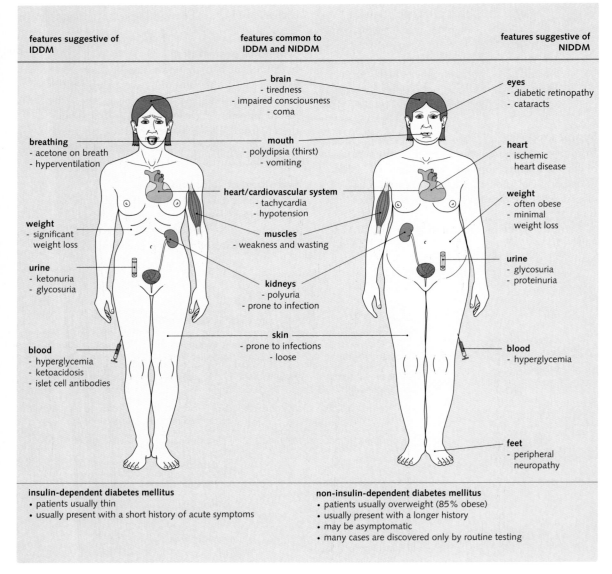

Fig. 5.12 Presentation of insulin-dependent diabetes mellitus (IDDM) and non-insulin-dependent diabetes mellitus (NIDDM).

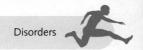

quick (over a number of weeks) so that complications have not developed by the time it presents. Diabetes should be suspected in young patients complaining of tiredness or with frequent skin infections (e.g., boils). Failure to treat IDDM with insulin can result in rapid death from cerebral edema following ketoacidosis.

Presentation of NIDDM

The onset of NIDDM is much slower than that of IDDM, with hyperglycemia developing over a number of years. By the time of presentation, the patient has often been exposed to excess glucose for so long that complications are already present; in fact, they may be the presenting feature (see Fig. 5.12). The earliest complications are retinopathy and peripheral neuropathy. NIDDM patients can present in a coma due to dehydration instead of ketoacidosis. Severe hypoglycemia and dehydration can result in hypovolemic (low blood volume) shock. In the worst cases this can result in **h**yper**o**smolar **n**on**k**etotic coma (HONK coma).

Ketoacidosis never occurs in NIDDM because some insulin activity is maintained:

- Anabolic actions (glucose uptake and metabolism) require high levels of insulin.
- Anticatabolic actions (inhibition of lipolysis and protein breakdown) require only low levels of insulin.

In NIDDM, insulin deficiency or resistance does not fall below this lower level so that the lipolysis and excess fatty acid release that cause ketoacidosis do not occur.

Complications of diabetes

Both types of diabetes can produce complications despite treatment; however, good glucose control lowers the risk of most complications. Chronic complications are grouped according to the size of blood vessel they affect:

- Macrovascular—large vessel disease due to accelerated atherosclerosis.
- Microvascular—small vessel disease due to hyaline arteriolosclerosis.

Macrovascular complications

Diabetes causes accelerated atherosclerosis due to chronically raised fatty acid levels (hyperlipidemia) following low insulin levels. Atheroma develops more rapidly and more severely than in nondiabetics, and it can block arteries, causing ischemia and a high risk of infarction. The major sites of macrovascular disease are shown in Fig. 5.13.

Microvascular complications

While atherosclerosis develops in major arteries, the smaller arterioles and capillaries are at risk of hyaline arteriolosclerosis. This is characterized by thickening of the vessel wall and basement membrane. The vessel lumen is reduced, causing localized ischemia. The vessel also becomes "leaky." This response may be a direct reaction to excess glucose. There are four main patterns of microvascular disease (Figs. 5.13 and 5.14). Diabetic retinopathy is the most common cause of blindness in the 30–65-year age group.

Diagnosis

Blood glucose levels are normally 3.5–5.5 mmol/L after an overnight fast. Diabetes is diagnosed if this fasting blood glucose is above 7.8 mmol/L on two occasions. Since NIDDM can develop gradually, a spectrum of disease is seen between normal blood glucose and diabetic blood glucose. A number of markers suggest the need for further observation:

- Glycosuria (glucose in urine).
- Fasting blood glucose of 6–7.8 mmol/L.
- Random blood glucose of >11.1 mmol/L.

To clarify the diagnosis, a glucose tolerance test is sometimes used. The fasting blood glucose is measured as normal, and the patient is then given a drink containing 75 g glucose. Blood glucose is measured 2 hours later, and diabetes is diagnosed if this second measurement is above 11.1 mmol/L.

Treatment

The treatment of diabetes aims to lower blood glucose and normalize metabolism with the least possible interference. Patient education is essential; ideally patients will regulate their own medication according to their lifestyle. There are three types of treatment:

- Diet alone (NIDDM).
- Diet and oral hypoglycemic agents (NIDDM).
- Diet and insulin (IDDM and NIDDM).

All patients with IDDM and many with NIDDM are treated with subcutaneous insulin injections to reduce acute and chronic complications.

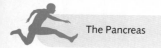

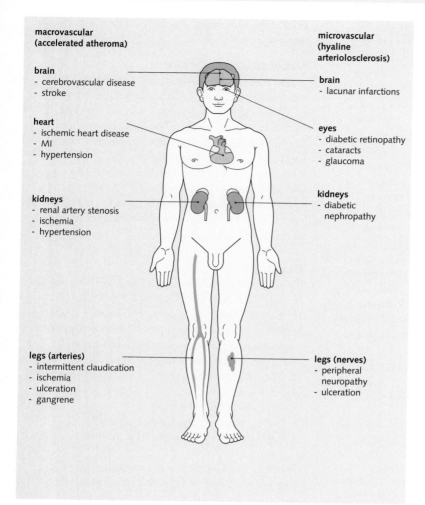

Fig. 5.13 Chronic complications of diabetes mellitus.

macrovascular
(accelerated atheroma)

brain
- cerebrovascular disease
- stroke

heart
- ischemic heart disease
- MI
- hypertension

kidneys
- renal artery stenosis
- ischemia
- hypertension

legs (arteries)
- intermittent claudication
- ischemia
- ulceration
- gangrene

microvascular
(hyaline
arteriolosclerosis)

brain
- lacunar infarctions

eyes
- diabetic retinopathy
- cataracts
- glaucoma

kidneys
- diabetic
  nephropathy

legs (nerves)
- peripheral
  neuropathy
- ulceration

Progressive changes caused by complications of diabetes mellitus			
Condition	**Early changes**	**Late changes**	**End result**
Retinopathy	Microaneurysms, hemorrhages, hard exudates	Soft exudates, neovascularization	Blindness
Nephropathy	Proteinuria, edema	Decline of glomerular filtration rate	Renal failure and death
Peripheral neuropathy	Reduced reflexes, reduced sensation (glove and stocking pattern)	Burning or aching sensation, joint deformity	Ulceration and amputation
Lacunar infarcts	Microinfarcts in the brain, asymptomatic	Progressive neurological deficits	Dementia and Parkinsonism

Fig. 5.14 Progressive changes caused by the complications of diabetes mellitus.

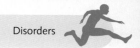

Patients with NIDDM are often treated with insulin in a similar manner to IDDM. This does not mean that they have developed IDDM. Insulin treatment helps to control blood glucose, which has been proven to reduce complications.

Diet
Regulation of diet is essential in all diabetics to help maintain blood glucose levels. Four principles govern this treatment:
- Avoid carbohydrates that can be rapidly absorbed (e.g., glucose) to prevent hyperglycemia.
- Eat regular, small meals to prevent hypoglycemia.
- Control calorie intake to lose/stabilize weight (especially NIDDM).
- Eat a low fat, healthy diet to reduce atherosclerosis.

In reality, more than 50% of patients fail to follow their diet and very few manage to achieve long-standing weight loss.

Oral hypoglycemic agents
NIDDM can be treated with oral medication to lower blood glucose. A number of medications are available:
- Sulfonylureas (e.g., gliclazide) stimulate β-cells by inhibiting the membrane-bound K^+ channel; the resulting depolarization causes insulin release (see Fig. 5.5). Side effects include weight gain and hypoglycemia.
- Biguanides (e.g., metformin) increase peripheral glucose uptake and reduce glucose output from the liver. Their mechanism of action is not understood. Side effects include nausea and diarrhea.
- Acarbose inhibits intestinal enzymes preventing the digestion of starch; blood glucose rises more slowly after a meal as a result. Side effects include flatulence and diarrhea.
- Thiazolidinediones (e.g., pioglitazone) are new drugs that reduce insulin resistance. They are usually used in combination with other drugs and

may involve a risk of heart failure and liver toxicity.

Subcutaneous insulin injections
Insulin must be injected because it is digested and thus inactivated if taken orally. Subcutaneous injections of insulin are used to treat all patients with IDDM and some with NIDDM. It is usually injected into the thigh, upper arm, or abdomen. Intensive monitored therapy to maintain low blood glucose has been proven to reduce long-term complications.

Many different types of insulin are available. In the past, porcine (pig) insulin was used, but recombinant human insulin is now favored because it reduces immunological reactions. Preparations of insulin vary in their duration of action. Clear insulin is short-acting and administered just before meals. Cloudy insulin has an intermediate or long effect; it replaces basal insulin secretion.

Patients regulate the type, dose, and frequency of injections to meet their requirements and lifestyle. This can vary on a day-to-day basis, or a regular dosing schedule can be followed.

Monitoring glucose control
Diabetics use monitoring to assess current blood glucose levels and long-term control. The following tests are available:
- Urine testing for glucose: this can be performed at home but it is unreliable.
- Capillary blood spot testing: this simple test gives an instant digital reading of blood glucose; it can be performed at home and is used to determine insulin or sugar doses.
- HbA_{1C}: glucose binds directly and irreversibly to hemoglobin to form HbA_{1C}. The proportion of HbA_{1C} in the blood gives a measure of glucose control over the previous two months. It is used quite commonly in clinical practice.
- Fructosamine: this is formed when glucose binds to serum albumin. It gives a measure of glucose control in the last two weeks but is rarely used in clinical practice.

Hypoglycemia
Treatment for diabetes mellitus may cause hypoglycemia in a number of situations:
- Low carbohydrate intake (e.g., missed meal).
- Unexpected exercise.

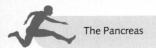

- Insulin overdose.
- Malabsorption.

Symptoms

Diabetics must know the symptoms of hypoglycemic attacks, and they should always carry a sugary snack in case they feel a "hypo" coming on. If action is not taken to prevent it, then recognizing the symptoms and signs of hypoglycemia can be life-saving; they are shown in Fig. 5.15. These symptoms are caused by raised epinephrine secretion and low cerebral glucose. Severe hypoglycemia can result in a coma. This is treated with intravenous infusion of 50 mL 50% dextrose and sugary drinks once the patient regains consciousness. Glucagon pens are now available for intramuscular injection in the event of a "hypo."

Screening to prevent complications

Along with preventing short-term hypo/hyperglycemia, diabetic clinics aim to minimize the long-term complications. Many of these complications are treatable if they are detected in their early stages, i.e., before symptoms develop.

Eyes

Retinopathy is a very common cause of blindness, and the early stages are completely treatable by laser photocoagulation. The eyes of diabetics should be tested and inspected regularly for signs of deterioration or retinopathy.

Kidneys

Urine samples should be checked regularly for microalbuminuria caused by early nephropathy

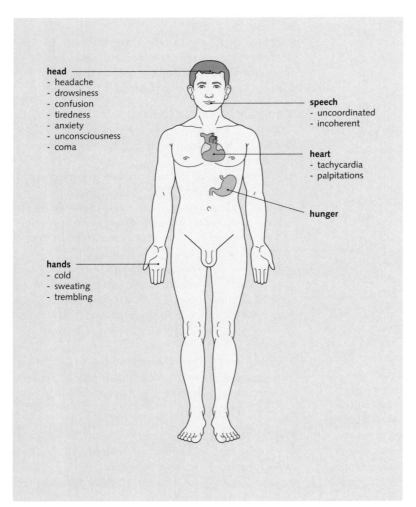

Fig. 5.15 Symptoms of hypoglycemia.

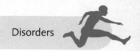

(kidney damage). If it is present, blood glucose should be regulated more aggressively. An angiotensin-converting enzyme (ACE) inhibitor can be used to prevent the resulting hypertension and to slow the progression to terminal renal failure.

Feet

The feet of elderly or immobile diabetics should be examined regularly by chiropodists. The combination of peripheral neuropathy and peripheral vascular disease can lead to injury, ulceration, infection and, eventually, gangrene. Poorly perfused gangrenous feet may need to be amputated. This can be prevented by early treatment and dressing or vascular surgery in severe cases.

Hypoglycemia in nondiabetic patients

Most people should be able to tolerate fasting for several days without developing hypoglycemia. If a patient is unable to do so, the mnemonic **EXPLAIN** lists the possible causes:

EX = **Ex**ogenous drugs (e.g., alcohol and insulin).

  P = **P**ituitary insufficiency, growth hormone deficiency.

  L = **L**iver failure or defective liver enzymes.

  A = **A**ddison's disease—deficiency of cortisol that raises blood glucose levels (also autoimmune causes).

  I = **I**nsulinomas—a type of islet-cell tumor (see below).

  N = **N**onpancreatic tumor—by ectopic insulin secretion or simply consuming glucose.

Endocrine pancreatic neoplasia

Tumors of the endocrine cells in the pancreas are called islet-cell tumors; they are usually benign and solitary, but they often secrete a specific hormone. Tumors are named according to the hormone they secrete:

- Insulinomas are the most common type of islet-cell tumor. The excess insulin that they secrete causes severe hypoglycemic attacks, which can lead to coma.
- Glucagonomas are very rare tumors that secrete glucagon. They are often asymptomatic, but they may cause diabetes mellitus.

Extremely infrequently islet-cell tumors can secrete other hormones such as gastrin in Zollinger–Ellison syndrome. This syndrome is characterized by recurrent, severe, and multiple peptic ulcers following excessive stomach acid secretion. Other rare tumors can produce vasoactive intestinal polypeptide (VIP) or adrenocorticotropic hormone (ACTH).

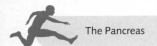

- Describe the anatomical location of the pancreas.
- Describe how the endocrine cells are arranged within the pancreas.
- List the hormones secreted by the pancreas along with the cell type responsible.
- Describe the development of the pancreas.
- How is the hormone insulin synthesized?
- Describe insulin receptors and how they function. What are the main differences from other types of receptors?
- Why is a basal level of insulin always secreted?
- State the dietary principles that should be followed by all diabetics.
- Describe the intracellular mechanism that allows high glucose levels to trigger insulin secretion.
- Describe the action of insulin on glucose uptake and metabolism.
- Describe the action of insulin on amino acid and fatty acid metabolism, including the processes it inhibits.
- List the actions of glucagon and the factors that stimulate its secretion.
- List three hormones that can raise blood glucose levels.
- Compare the two types of diabetes mellitus.
- Explain how ketoacidosis develops in IDDM and why this does not occur in NIDDM.
- List the symptoms caused by hyperglycemia and starvation. How does dehydration develop?
- Describe the complications of diabetes mellitus along with preventive screening.
- How is diabetes mellitus diagnosed and monitored?
- List the symptoms of hypoglycemia. How can it be prevented?
- Briefly describe the tumors that can develop in the endocrine cells of the pancreas.

6. Up and Coming Hormones

This chapter describes several tissues whose endocrine functions are still under study:

- Gastrointestinal (GI) tract—secretes many hormones that regulate digestive function. Some act on distant organs by traveling through the blood, while others act locally as mediators.
- Pineal gland—secretes melatonin, which regulates circadian rhythms.
- Adipose tissue—secretes leptin, which regulates food intake and fertility.

The GI tract and adipose tissue are examples of diffuse endocrine tissues because they are located throughout the body.

Endocrine role of the gastrointestinal tract

Endocrine cells that are distributed along the length of the GI tract are called enteroendocrine cells and are a type of APUD cell (see below). They secrete several different peptide hormones that coordinate the digestion and absorption of food.

Some GI tract peptides (e.g., vasoactive intestinal peptide [VIP], cholecystokinin [CCK], gastrin) also act as neurotransmitters in the CNS and the neurons that innervate the GI tract (called the enteric nervous system). This overlap demonstrates the close relationship and common origin of the endocrine and nervous systems. The following bodily functions are regulated in the CNS by these peptide neurotransmitters:

- Biological rhythms—VIP.
- Satiety (fullness after food)—CCK.
- Thermoregulation—bombesin.
- Growth—somatostatin.

The APUD concept

APUD cells are a group of endocrine cells that secrete small peptide hormones in many tissues throughout the body. They are linked by three features:

- Similar appearance under an electron microscope (e.g., neurosecretory granules).
- Similar biochemical pathway for amine or peptide hormone synthesis.
- Embryological origin from the endodermal GI tract.

> **Important terms:**
> **APUD cells:** peptide-secreting endocrine cells found throughout the body
> **Circadian rhythm:** variations in physiological processes that are repeated over a 24-hour cycle
> **Pineal gland:** melatonin-secreting gland found in the brain, important for regulating circadian rhythms
> **Adipose tissue:** cells that store fat

They are also called neuroendocrine cells owing to their secretion of both neurotransmitters and "hormones."

The name APUD is an abbreviation of the method by which the peptide hormones are synthesized: it stands for **a**mine **p**recursor **u**ptake and **d**ecarboxylation. This means that APUD cells convert actively absorbed amine precursors into amino acids, which are used to make the peptide hormones.

The following cells are examples of APUD cells:

- Islets of Langerhans cells that secrete insulin and glucagon.
- Enteroendocrine cells (see below).
- Parafollicular cells that secrete calcitonin; they are found in the thyroid gland.
- Juxtaglomerular complex that secretes renin; they are found in the kidneys.
- Neuroendocrine cells of the respiratory tract that secrete 5-hydroxytryptamine (5-HT; serotonin) and calcitonin.

Gastrointestinal tract peptides

The major peptides secreted by the enteroendocrine cells of the GI tract are described below. Figures 6.1 and 6.2 show the location of GI tract peptide

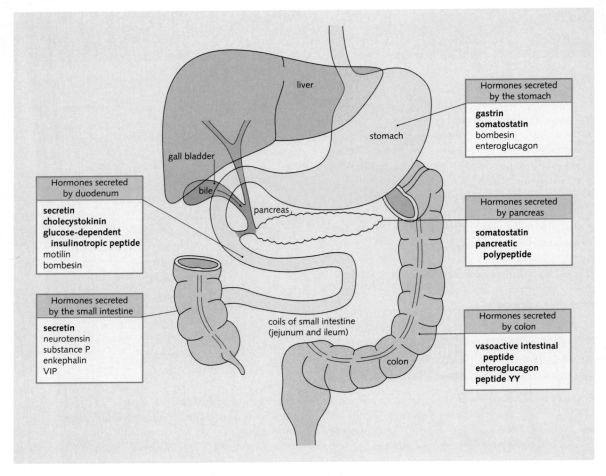

Fig. 6.1 Sites at which the gastrointestinal tract peptides are secreted.

Hormones secreted by the stomach

gastrin
somatostatin
bombesin
enteroglucagon

Hormones secreted by duodenum

secretin
cholecystokinin
glucose-dependent insulinotropic peptide
motilin
bombesin

Hormones secreted by pancreas

somatostatin
pancreatic polypeptide

Hormones secreted by the small intestine

secretin
neurotensin
substance P
enkephalin
VIP

Hormones secreted by colon

vasoactive intestinal peptide
enteroglucagon
peptide YY

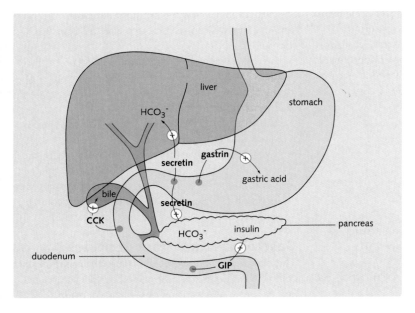

Fig. 6.2 Major actions of four gastrointestinal tract hormones. (CCK, cholecystokinin; GIP, glucose-dependent insulinotropic peptide.)

release and the major actions of four GI tract hormones. The actions of other peptides are shown in Fig. 6.3.

Delivery

GI tract peptides reach their target cells by two means:

- Endocrine, via the blood.
- Paracrine, acting locally to affect nearby cells.

Some peptides act in both manners (e.g., somatostatin).

Gastrin

Gastrin is secreted by enteroendocrine cells (G cells) in the pylorus of the stomach after a meal. It is secreted in response to:

- Peptides or amino acids in the stomach.
- Vagal stimulation (i.e., parasympathetic).
- Distension of the stomach.

It acts to increase protein breakdown, specifically by:

- Stimulating the parietal cells of the stomach to secrete hydrochloric acid and intrinsic factor.
- Stimulating the chief cells of the stomach to secrete pepsin.
- Increasing gastric motility.
- Stimulating secretion of insulin, glucagon, and secretin.
- Relaxing the pyloric and ileocecal sphincters.

Secretin

Secretin is secreted by the duodenum and the rest of the small intestines in response to acid secreted by

The sites of secretion, stimuli for secretion, and actions of the minor gut peptides			
Gut peptide	**Site of secretion**	**Stimulus for secretion**	**Action of peptide**
Enteroglucagon	A cells in the stomach and L cells in the colon	Presence of glucose and fat in the stomach	Reduces gastric acid secretion and gut motility
Bombesin	P cells in the stomach and duodenum	Fasting	Stimulates gastrin release
Motilin	EC cells in the duodenum	Absence of food in the duodenum	Speeds gastric emptying and stimulates colonic motility
Vasoactive intestinal polypeptide (VIP)	D1 cells and neurons in the small intestine and colon	Gut distension	Stimulates local gut secretion, motility, and blood flow
Peptide YY (related to pancreatic polypeptide)	PYY cells of the colon	Presence of intestinal fat	Inhibits gastric motility and acid secretion (peptide YY is elevated in celiac disease and cystic fibrosis)
Substance P	Enteric neurons in the small intestine	Cholecystokinin (CCK), 5-hydroxy-tryptamine (5-HT)	Stimulates gut motility, secretion, and immune response; may have a role in inflammatory bowel disease
Enkephalin	Enteric neurons in the small intestine	Unknown	Inhibits gut motility and secretion
Neurotensin	N cells of the small intestine	Presence of intestinal fat	Stimulates local gut motility, secretion, and immune response

Fig. 6.3 Actions of the minor gastrointestinal tract peptides. The other peptides are described in the text.

the stomach. It neutralizes the acid produced by gastrin release by:

- Stimulating pancreatic and liver secretion of bicarbonate.
- Inhibiting acid secretion from the parietal cells of the stomach.
- Increasing the response to cholecystokinin (CCK).

Cholecystokinin

CCK is secreted in the duodenum in the presence of fat or amino acids. It increases the breakdown of fat by:

- Causing contraction of the gallbladder and release of bile into the duodenum.
- Stimulating pancreatic enzyme secretion (e.g., lipase).
- Causing some bicarbonate release from the pancreas.
- Producing a sensation of fullness.

The concept of hormones was first put forward by the English physiologists Bayliss and Starling in 1902. They deduced that a blood-borne signal secreted by the duodenum acted on the pancreas. They called this signal secretin, and the name is still used today.

Glucose-dependent insulinotropic peptide

Glucose-dependent insulinotropic peptide (GIP) used to be called gastric inhibitory peptide (also GIP), but this was inaccurate and too easy to pronounce. It is secreted by the lining of the duodenum in response to fats and carbohydrates. It acts to:

- Stimulate insulin secretion if blood glucose is high.
- Inhibit gastric acid production and gastric motility.

Somatostatin

Somatostatin is secreted mainly by the δ-cells of the islets of Langerhans in the pancreas but also by the stomach and GI tract neurons. It is also secreted by the hypothalamus, where it is called growth hormone-inhibiting hormone (GHIH). Secretion is stimulated by:

- Acidity and amino acids in the stomach.
- High blood glucose.
- CCK.

Somatostatin acts to slow down digestion by inhibiting:

- Secretion of all other GI tract and pancreatic hormones.
- Secretion of pancreatic enzymes and bile.
- Gastric motility.

Pancreatic polypeptide

Pancreatic polypeptide is secreted by the F cells of the islets of Langerhans in the pancreas in response to protein in the stomach or low blood glucose. Its actions remain unclear, but it slows the absorption of food by:

- Inhibiting gallbladder contraction.
- Inhibiting pancreatic enzyme secretion.

Insulin and glucagon

Insulin and glucagon are both peptides secreted by enteroendocrine cells in the pancreas. The important functions they perform are described in Chapter 5.

Pineal gland

Structure
Macrostructure

The pineal gland secretes the hormone melatonin which regulates circadian rhythms. It is a small gland found at the posterior end of the corpus callosum, forming a section of the roof in the posterior wall of the third ventricle (Fig. 6.4).

The pineal gland begins to calcify after puberty making it a useful midline marker in x-rays and computed tomography (CT) scans.

The French philosopher Descartes (1594–1650) believed that the pineal gland was the "seat of the soul" that unified the functions of body and mind.

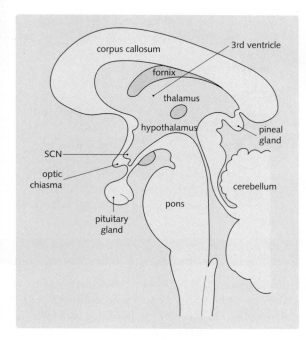

Fig. 6.4 Median section of the midbrain and brainstem showing the anatomical location of the pineal gland and suprachiasmatic nucleus (SCN).

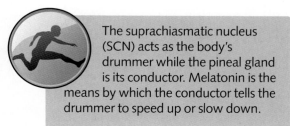

The suprachiasmatic nucleus (SCN) acts as the body's drummer while the pineal gland is its conductor. Melatonin is the means by which the conductor tells the drummer to speed up or slow down.

Microstructure

The gland is composed of two types of neural cells:
- Pinealocytes—specialized secretory neurons.
- Glial support cells.

In keeping with all endocrine organs, it has a very rich blood supply that forms a network of capillaries surrounded by the pinealocytes. It receives innervation from many parts of the brain, but the main connections are with the:
- Suprachiasmatic nucleus (SCN).
- Retina.
- Sympathetic system.
- Parasympathetic system.

Function

The pineal gland synthesizes and secretes the hormone melatonin. This is not the same as the brown skin pigment called melanin. Melatonin is a modified form of the amino acid tryptophan, which is first converted to 5-HT, then to melatonin. Most modified amino acid hormones are derived from tyrosine.

Regulation

The main control of melatonin release is from the SCN. This nucleus is located in the hypothalamus, above the optic chiasma as its name suggests. It is essentially the "body clock" which regulates body rhythms including:
- Day and night (circadian rhythm).
- Seasonal rhythms (e.g., mating cycles).

The GI tract hormone vasoactive intestinal polypeptide (VIP) is also secreted by the cells of the SCN as a neurotransmitter.

Melatonin secretion is also regulated by light and dark. Stimulation from the retina (i.e., light) inhibits melatonin secretion, so melatonin is secreted in response to darkness. The pineal gland allows physical stimulation of light to be converted into the chemical signal melatonin.

Effects of melatonin

Melatonin has three main effects:
- It induces sleep (hypnotic effect).
- It resets the SCN.
- It influences the hypothalamus, especially the reproductive functions.

Circadian rhythms influence almost every cell in the body. Hormones secreted from the hypothalamus, pituitary gland, and gonads all respond dramatically to these rhythms—e.g., corticotropin-releasing hormone (CRH) and adrenocorticotropic hormone (ACTH) secretion peak early in the morning. The regulation and actions of melatonin are shown in Fig. 6.5.

Jet lag and melatonin treatment

The pineal gland has evolved to allow adaptation to changing day length (i.e., seasons). However, resetting of the SCN is best demonstrated by jet flight in the following way:

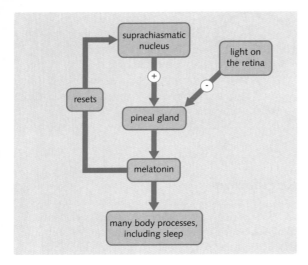

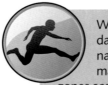

Fig. 6.5 Regulation of melatonin and its actions.

- When people leave their home country, the SCN and pineal gland are synchronized: every night the SCN and darkness both stimulate melatonin production inducing sleep.
- If a person flies across time zones, the SCN remains set at the previous time zone so that melatonin production (and, therefore, tiredness) does not change.
- The light input into the pineal gland gradually adapts melatonin secretion to fit the new time zone. It can alter secretion by a couple of hours each day.
- Melatonin receptors in the SCN allow the clock to adjust to the time zone so that the pineal gland and SCN are once again synchronized.

The sensation of retaining the previous time zone until resetting is complete is commonly called jet lag. The person feels tired and sleepy at times appropriate to the previous time zone, and they may take several days to adapt. A similar effect is seen in shift work; this is especially important in medical employment, during which physicians and staff workers often change their daily work schedules.

Taking oral melatonin can shorten the period of jet lag or adaptation to a new shift. Melatonin should be taken at the times of darkness in the new time zone while on the plane and for several days at the destination. For shift work, the melatonin should be taken during the period of desired sleep. The SCN is reset more quickly, and the body becomes resynchronized.

Melatonin is also given to some disabled children to maintain normal day and night cycles. It is given at night to induce sleep.

Without the signals of light and dark, the body clock has a natural cycle of 25 hours. This makes adaptation to later time zones easier and accounts for jet lag being worse when flying west to east.

Endocrine role of adipose tissue

Adipose tissue has recently been identified as an endocrine tissue that secretes a polypeptide hormone called leptin. The levels of this hormone correlate well with the percentage of adipose tissue, creating an endocrine indicator of energy stores. This signal is transported across the blood–brain barrier to act on the hypothalamus. It has two effects:
- It inhibits food intake.
- It permits gonadotropin-releasing hormone (GnRH) production.

The inhibition of food intake has prompted a lot of interest in leptin as a cure for obesity. Leptin is a protein that is digested if taken orally; like insulin, it must be administered by subcutaneous injection. At the highest doses leptin does cause some weight loss, although the effect is not impressive or effective in all patients.

Leptin resistance caused by the blood–brain barrier may prevent remarkable weight loss. It has been suggested that only a fixed amount of leptin can be transported across this barrier so that excess leptin in the blood does not increase leptin in the CNS above a fixed level. Disorders in this barrier may also account for some cases of obesity. Inherited leptin deficiency is an incredibly rare recessive disorder that causes gross obesity and infertility.

The name leptin is derived from the Greek word *leptos*, meaning thin.

The action of leptin on GnRH release (Fig. 6.6) explains the infertility of underweight women. This is a protective response to prevent pregnancy in the undernourished. Leptin is also secreted prepubertally and it plays a role in the onset of puberty. Body weight is a better predictor of the onset of menstruation than age.

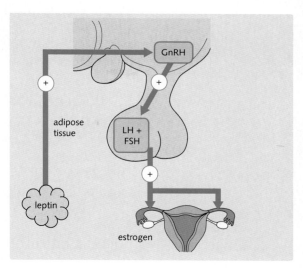

Fig. 6.6 The action of leptin on fertility. (FSH, follicle-stimulating hormone; GnRH, gonadotropin-releasing hormone; LH, luteinizing hormone.)

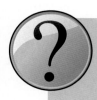

- Define an APUD cell. List three examples with the hormones they secrete.
- Describe the actions of gastrin, cholecystokinin, and secretin.
- Describe the anatomical location of the pineal gland. What types of cells are present?
- What type of hormone is melatonin? How is it synthesized?
- What signals trigger the release of melatonin?
- Describe the function of the suprachiasmatic nucleus (SCN). How does melatonin affect these cells?
- Describe jet lag from an endocrine point of view.
- What type of hormone is leptin?
- Why are severely underweight women infertile?
- Define leptin resistance. How is this believed to occur?

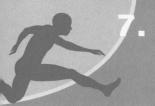

7. Endocrine Control of Fluid Balance

Water is essential for every single cell in the body, so the regulation of water levels is very important. The loss and gain of water from the body is called fluid balance. The regulation of fluid balance takes place mainly in the kidneys, where hormones control the volume and concentration of water that is excreted. The excretion of water is largely controlled by the regulation of sodium absorption. Since sodium is osmotically active, water follows it across membranes. There are many hormones involved in this process. However, the main three are:

- Antidiuretic hormone (ADH)—from the posterior pituitary gland (Fig. 7.1).
- Angiotensin II—from the kidney (Fig. 7.2).
- Aldosterone—from the adrenal cortex (Fig. 7.2).

Important terms:
Peripheral resistance: resistance created by arterioles that can be increased by reducing their diameter; blood pressure increases as resistance rises
Vasoconstriction: contraction of arterioles to raise peripheral resistance
Osmolarity: the concentration of the solutes or electrolytes in the blood
Hypovolemia: low blood volume
Diuretic: a substance that increases water loss from the kidneys
Osmotically active: the ability to attract water across a cell membrane to areas of higher concentration

Blood pressure is also affected by fluid balance because changes in blood volume affect the pressure in arteries. Many of the hormones that regulate fluid balance also control the diameter of arteries, allowing blood pressure to be maintained despite loss or gain of water.

After reading this chapter you should be able to:
- Highlight the need for fluid balance.
- Explain the actions of antidiuretic hormone.
- Describe the actions of the renin–angiotensin II system.
- Understand the actions of aldosterone.
- Discuss other factors that affect fluid balance.

Fluid balance

The importance of water
Water is found inside and outside of cells and also in the blood as plasma. Because it is essential for the normal function of all cells, it must be tightly regulated. About 50 L water is found in the average human, accounting for 70% of body weight.

The importance of sodium
Fluid balance is intimately linked to sodium balance. Sodium ions are osmotically active and present in large quantities within the body. Water tends to passively follow movements of sodium ions. The normal plasma concentration of sodium ions is 135–145 mmol/L. In the kidney, water excretion is largely controlled by regulating sodium excretion or reabsorption.

Fluid balance and circulation
Variations in fluid balance rapidly affect blood volume and, therefore, blood pressure. Changes in fluid balance can be compensated for by variations in:
- Cardiac output (i.e., stroke volume and rate).
- Peripheral resistance (i.e., vasodilatation or vasoconstriction).

Regulation of fluid balance
Water intake
Water intake is controlled by the sensation of thirst. Thirst is determined by osmoreceptors in the hypothalamus that detect the osmolarity of plasma. Some hormones involved in fluid balance can also cause this feeling directly. Water is also gained from food and metabolism (Fig. 7.3).

Water excretion
Water excretion is controlled mainly by the kidney. The kidney filters the entire blood volume once

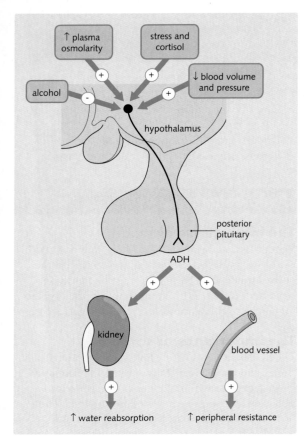

Fig. 7.1 Hormonal regulation of plasma osmolarity by antidiuretic hormone (ADH).

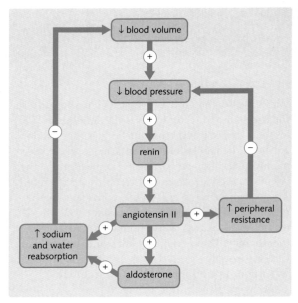

Fig. 7.2 Hormonal regulation of blood volume by renin, angiotensin II, and aldosterone.

Expected intake and output of water over a 24-hour period	
Water intake (mL)	**Water loss (mL)**
Drinking: 1500 Food: 500 Metabolism: 400	Urine: 1500 Respiration: 400 Skin evaporation: 400 Feces: 100
Total: 2400	Total: 2400

Fig. 7.3 Expected intake and output of water over a 24-hour period.

every 5 minutes. Water and sodium are filtered into the kidney tubules by the glomeruli, but most is reabsorbed into the blood. Sodium ions are actively reabsorbed, while water passively follows the sodium by osmosis. Any sodium or water that is not reabsorbed is excreted in the urine.

Fluid balance can be regulated in the kidneys by altering two factors:
- Sodium reabsorption.
- Permeability of the tubules to water.

Water is also lost by the processes shown in Fig. 7.3, but by far the majority of water loss occurs through urine output from the kidney.

Factors involved in fluid balance

Fluid balance is regulated by controlling the intake and excretion of water and sodium. Hormones regulate this balance by acting on:

- Thirst—stimulated in the hypothalamus.
- Volume and concentration of water excreted in the urine.
- Peripheral resistance, which affects blood pressure.

Three main hormones regulate fluid balance; their sites and actions on the kidney nephron are shown in Fig. 7.4:
- Antidiuretic hormone (ADH; vasopressin)—conserves water.
- Angiotensin II—conserves sodium and, therefore, water.
- Aldosterone—conserves sodium and, therefore, water.

Fig. 7.4 Location and type of action by the three major hormones in the kidney nephron. (ADH, antidiuretic hormone.)

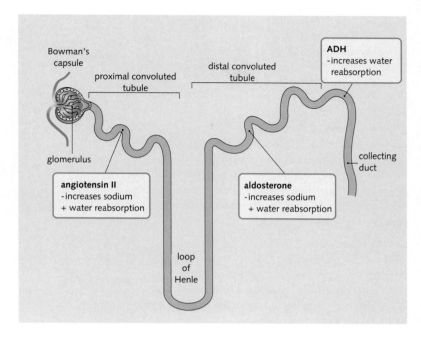

The actions of these three hormones are modified by other hormones, nerves, and chemical factors, including:

- Atrial natriuretic factor (ANF).
- Renal sympathetic nerves and catecholamines.
- Kinins.
- Prostaglandins.
- Dopamine.

Hormones involved in fluid balance

Antidiuretic hormone

ADH (or vasopressin) acts on the kidney to conserve water. It increases the permeability of the collecting ducts so that more water is reabsorbed, resulting in the production of more concentrated urine. It also causes constriction of the arterioles to raise peripheral resistance—hence vasopressin, the old name for this hormone. ADH regulates fluid balance by influencing the movement of water directly, not through sodium movement. The regulation and actions of ADH are shown in Fig. 7.1.

Synthesis and secretion

ADH is a polypeptide hormone synthesized by neurosecretory cells in the supraoptic nucleus of the hypothalamus. It is transported along their axons to the posterior pituitary gland, where it is stored in vesicles. This process is described in more detail in Chapter 2.

ADH is secreted by the posterior pituitary gland in response to:

- High plasma osmolarity (concentrated blood).
- Low blood volume.

It is rapidly degraded by the liver and kidney.

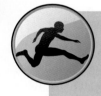

ADH secretion is inhibited by alcohol, causing large volumes of dilute urine to be excreted and resulting in dehydration the next morning.

Intracellular actions

ADH acts on G-protein-linked vasopressin receptors (V receptors) found on the cell surface of target cells. These target cells are found in two tissue types:

- Kidney—ADH acts on V_2 receptors on collecting duct cells, causing water transport proteins (aquaporins) to be inserted in the luminal membrane of collecting duct cells. This process uses cAMP as a second messenger.

- Blood vessels—ADH acts on V_1 receptors causing smooth muscle contraction (i.e., vasoconstriction). Inositol triphosphate (IP_3) acts as a second messenger causing calcium levels to rise, resulting in vasoconstriction.

Effects

On the kidneys

ADH is secreted in response to high blood osmolarity. It increases the reabsorption of water in the kidney by increasing the permeability of the collecting duct. This prevents the excretion of water whilst sodium remains unchanged, so that the blood osmolarity decreases and concentrated urine is produced.

On the blood vessels

ADH is also secreted in response to low blood volume. It causes vasoconstriction of the arterioles, which increases peripheral resistance and raises blood pressure. This action normally has little effect on blood pressure regulation, but it is important following severe hemorrhage that significantly reduces blood volume.

Deficiency and excess

ADH deficiency causes diabetes insipidus, in which excess dilute urine is produced causing fluid loss (polyuria), dehydration, polydipsia, and blood with high osmolarity.

ADH excess is called the syndrome of inappropriate ADH secretion (SIADH). It results in water retention.

Both of these conditions are described in more detail in Chapter 2.

The rennin–angiotensin II system

The actions of renin and angiotensin II are intimately linked so they are described together. The renin–angiotensin II system acts on the kidney to conserve sodium and water. Renin is produced by the kidney, and it causes the production of angiotensin II. Angiotensin II causes reabsorption of sodium in the proximal tubules of the kidney and water follows this movement. Angiotensin II also increases peripheral resistance and aldosterone release. The regulation and actions of renin and angiotensin II are shown in Fig. 7.4.

Synthesis and secretion of renin

Renin is a small peptide enzyme secreted by the cells of the juxtaglomerular complex. This structure is made of three cell types (Fig. 7.5):

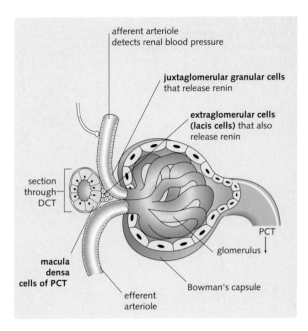

Fig. 7.5 Structure of the juxtaglomerular complex. (PCT, proximal convoluted tubule; DCT, distal convoluted tubule, lying very close to the afferent and efferent arterioles.)

- Macula densa—part of the distal tubule of the nephron that detects sodium.
- Juxtaglomerular cells—part of the afferent glomerular arteriole that releases renin.
- Extraglomerular mesangial cells—glomerular support cells that control blood flow in the afferent glomerular arteriole.

The function of this structure is complex; however, it can detect both sodium in the distal convoluted tubule and blood pressure. The juxtaglomerular cells secrete renin in response to low blood pressure.

Effects of renin

Renin is an enzyme that acts on a plasma protein called angiotensinogen, synthesized by the liver. It cleaves this protein to form angiotensin I. This inactive form is rapidly converted to the active form angiotensin II by the action of angiotensin-converting enzyme (ACE) in the blood. ACE is a major site of action for antihypertensive drugs called ACE inhibitors.

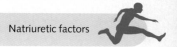

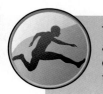

The main site of ACE action and angiotensin II synthesis is the endothelium of the capillaries in the lung.

Effects of angiotensin II

Angiotensin II has five important actions to increase blood volume and pressure:

- Stimulating sodium pumps in the proximal tubule to increase sodium reabsorption, causing water reabsorption.
- Peripheral vasoconstriction to raise blood pressure.
- Stimulating sensation of thirst in the hypothalamus.
- Stimulating aldosterone release from the adrenal cortex.
- Inhibiting renin release (negative feedback).

Thus, angiotensin II conserves sodium and water to increase blood volume while raising the blood pressure.

ACE inhibitors inhibit production of angiotensin II, causing lower blood volume and reduced peripheral resistance. Both actions decrease blood pressure; thus these drugs are used to treat hypertension and heart failure.

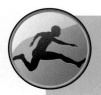

The primary functions of the rennin–angiotensin II system are to keep blood volume and pressure constant.

Aldosterone

Aldosterone is a mineralocorticoid steroid hormone synthesized by the zona glomerulosa cells of the adrenal cortex. Since the main stimulus for secretion is angiotensin II, it is often considered part of the renin–angiotensin II system. Aldosterone causes the conservation of sodium and water. See Chapter 4 for a complete description of aldosterone and the associated disorders. The regulation and actions of aldosterone are shown in Figs. 7.2 and 7.4.

Intracellular actions

Aldosterone acts on intracellular mineralocorticoid receptors in the distal convoluted tube of the kidney. It causes increased expression of the Na^+/K^+ ATPase, which allows sodium to be reabsorbed in exchange for potassium. Water follows the movement of sodium as the internal concentration increases and is reabsorbed.

Effects

Aldosterone is secreted in response to high potassium or reduced blood volume through the action of renin and angiotensin II. It causes sodium and water to be conserved to help rectify these changes.

Natriuretic factors

Natriuretic factors have a diuretic effect, the opposite effect of ADH, angiotensin II, and aldosterone. They increase sodium excretion so that water excretion is also increased. This causes blood volume to decrease, and blood pressure is lowered. Natriuretic factors act as an "escape mechanism" to prevent excess water retention.

Atrial natriuretic factor

ANF is a polypeptide hormone synthesized by the muscle cells of the atrium of the heart. It is secreted in response to high blood volume, which is detected by the stretching of cardiac muscle.

The main actions of ANF are:

- Decrease of sodium reabsorption by kidneys.
- Inhibition of renin secretion.
- Inhibition of aldosterone secretion.
- Vasodilation, causing a drop in blood pressure.

Kinins

Kinins are polypeptides formed in the blood by the action of the enzyme kallikrein on plasma globulins. They act in the kidney to:

- Inhibit the action of ADH.
- Decrease sodium reabsorption.
- Stimulate prostaglandin synthesis in the kidney.
- Stimulate vasodilation in the kidney.
- Relax vascular smooth muscle via nitric oxide to decrease blood pressure.

Renal prostaglandins

Renal prostaglandins are locally acting lipid molecules synthesized by kidney cells. They act in the kidney to:

- Inhibit the action of ADH and aldosterone.
- Stimulate vasodilatation in the kidney.

Dopamine

Dopamine is an amine synthesized in the proximal tubule cells. It acts in the kidneys to:

- Decrease sodium reabsorption.
- Induce vasodilatation in the kidney.

Disorders of fluid balance

A deficiency of water is called dehydration; it may or may not be accompanied by sodium deficiency. The causes and effects of dehydration are shown in Fig. 7.6.

An excess of water is called fluid retention; it may or may not be accompanied by an excess of sodium. The causes and effects of fluid retention are shown in Fig. 7.7.

Causes and effects of dehydration		Deficient sodium and water	Deficient water
Cause	Deficient input	Decreased ingestion, e.g., unconscious	Unable to find water, hypothalamic thirst disorder
	Excess output	Diarrhea, vomiting, burns, hemorrhage, aldosterone deficiency	Diabetes insipidus and mellitus
Effect	Plasma osmolarity	No change	Raised
	Symptoms	Thirst, postural dizziness, weakness, collapse, headache, apathy, confusion, coma	
	Signs	Hypotension, tachycardia, slow capillary refill, reduced skin turgor, cool peripheries, sunken eyes, dry membranes, weight loss	

Fig. 7.6 The causes and effects of dehydration.

Causes and effects of fluid retention		Excess sodium and water	Excess water
Cause	Excess input	Excess fluid transfusion	Excess drinking, e.g., psychological
	Deficient output	Cardiac or renal failure	Acute renal failure or SIADH
Effect	Plasma osmolarity	No change, causes edema	Decreased, no edema
	Symptoms	Nausea, vomiting, anorexia, muscle weakness, headache, apathy, confusion, fits, coma	
	Signs	Hypertension, raised JVP, displaced apex beat	

Fig. 7.7 The causes and effects of water retention.

- Describe the processes by which water can be lost or gained from the body. Which two processes are most important in the regulation of fluid balance?
- How do blood volume and peripheral resistance influence blood pressure?
- Explain the regulation and secretion of ADH.
- List the actions of ADH.
- Describe the regulation and secretion of renin and angiotensin II. How do ACE inhibitors act?
- Describe the actions of renin and angiotensin II.
- Explain the regulation and action of aldosterone.
- Name three peptides that affect fluid balance along with their actions.
- List the common causes of dehydration and the signs and symptoms that result.
- What are the common causes of water retention and the signs and symptoms that result?

8. Endocrine Control of Calcium Homeostasis

Calcium is essential for many important processes in the body. Bone formation, nerve depolarization, and muscle contraction, including cardiac muscle, all require calcium to function normally. Blood levels must be carefully regulated, otherwise cardiac arrest can occur. Calcium regulation is not controlled by the hypothalamus or pituitary gland.

Blood calcium levels are regulated by three hormones (Fig. 8.1):

- Parathyroid hormone (PTH)—increases blood calcium levels.
- Vitamin D—stimulates calcium absorption from the gastrointestinal tract.
- Calcitonin—causes calcium excretion and lowers blood levels.

PTH is the most important of these hormones; it regulates moment-to-moment control of plasma calcium levels. Low plasma calcium triggers the secretion of PTH. Three sites respond to PTH to increase calcium levels: kidneys, bones, and intestines.

An excess of PTH causes hypercalcemia, whereas PTH deficiency results in hypocalcemia. Other causes of hypocalcemia (e.g., chronic renal failure) cause a rise in PTH. Excess PTH results in decalcified, weak bones.

After reading this chapter you should be able to:

- Highlight the physiological requirement for calcium.
- Understand the regulation of calcium levels.
- Explain how the three hormones control this regulation.
- Describe the common disorders of calcium metabolism.

> **Important terms:**
> **Hyperparathyroidism:** an excess of parathyroid hormone
> **Osteoclast:** a cell that breaks down bone releasing calcium
> **Osteoblast:** a cell that deposits bone using calcium
> **Reabsorption:** when substances are filtered out of the blood from the kidney prior to excretion

The role of calcium

Calcium is a mineral obtained in the diet and excreted by the kidneys. The adult body contains about 1.2 kg calcium, the vast majority (99%) of which is contained in bones so that it does not contribute to rapid, homeostatic control. A small reservoir of calcium in bone is available for rapid exchange and is mainly under the control of PTH. The remaining calcium is present in the plasma, extracellular fluid, and intracellular compartments of cells.

Although only a small proportion of the body's calcium is available to cells, it performs many vital functions, especially in the neuromuscular system. The main processes that require calcium are:

- Bone formation and maintenance.
- Muscle contraction, including cardiac muscle.
- All processes that involve exocytosis, including synaptic transmission and hormone release.

The processes requiring calcium are described in Fig. 8.2.

Mechanisms involved in calcium homeostasis

Calcium intake

About 1 g calcium is required in the diet every day. It is found in many foods, especially dairy products. Only 30% of dietary calcium is absorbed by the upper small intestine, although this figure can vary with a number of factors:

- Diet—lactose in milk increases absorption, while phytic acid in brown bread decreases absorption.
- Age—absorption is increased in the young and decreased in the elderly.
- Hormones—vitamin D increases absorption.
- Pregnancy and lactation—both increase absorption.

Calcium balance

Calcium balance is calculated as absorbed calcium minus excreted calcium. This balance is affected by age and some diseases:

- Children usually have a positive calcium balance; this allows bones to grow.
- In adults, input and output should be the same.
- Postmenopausal women tend to have a negative calcium balance (i.e., calcium is lost).

Control of plasma calcium

Since calcium is essential, plasma levels must be tightly regulated. The normal range is 2.12–2.65 mmol/L. Since dietary intake is variable, the body must be able to adapt to raised or reduced plasma calcium. Calcium regulation involves the loss or gain of calcium from three tissues: kidneys, intestines, and bones.

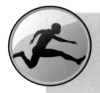

At any time, about 20% of bones are being broken down and rebuilt to repair numerous microfractures.

The movements and distribution of calcium in the body are shown in Fig. 8.3. The movements are regulated by the three hormones discussed below.

Forty per cent of plasma calcium is bound to albumin. Diseases that lower plasma albumin can increase unbound (i.e., active) calcium levels, causing symptoms of hypercalcemia. When measuring plasma calcium levels, it is total blood calcium that is measured. Albumin levels must be taken into account to calculate unbound, corrected calcium levels.

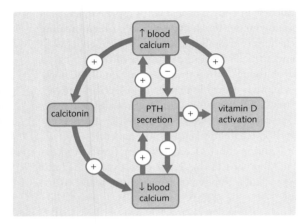

Fig. 8.1 Hormonal regulation of blood calcium by parathyroid hormone (PTH), vitamin D, and calcitonin.

Hormones involved in calcium homeostasis

Three hormones regulate calcium levels in the blood and tissues:

Processes that require calcium	
System	Role of calcium
Bone formation	Calcium is a vital mineral component of bone; it makes the bone strong and rigid
Blood clotting	Many clotting factors are activated by calcium
Muscle contraction	Calcium binds to troponin, which allows myosin to bind to actin
Intracellular signaling	Calcium regulates the activity of a number of intracellular proteins in response to the second messenger IP_3
Nervous system	Calcium is essential for membrane potential and depolarization; synapses use calcium to release neurotransmitters
Endocrine system	All processes that involve exocytosis (e.g., hormone secretion) require calcium
Cardiovascular system	Calcium regulates the membrane potential and contraction of muscle cells

Fig. 8.2 Processes that require calcium.

- Parathyroid hormone from the parathyroid gland.
- Vitamin D (cholecalciferol) from the diet and skin.
- Calcitonin from the thyroid gland.

Their effects are summarized in Figs. 8.1 and 8.4.

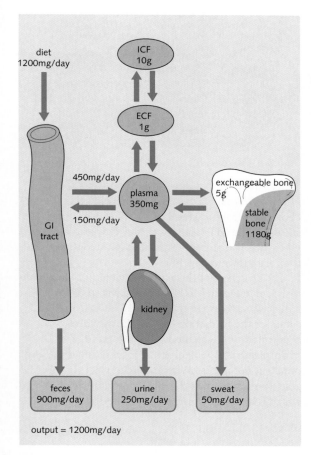

Fig. 8.3 Normal distribution and movements of calcium in the body. (ICF, intracellular fluid; ECF, extracellular fluid.)

Parathyroid hormone (PTH)

PTH is essential to life; it is synthesized by the chief cells in the parathyroid glands. These four small glands are found behind the thyroid gland in the neck. Their development and anatomy are described in Chapter 3.

PTH is released in response to low blood calcium, and its actions are aimed at raising calcium levels back to their normal physiological concentration. Once blood calcium levels are restored, further PTH release is inhibited.

Synthesis and receptors

PTH is a polypeptide hormone synthesized as pre-proparathyroid hormone. Two cleavage reactions result in PTH, a protein of 84 amino acid residues. This hormone is stored in cell vesicles until low plasma calcium triggers its release.

PTH acts via G-protein-linked receptors on the cell surface. These receptors are found on osteoblasts, renal tubule cells, and cells in the intestinal epithelium. The receptors couple to Gs/adenylyl cyclase, which generates cyclic AMP (cAMP) as a second messenger to regulate the phosphorylation of intracellular proteins via protein kinase A (PKA). Key intracellular proteins respond to PKA by favoring calcium movement back to the plasma in a cell-specific manner.

Actions

PTH is the most important regulator of blood calcium levels; it is essential to life. The actions of PTH on calcium regulation are shown in Fig. 8.5.

On the kidneys

PTH has three major effects:
- Increase of calcium ion reabsorption by stimulating active uptake in the distal convoluted tubule.

Fig. 8.4 Summary of the actions of parathyroid hormone (PTH), calcitonin, and vitamin D on calcium regulation.

Actions of the hormones involved in calcium homeostasis			
	PTH	Vitamin D	Calcitonin
Secreted/activated in response to:	Low blood calcium	PTH	High blood calcium
Kidneys	Calcium reabsorbed; vitamin D activated	Calcium reabsorbed	Calcium excreted
Bones	Calcium released	Calcium trapped	Calcium trapped
Intestines	Negligible	Calcium absorbed	Negligible

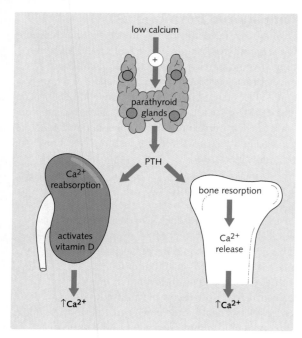

Fig. 8.5 Actions of parathyroid hormone (PTH) on the kidney and bone.

- Increase of phosphate ion excretion by inhibiting uptake in the proximal and distal convoluted tubules.
- Stimulation of 1α-hydroxylase, an enzyme that activates vitamin D.

On the bones

PTH acts primarily on the osteoblasts in bone. However, these cells indirectly regulate osteoclast activity via paracrine actions of prostaglandins. In general, PTH causes the resorption of bone, releasing calcium and phosphate ions. The actions are:

- Direct inhibition of osteoblast collagen synthesis.
- Indirect stimulation of osteoclast activity.
- Increased collagenase synthesis to resorb the bone.
- Increased hydrogen ion release from osteoclasts to acidify the resorptive zone and enhance calcium release.

On the intestines

PTH may have a direct action on calcium absorption in the upper small intestines, but this is unproven. The major effects are indirect, through the activation of vitamin D.

Vitamin D

Vitamin D is absorbed by the small intestine as part of the diet or is synthesized from cholesterol in the skin. Vitamin D synthesis requires ultraviolet (UV) light, usually derived from the sun. Vitamin D raises blood calcium and phosphate levels mainly through slow, sustained actions on the intestines.

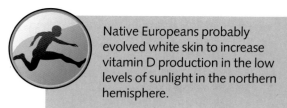

Native Europeans probably evolved white skin to increase vitamin D production in the low levels of sunlight in the northern hemisphere.

Activation

Human vitamin D is an inactive steroid called cholecalciferol (or vitamin D_3); this fat-soluble steroid is stored in adipose tissue. Two reactions must take place in different organs to activate vitamin D; they are shown in Fig. 8.6.

The structure of the activated vitamin D molecule is shown in Fig. 8.7. It can be inactivated by 24-hydroxylase found in the kidney. This enzyme catalyses the formation of 1,24,25-trihydroxy-cholecalciferol, which is rapidly excreted. The 24-hydroxylase is also highly active when calcium uptake is not necessary from the GI tract. In this case, formation of 24,25-dihydroxyvitamin D_3, which is biologially inactive, is favored.

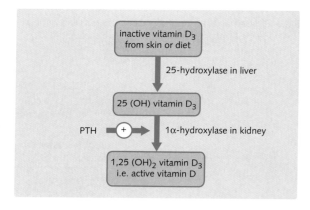

Fig. 8.6 Activation of vitamin D. (25 (OH) vitamin D_3, 25-hydroxyvitamin D_3; 1,25 (OH)$_2$ vitamin D_3, 1,25-dihydroxyvitamin D_3.)

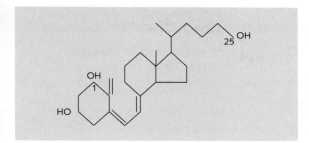

Fig. 8.7 Structure of 1,25-dihydroxyvitamin D$_3$, the active form of vitamin D.

All forms of vitamin D are transported in the blood by a specific plasma protein or within chylomicrons. Vitamin D is fat-soluble (lipophilic) so that it crosses cell membranes and acts via specific intracellular receptors in a manner similar to a typical steroid hormone.

Actions

The actions of vitamin D on calcium regulation are shown in Fig. 8.8.

On the kidney

Activated vitamin D has three effects:

- Increase of calcium reabsorption in the proximal and distal convoluted tubule.
- Increase of phosphate reabsorption in the proximal convoluted tubule.
- Inhibition of 1α-hydroxylase activity. This is a form of negative feedback.

On the bones

Vitamin D directly stimulates osteoblast activity to increase bone mass and calcification. Disorders of vitamin D absorption or activation can cause weak bones (rickets in children or osteomalacia in adults). If this is due to kidney disease, it is called renal osteodystrophy (discussed later).

On the intestines

The main action of vitamin D is stimulation of dietary calcium and phosphate absorption in the duodenum and jejunum. The exact mechanism is unclear, but vitamin D increases the synthesis of calcium-binding proteins in the intestinal cells. This action on the intestines takes a long time to produce an effect, so it does not raise calcium levels acutely.

Calcitonin

Calcitonin is secreted by the parafollicular cells (C cells) in the thyroid gland. The development and anatomy of this gland is described in Chapter 3. Calcitonin is secreted in response to high blood calcium, and it lowers calcium levels. It is not

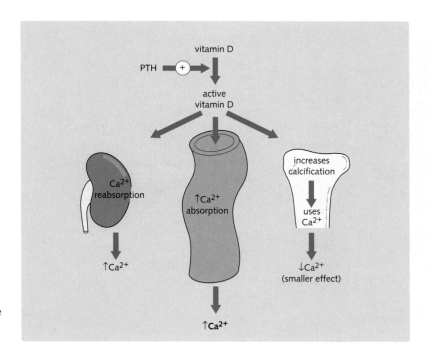

Fig. 8.8 Actions of vitamin D on the gastrointestinal tract, bone, and kidney.

essential to life, but it acts to fine-tune blood calcium levels.

Synthesis and receptors

Calcitonin is a polypeptide hormone that is formed by the breakdown of a larger prohormone. Calcitonin is stored in secretory vesicles, from which it is released when blood calcium levels rise.

Calcitonin acts on G-protein-coupled receptors that release cAMP to cause specific cellular effects.

Actions

The actions of calcitonin on calcium regulation are shown in Fig. 8.9.

On the kidney

Calcitonin inhibits the reabsorption of calcium and phosphate, thus favoring excretion of both ions.

On the bones

Calcitonin acts primarily on osteoclasts in the bone. It inhibits these cells to prevent all stages of bone resorption, preventing calcium and phosphate release into the blood.

Calcitonin is not essential for calcium regulation, and there are no clinical consequences of calcitonin deficiency or excess. Neither removal of the thyroid gland with its parafollicular cells at thyroidectomy nor calcitonin-secreting medullary cell malignancy affect calcium balance significantly.

Disorders of calcium regulation

Since PTH is the most important hormone in calcium homeostasis, disorders of this system are grouped according to their effect on PTH release. The two groups are:

- Hyperparathyroidism (excess of PTH).
- Hypoparathyroidism (deficiency of PTH).

Primary hyperparathyroidism

Primary hyperparathyroidism is excessive PTH release. All the actions of PTH raise calcium levels so hypercalcemia (excess blood calcium) results. Hypercalcemia and excess PTH cause the symptoms shown in Fig. 8.10. Prolonged hyperparathyroidism causes bone demineralization and softening, called osteomalacia in adults and rickets in children. The symptoms and signs of these diseases are shown in Fig. 8.11.

When evaluating a patient with suspected hypercalcemia, remember: "Bones, stones, abdominal groans, and psychic moans."

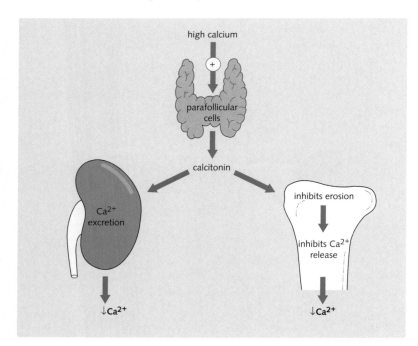

Fig. 8.9 Actions of calcitonin on the kidney and bone.

Fig. 8.10 Symptoms and signs of hypercalcemia.

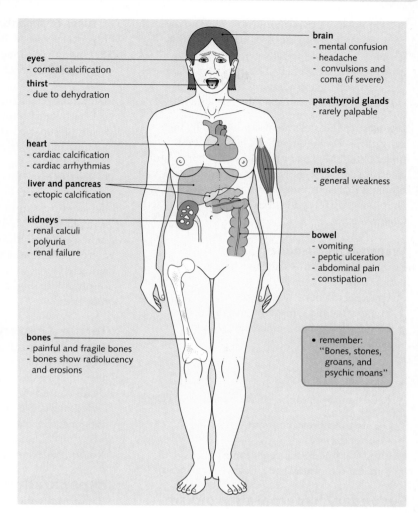

eyes
- corneal calcification

thirst
- due to dehydration

heart
- cardiac calcification
- cardiac arrhythmias

liver and pancreas
- ectopic calcification

kidneys
- renal calculi
- polyuria
- renal failure

bones
- painful and fragile bones
- bones show radiolucency and erosions

brain
- mental confusion
- headache
- convulsions and coma (if severe)

parathyroid glands
- rarely palpable

muscles
- general weakness

bowel
- vomiting
- peptic ulceration
- abdominal pain
- constipation

- remember: "Bones, stones, groans, and psychic moans"

Symptoms and signs caused by rickets and osteomalacia	
Rickets (childhood)	**Osteomalacia (adulthood)**
"Knock-knees" or "bow-legs" caused by bending of the long bones	Bone pain
Chest deformities, back deformities (e.g., kyphosis) and protruding forehead	Bones appear "thin" on x-ray, with localized lucencies (called Losser's zones)
Features of hypocalcemia	Fractures (common in the neck of the femur)
	Features of hypocalcemia (e.g., proximal myopathy causes waddling gait)

Fig. 8.11 Symptoms and signs caused by rickets and osteomalacia.

Primary hyperparathyroidism is a relatively common endocrine disorder (about 1 in 1000 people), and it is especially common in postmenopausal women. The main causes are:
- Parathyroid gland adenoma (80%).
- Diffuse parathyroid gland hyperplasia (20%).

Neoplastic chief cells are not inhibited by high calcium, and consequently PTH secretion is unregulated. Malignant tumors of the parathyroid gland are very rare, but they can be associated with other endocrine tumors in multiple endocrine neoplasia (MEN) syndromes. These are discussed in Chapter 10.

Diagnosis and treatment
Primary hyperparathyroidism is suspected if a patient has:
- Unexpected bone weakness.
- Hypercalcemia symptoms and signs.
- Hypercalcemia on a blood test with low phosphate levels.

It is investigated by:
- Measuring blood PTH.
- Radioisotope scanning of the parathyroid glands.

There are three treatment options:
- Restrict dietary calcium.
- Drug treatment (e.g., calcitonin).
- Surgical removal of the parathyroid gland(s).

Secondary hyperparathyroidism
Many diseases can cause hypocalcemia (e.g., chronic renal failure), which stimulates PTH secretion as a compensatory response. If hypocalcemia is prolonged, the parathyroid glands can enlarge by hyperplasia to secrete excess PTH. This is called secondary hyperparathyroidism.

Osteomalacia is also a feature of secondary hyperparathyroidism because of the excess PTH. Hypocalcemia and excess PTH cause the symptoms shown in Fig. 8.12.

Plasma calcium levels determine the threshold of action potentials. Low calcium causes a low threshold, resulting in tingling sensations and muscle contractions.

Causes of secondary hyperparathyroidism
Hypocalcemia can be caused by:
- Chronic renal failure.
- Vitamin D deficiency.

In chronic renal failure, the kidneys fail to reabsorb calcium. Renal osteodystrophy can also develop as a result of impaired 1α-hydroxylase activity. The kidneys fail to activate vitamin D, consequently PTH secretion increases. The bones are demineralized, hence the name osteodystrophy.

Vitamin D deficiency can occur if the diet is deficient in vitamin D or the skin does not receive sunlight (e.g., elderly people who stay indoors and only see the sun through glass, or women in cultures who cover their skin). Deficiency of activated vitamin D causes hypocalcemia as a result of impaired calcium absorption in the intestines.

Tertiary hyperparathyroidism
Tertiary hyperparathyroidism is a complication of secondary hyperparathyroidism. Very rarely, an adenoma can develop in the hyperplastic parathyroid glands caused by prolonged hypocalcemia. If the underlying cause of hypocalcemia is corrected, then hypercalcemia can develop due to excess PTH secretion. This complication is diagnosed and treated as a primary parathyroid adenoma.

Hypoparathyroidism
Hypoparathyroidism is the deficiency of PTH resulting in hypocalcemia. It causes the usual symptoms of hypocalcemia (Fig. 8.12) but without osteomalacia. The main causes are listed below:
- Complication of thyroid or parathyroid surgery.
- Idiopathic hypoparathyroidism—an autoimmune disorder.
- Pseudohypoparathyroidism—congenital PTH resistance.

Osteoporosis
Osteoporosis is caused by reduced osteoblast activity and diminished remodeling. New bone is not formed, microfractures cannot be repaired, and the bones become thin and brittle. Osteoporosis is caused by a deficiency of estrogen or testosterone. It is very common in postmenopausal women, and signs of bone degeneration are seen in 100% of 80-year-old women.

Fig. 8.12 Symptoms and signs of hypocalcemia.

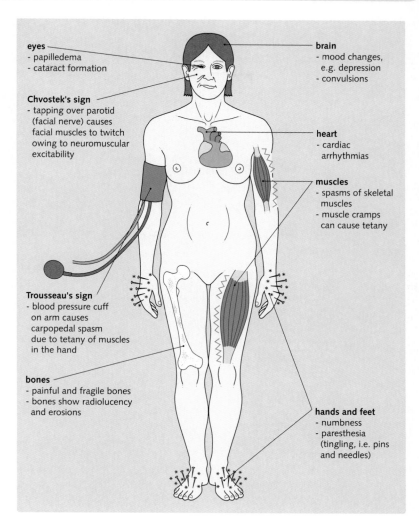

eyes
- papilledema
- cataract formation

Chvostek's sign
- tapping over parotid (facial nerve) causes facial muscles to twitch owing to neuromuscular excitability

Trousseau's sign
- blood pressure cuff on arm causes carpopedal spasm due to tetany of muscles in the hand

bones
- painful and fragile bones
- bones show radiolucency and erosions

brain
- mood changes, e.g. depression
- convulsions

heart
- cardiac arrhythmias

muscles
- spasms of skeletal muscles
- muscle cramps can cause tetany

hands and feet
- numbness
- paresthesia (tingling, i.e. pins and needles)

The main treatments of osteoporosis are dietary calcium and vitamin D supplements and hormone replacement therapy (HRT; see Chapter 12). Calcitonin can be used; however, it is very expensive and it must be injected subcutaneously.

- Explain what happens when blood calcium levels rise.
- Explain what happens when blood calcium levels fall.
- Describe the action of parathyroid hormone on the kidneys, bones, and intestines.
- Describe the action of vitamin D on the kidneys, bones, and intestines.
- How is vitamin D activated? Which hormone controls this process?
- Describe the action of calcitonin on the kidneys, bones, and intestines.
- What is the difference between primary, secondary, and tertiary hyperparathyroidism? What disorders commonly cause these conditions?
- List the symptoms caused by primary hyperparathyroidism. Do calcium levels rise or fall?
- List the symptoms caused by secondary hyperparathyroidism. Do calcium levels rise or fall?
- List the symptoms and causes of hypoparathyroidism.

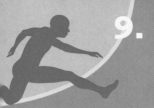

9. Endocrine Control of Growth

Growth hormone (GH) is often described as a pituitary hormone that acts directly on tissues instead of stimulating peripheral endocrine tissues like other anterior pituitary hormones. This view has been challenged by the discovery of insulin-like growth factors (IGFs) secreted by the liver in response to GH. The regulation of growth therefore follows the conventional pattern starting in the hypothalamus (described in Chapter 2).

Growth is a process that takes place at many levels. It can be defined as an increase in:
- Anabolism (e.g., protein synthesis).
- Cell size and number.
- Cell maturation and maintenance.
- Organ size.
- Body size or weight.

> Important terms:
> **Anabolism:** the process of building large molecules from smaller ones
> **Epiphysis:** the end of a long bone (plural, epiphyses)
> **Epiphyseal growth plate:** an area of cartilage between the epiphysis and shaft of the bone that proliferates during childhood, resulting in elongation of the bone
> **Growth factor:** any chemical that stimulates cellular growth
> **Cell maturation:** when a cell differentiates to reach its final form

Acting through IGFs, GH stimulates all the processes listed above. By promoting anabolic processes, the cell increases in size. This promotes cell division and maturation causing the organ to grow. The cellular actions of GH begin before birth and continue throughout life, though the rate varies. The fastest rate of growth is in the fetus and neonate; however, a growth spurt also occurs during puberty.

The growth of the body is limited by the epiphyses (growth plates) at the ends of the long bones. GH stimulates these plates to grow, causing the bones to lengthen and body height to increase. It also stimulates fusion of these growth plates preventing further growth.

After reading this chapter you should be able to:
- Understand the regulation of growth hormone.
- List the actions of insulin-like growth factors.
- Discuss other factors that affect growth.
- Explain how height is determined.
- Describe the disorders of excess or deficient growth hormone.

Direct control of growth

Growth hormone (GH)
GH (also called somatotropin) is a polypeptide that is secreted by the somatotroph cells in the anterior pituitary gland. Like many pituitary hormones, it is synthesized as a precursor molecule (pre-progrowth hormone). Two cleavages release the active hormone. For more information about the anterior pituitary see Chapter 2.

Regulation of secretion
GH secretion is regulated by two hypothalamic releasing factors:
- Growth hormone-releasing hormone (GHRH).
- Somatostatin (also called growth hormone-inhibiting hormone or GHIH).

GHRH is released in a pulsatile manner, especially during deep sleep or hypoglycemia, and GH release follows this pattern. Secretion of GH from the anterior pituitary gland is also regulated by the negative feedback of IGF-1 and other growth factors (Fig. 9.1).

Effects
GH promotes the growth and maintenance of most cells. It has an anabolic effect:
- Stimulates the uptake of amino acids.
- Stimulates the synthesis of proteins.

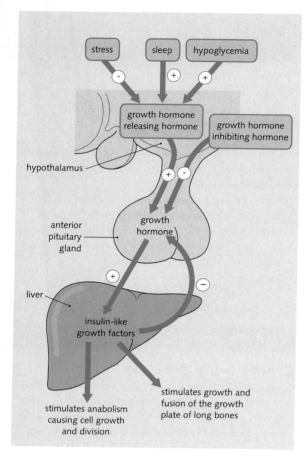

Fig. 9.1 Hormonal regulation of growth hormone.

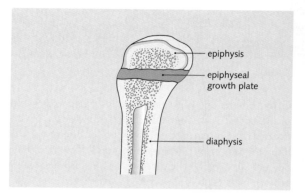

Fig. 9.2 The regions of a growing bone.

The majority of actions associated with GH are actually mediated by IGFs. GH promotes their synthesis, mainly in the liver but also in other tissues.

GH is transported in the blood bound to GH-binding protein. It acts via G-protein and Janus kinase (JAK) receptors on the cell surface of target cells.

Insulin-like growth factors

Insulin-like growth factors (IGFs or somatomedins) are polypeptide hormones that exist in two forms: IGF-1 and IGF-2. They resemble insulin in structure and they act through similar receptors. IGF-1 is more important as a stimulator of growth. IGFs are transported in the blood by a number of IGF-binding proteins.

Metabolic actions

Both IGF hormones have some insulin-like actions, e.g., increasing amino acid uptake and protein

synthesis. However, they also oppose the actions of insulin on glucose by preventing glucose uptake and causing glycogen breakdown to raise blood glucose.

Growth actions

The increase in protein synthesis caused by the metabolic effects of IGF hormones causes cells to grow. This stimulates cell division and maturation causing organs and soft tissues to enlarge.

The growth of the long bones depends on the state of the epiphyseal growth plate. This plate is a layer of chondrocytes (cartilage cells) located between the end (epiphysis) and shaft (diaphysis) of the bone (Fig. 9.2). Before puberty, IGFs stimulate these chondrocytes to grow, divide, and mature into osteocytes (bone cells), allowing the bone to lengthen while maintaining a population of chondrocytes in the plate for further growth. During puberty, IGFs and sex steroids stimulate the chondrocytes within the plate to mature into osteocytes so that the epiphysis and diaphysis become fused together. When the bone is no longer able to lengthen with further IGF stimulation, final adult height is reached.

Other growth factors

Growth in specific tissues is also stimulated by a number of growth factors, many of which are small peptides that act in a paracrine (local) manner. Their relationship to GH is not known. The actions and secretion of several such peptides are described in Fig. 9.3.

Growth factor	Mode of delivery	Action on growth and development	Method and control of secretion
		The secretion of growth factors and their effects	
Nerve growth factor (NGF)	Paracrine	Induces neuron growth and helps to guide growing sympathetic nerves to organs they will innervate (may also act on the brain and aid memory retention)	Secreted by cells in path of growing axon; regulation of secretion not yet understood
Epidermal growth factor (EGF)	Paracrine and endocrine	Promotes cell proliferation in the epidermis, maturation of lung epithelium, and skin keratinization	Secreted by many cell types, i.e., not only epidermal cells (EGF is also found in breast milk); regulation of secretion not yet understood
Transforming growth factors (TGF-α, TGF-β)	Paracrine	Stimulate growth of fibroblast cells; TGF-α acts similarly to EGF; TGF-β especially affects chondrocytes, osteoblasts, and osteoclasts	Secreted by most cell types but especially platelets and cells in placenta and bone; regulation of secretion not yet understood
Fibroblast growth factor (FGF)	Paracrine	Mitogenic effect in several cell types; may induce angiogenesis (formation of new blood vessels), which is essential for growth and wound healing	Secreted by most cell types; regulation of secretion not yet understood
Platelet-derived growth factor (PDGF)	Paracrine	Potent cell-growth promoter; chemotactic factor (involved in inflammatory response)	Secreted by activated blood platelets during blood vessel injury
Erythropoietin	Endocrine	Stimulates the production of erythrocyte precursor cells	Secreted by the kidney in response to falling tissue oxygen concentration
Interleukins (IL) (at least 13 known)	Autocrine and paracrine	IL-1 stimulates B-cell proliferation and helper T cells to produce IL-2; IL-2 autoactivates helper T cells and activates cytotoxic T cells	IL-1 is secreted by activated macrophages; IL-2 is secreted by activated helper T cells

Fig. 9.3 The secretion of growth factors and their effects.

Indirect control of growth

Many factors apart from GH control growth, including:

- Genetics—tall parents often have tall children.
- Adequate nutrition—however, excess nutrition does not increase height.
- Health—chronic disease affects height.
- Other hormones.

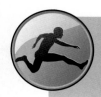

Height is often used as a marker for nutrition when examining historical records or ancient skeletons.

Other hormones

Growth problems can be caused by the abnormal secretion of a number of hormones, including:

- Insulin.
- Antidiuretic hormone (ADH).
- Parathyroid hormone and vitamin D.
- Cortisol.
- Sex steroids.
- Thyroid hormones.

Thyroid hormone is described in Chapter 3; it stimulates cell metabolism promoting cell growth and division, especially in the skeleton and developing central nervous system (CNS). It also stimulates GH secretion from the pituitary.

Cortisol is described in Chapter 4. It inhibits pituitary GH secretion; thus chronic ill health or stress can suppress growth.

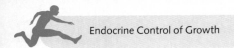

Normal growth can occur only if the internal environment and nutrition are suitable.

Fetal growth

In the fetus, a hormone called placental lactogen is secreted from the placenta. It stimulates fetal cartilage development, and it acts in a similar manner to prolactin on the maternal mammary glands.

Thyroid hormones are essential for the development of the skeleton and CNS. A deficiency in the fetus or neonate results in cretinism.

Puberty

Sexual maturation and the pubertal growth spurt are described in Chapter 11. The main hormones involved are:

- Gonadotropins—luteinizing hormone (LH) and follicle-stimulating hormone (FSH).
- Sex steroids—estrogen and testosterone.

Determination of height

A person's final height is determined simply by the rate and duration of growth. While the rate is determined by the growth hormones and factors already described, the duration is determined by their action on the bones.

During puberty, the epiphyseal growth plates at the end of the long bones begin to fuse. This fusion prevents further growth and, therefore, further height gain. Total fusion occurs between 18 and 20 years of age in males and earlier in females.

The fusion of the epiphyseal plates is stimulated primarily by GH and sex steroids; however, thyroid hormones also promote this effect. A simple increase in GH during puberty is not sufficient to increase final height since the bones simply mature faster and stop growing.

Only the bones that grow in this manner are prevented from responding to further GH. The jaw and skull can continue to grow past puberty; this effect is seen in GH excess. Ultimately, height is determined by multiple genetic factors.

Disorders of growth

Excess of growth hormone

The rare excess of GH in children is called gigantism. The secretion occurs before puberty and fusion of the epiphyses, so the child is very tall for their age. Since the epiphyses also fuse at an earlier age, the child may have an unremarkable height in adulthood. Diabetes is very common in this group because of the opposing actions of GH and insulin on blood glucose.

An excess of GH is slightly more common in adults, in whom it is called acromegaly. The signs and symptoms are shown in Fig. 9.4. See also Fig. 17.7. The long bones can no longer lengthen, so there is no increase in height. However, the soft tissues and other bones can still grow, causing the distinctive features of this condition.

The excess of GH in any age group is usually caused by a somatotroph adenoma of the anterior pituitary gland. This can also cause other symptoms by compressing surrounding structures (see Chapter 2).

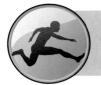

Tall stature is most often caused by tall parents; an excess of growth hormone is very rare.

Diagnosis and treatment

Excess GH can be diagnosed by high IGF-1 levels, but the best test is to measure GH levels following an oral glucose tolerance test. GH levels should fall with the rise in glucose. Computed tomography (CT) or magnetic resonance imaging (MRI) scans can be used to confirm the presence of a functional pituitary adenoma.

Somatotroph adenomas are removed surgically. Following the operation, the patient must be routinely monitored for GH levels and other pituitary hormones throughout life. If surgery is not appropriate, bromocriptine or octreotide (a GHIH analog) can be used.

Deficiency of growth hormone

The deficiency of GH in children is called dwarfism. It is detected by short stature along with either:

- Dropping between growth chart centiles (i.e., not following expected course).
- Being significantly shorter than mean parental height (MPH).

Fig. 9.4 The symptoms and signs of acromegaly.

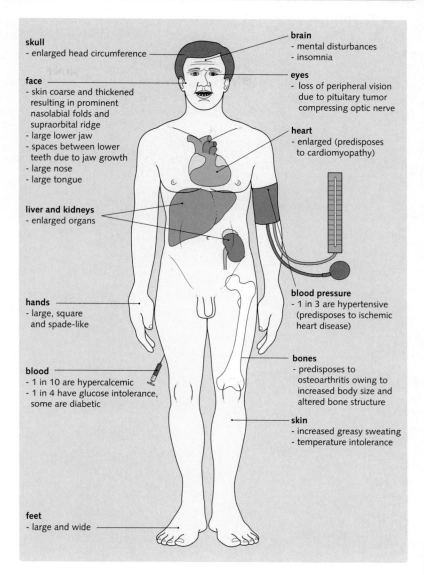

skull
- enlarged head circumference

face
- skin coarse and thickened resulting in prominent nasolabial folds and supraorbital ridge
- large lower jaw
- spaces between lower teeth due to jaw growth
- large nose
- large tongue

liver and kidneys
- enlarged organs

hands
- large, square and spade-like

blood
- 1 in 10 are hypercalcemic
- 1 in 4 have glucose intolerance, some are diabetic

feet
- large and wide

brain
- mental disturbances
- insomnia

eyes
- loss of peripheral vision due to pituitary tumor compressing optic nerve

heart
- enlarged (predisposes to cardiomyopathy)

blood pressure
- 1 in 3 are hypertensive (predisposes to ischemic heart disease)

bones
- predisposes to osteoarthritis owing to increased body size and altered bone structure

skin
- increased greasy sweating
- temperature intolerance

MPH is the average of the parents' height plus 7 cm in boys or minus 7 cm in girls. Final height is usually within 10 cm in either direction of the MPH.

The most common cause of dwarfism is a deficiency of GHRH from the hypothalamus; craniopharyngiomas can also be responsible. See Chapter 2 for more details.

Diagnosis and treatment

GH deficiency is diagnosed using a stimulation test. GH levels are measured after exercise or a dose of clonidine, both of which should raise GH levels. Insulin-induced hypoglycemia is no longer routinely used in children owing to the potential risk of severe hypoglycemia. GH deficiency is treated with subcutaneous injections of synthetic GH before bedtime every night.

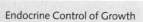

- Describe the regulation of growth hormone and IGF secretion.
- What factors stimulate the secretion of growth hormone?
- Describe the actions of IGFs on cells.
- Describe the actions of IGFs on the growth plate of bones.
- What other factors affect growth?
- Name four peptide growth factors, the tissue that secretes them, and where they have an effect.
- How is height determined?
- How is the mean parental height calculated? What are the boundaries of "normal" height from the MPH?
- List the symptoms of acromegaly.
- How is acromegaly diagnosed?

10. Endocrine Disorders of Neoplastic Origin

The "disorders" sections of several chapters have mentioned several multiple endocrine neoplasia (MEN) syndromes and ectopic hormones. This chapter describes these conditions in more detail.

MEN syndromes are endocrine tumors that originate in multiple sites. There are three patterns, called MEN-I, MEN-IIa, and MEN-IIb. These syndromes are rare, but they can cause tumors in young adults. They are usually inherited.

The term "ectopic hormone" is used to describe hormone secretion from tissues that do not usually secrete that specific hormone. Many tumors secrete ectopic hormones, often in tissues that are significant components of the endocrine system.

After reading this chapter you should be able to:
- Discuss the theories of MEN etiology.
- List the tumors caused by the three MEN syndromes.
- List the most common ectopic hormones.
- Describe the theories of ectopic hormone production.

 MEN syndromes are rare, but they may be life-threatening.

Multiple endocrine neoplasia syndromes

MEN syndromes are patterns of endocrine tumors that often occur at the same time. The tumors are rare, usually aggressive, and arise in multiple tissues; they occur earlier than single sporadic tumors. The underlying cause is probably genetic since these syndromes have a very strong (but not complete) autosomal dominant family history.

It is not known why MEN tumors commonly occur at the same time, but there are three theories:

- The affected tissues may share a common embryological origin that is affected by an abnormality.
- A circulating abnormal growth factor induces excess cell division in a number of endocrine tissues.
- A genetic abnormality is expressed in certain endocrine cells, resulting in tumor growth.

Three patterns of MEN have been described: MEN-I, MEN-IIa, and MEN-IIb (Fig. 10.1).

MEN-I (Wermer's syndrome)
The most common tumors are:
- Parathyroid hyperplasia.
- Pancreatic islet-cell tumors.
- Pituitary adenoma.

The pancreatic islet-cell tumors may secrete ectopic hormones—e.g., gastrin in Zollinger–Ellison syndrome (see Chapter 5). Thirty percent of the very rare Zollinger–Ellison tumors are caused by MEN-I. Less commonly MEN-I is associated with:
- Parathyroid adenoma.
- Hyperplasia of thyroid parafollicular cells.
- Adrenal cortical hyperplasia.

MEN-IIa (Sipple's syndrome)
The main tumors of the MEN-IIa syndrome are:
- Pheochromocytoma (often bilateral).
- Medullary cell carcinoma of the thyroid (often multifocal).

Occasionally parathyroid hyperplasia can develop.

MEN-IIb
The very rare MEN-IIb is sometimes called MEN-III. However, the tumors that develop are similar to MEN-IIa. Two other types of tumor develop in the skin and submucosa throughout the body:
- Neuromas (tumors of neurons).
- Ganglioneuromas (tumors of neuronal ganglia).

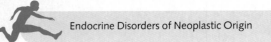
Tumors and hormones associated with the three MEN syndromes		
Syndrome	Associated tumors	Hormones secreted
MEN-I	Parathyroid hyperplasia, pancreatic islet-cell, pituitary adenomas	PTH, insulin, prolactin
MEN-IIa	Medullary carcinoma of the thyroid, pheochromocytomas	Calcitonin, epinephrine
MEN-IIb	Medullary carcinoma of the thyroid, pheochromocytomas, neuromas	Calcitonin, epinephrine

Fig. 10.1 The principal tumors and hormones secreted in the three multiple endocrine neoplasia (MEN) syndromes.

Examples of syndromes caused by ectopic hormone secretion		
Syndrome	Hormone secreted by tumor cells	Tumor
Hypercalcemia	Parathyroid hormone (PTH) or PTH-like peptide	Squamous-cell carcinoma of the lung, breast carcinoma
Hyponatremia	ADH	Oat-cell carcinoma of the bronchus, some intestinal tumors
Hypokalemia (symptoms of Cushing's syndrome caused by ACTH excess take longer to develop)	ACTH and ACTH-like peptides	Oat-cell carcinoma of the bronchus, medullary carcinoma of the thyroid, thymic carcinoma, islet-cell tumors
Gynecomastia	Human placental lactogen	Carcinoma of the bronchus, liver, or kidney
Galactorrhea	Prolactin	Carcinoma of the bronchus, hypernephroma
Polycythemia	Erythropoietin	Hypernephroma, carcinoma of the uterus
Hypoglycemia	Insulin (rare)	Hepatomas, large mesenchymal tumors
No syndrome	Calcitonin	Oat-cell carcinoma of the lung

Fig. 10.2 Examples of syndromes caused by ectopic hormones. (ACTH, adrenocorticotropic hormone; ADH, antidiuretic hormone; PTH, parathyroid hormone.)

Ectopic hormone syndromes

Ectopic hormones

Ectopic means out of place. The term ectopic hormone is used when a tissue secretes a hormone that it does not normally secrete. The hormone is released in an uncontrolled manner by a tumor (benign or malignant). The tumor can be:
- Endocrine tissue secreting unusual hormones.
- Nonendocrine tissue secreting any hormone.

Symptoms are usually caused by the excess of the ectopic hormone while the tumor is still small. Examples of syndromes caused by ectopic hormone secretion are listed in Fig. 10.2.

Treatment

The tumors are treated in a similar manner to any symptomatic tumor:
- Surgical removal.
- Irradiation.
- Chemotherapy.

Etiology of ectopic hormones

The exact mechanism behind ectopic hormone release is not fully understood, and it may vary among tumors. There are two main theories:

- The tumor originates from cells that normally secrete small amounts of hormones—e.g., cells of the bronchial mucosa normally secrete adrenocorticotropic hormone (ACTH) and anaplastic carcinoma of the lung secretes ectopic ACTH.
- Mutations associated with the transformation to neoplasia activate dormant genes resulting in ectopic hormone production.

Types of ectopic hormones

Ectopic hormones are almost always peptide hormones because their synthesis requires expression of only a single gene. Steroid hormones synthesis requires the expression of a complicated series of enzymes.

The ectopic hormone is often not an exact version of a normal hormone (e.g., breast cancer cells secrete PTH-like peptide). This would fit the second theory of etiology since the normal processing enzymes may not be present.

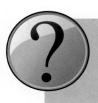

- Describe the theories of MEN tumor formation.
- List the common tumors associated with each of the MEN syndromes.
- What features of an endocrine tumor suggest a MEN syndrome?
- Describe the theories behind ectopic hormone secretion.
- List four tumors known to secrete ectopic hormones, along with the relevant hormone.

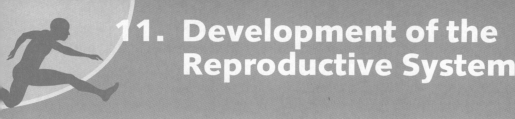

The development of the reproductive system begins 4 weeks after conception and continues through puberty. The majority of the structures are derived from the middle embryological layer called the mesoderm; however, the cells that give rise to the gametes (sperm and oocytes) are derived from the endodermal yolk sac.

Between weeks 4 and 7 there are no clear differences between the male and female development. Differences begin to appear by the 7th week when the indifferent genitalia develop to form distinct reproductive systems for each sex.

Sexual development is arrested soon after birth until puberty. At puberty the gonads are reactivated by luteinizing hormone (LH) and follicle-stimulating hormone (FSH) secretion, and sex steroids (e.g., estrogen and testosterone) are produced. These cause secondary sexual development and the attainment of sexual maturity.

After reading this chapter you should be able to:
- Discuss how gender is determined.
- Visualize the embryological development of the male and female reproductive systems.
- Describe the changes that occur in males and females at puberty.

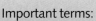

Important terms:
Ectoderm: outer embryological layer that forms the skin and nervous system
Mesoderm: middle embryological layer that forms the reproductive, cardiovascular, and musculoskeletal systems
Endoderm: inner embryological layer that forms the intestines and the germ cells
Mesenchyme: support tissue derived from the mesoderm
Gonads: the ovaries or testes

Embryological development of gender

Genetic determination of gender
The gender of a fetus is determined at conception by the sex chromosome in the sperm that fertilizes the oocyte (chromosome 23, which can be either X or Y). A single gene on the Y chromosome, called the sex-determining region (SRY), is responsible for the male (XY) phenotype. The protein transcribed by this is called testis-determining factor (TDF). The absence of this gene and protein results in a female (XX) phenotype.

Early indifferent development
Gonads
The SRY gene is not activated until the 7th week of gestation. For the first 6 weeks, development is identical in both sexes. The gonads begin to form during the 5th week. Three types of cells form the gonads (Fig. 11.1):
- Mesenchyme, developing support tissue from the mesoderm.
- Mesothelium, a type of mesenchyme that forms the lining of body cavities (e.g., peritoneal lining).
- Primordial germ cells, the developing gamete-producing cells.

The mesothelium and mesenchyme proliferate to form a bulge called the gonadal or genital ridge. This is found at the back of the developing abdominal cavity embedded in the mesonephroi; these are ridges of tissue that act as primitive kidneys until the permanent kidneys develop.

The mesonephroi (singular, mesonephros) are evolutionary remnants of primitive kidneys similar to those found in amphibians. They regress when the permanent kidneys form.

The origins and fates of the cells that form the gonads			
Cells	Origins	Structure at 6 weeks	Adult structure
Mesothelial cells	Mesodermal lining of the peritoneum	Cortex of the gonadal ridge and primary sex cords	Ovarian follicles or seminiferous tubules
Mesenchymal cells	Surrounding mesoderm	Medulla of the gonadal ridge	Leydig cells in the testes, and supporting stroma in the ovaries
Primordial germ cells	Migrate from the endodermal lining of the yolk sac	Primary sex cords	Gamete-producing male spermatogonia and female oocytes

Fig. 11.1 The origins and fates of the cells that form the gonads.

The mesenchyme forms an inner medulla while the mesothelium forms an outer cortex. The cortex has finger-like projections that reach into the medulla; these are called primary sex cords. The primordial germ cells enter the genital ridge and join the primary sex cords. The indifferent gonads are now complete (Fig. 11.2).

Genital ducts
While the indifferent gonads are developing, two genital ducts are formed from the mesoderm (Fig. 11.3):
- Mesonephric (wolffian) duct—this duct drains the urine from the mesonephroi; it forms the male genital ducts (e.g., epididymis, vas deferens).
- Paramesonephric (müllerian) duct—this funnel-ended duct lies proximally to the mesonephric duct; it forms the female genital ducts (e.g., fallopian tubes, uterus).

External genitalia
The external genitalia also begin to develop around the 4th week. Initially, five mesenchymal swellings covered with ectoderm develop round the cloacal membrane; this membrane covers the end of the hindgut and urethra, both of which are endodermal structures. These five swellings are also shown in Fig. 11.4:
- One genital tubercle.
- Two urogenital folds.
- Two labioscrotal folds.

The genital tubercle enlarges to form the phallus. The cloacal membrane divides into two and then ruptures to form:

- Urogenital orifice, although the vagina remains covered by the hymen.
- Anus.

A ligament forms between the indifferent gonad and the labioscrotal swellings through the inguinal canal. It is called the gubernaculum. It guides the descent of the testes into the scrotum and forms the round ligaments of the uterus and ovaries.

Male development
The testes
As the 6th week ends the SRY gene is transcribed and testis-determining factor (TDF) is produced. This factor acts on the mesothelial primary sex cords, which differentiate into the seminiferous cords. These separate from the surrounding mesenchyme to form the seminiferous tubules. The fate of the three cell types in the testes is shown in Fig. 11.2:
- Mesenchyme gives rise to interstitial (Leydig) cells.
- Mesothelium forms Sertoli cells.
- Primordial germ cells form spermatogonia.

The testes enlarge and separate from the mesonephros. They follow the path of the gubernaculum to reach the scrotum via the inguinal canal. The layers of the abdominal wall travel ahead of the testis into the inguinal canal, passing into the scrotum to form the layers of the scrotal wall and spermatic cord. A thin fold of peritoneum also descends; however, its connection with the abdomen (called the processus vaginalis) is lost. The small peritoneal sac remains in the scrotum as the tunica vaginalis. The testes finish their descent around the

Fig. 11.2 The development of the male and female gonads.

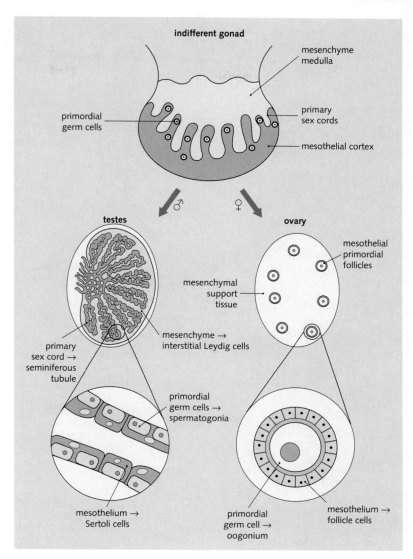

7th month; they retain their abdominal blood vessels and lymphatic drainage. This migration and the formation of the scrotum are shown in Fig. 11.5.

Internal genitalia

The Leydig cells of the testes begin to secrete androgens (e.g., DHT, testosterone) from the 8th week. These androgens stimulate the further development of the wolffian ducts, which differentiate into the:
- Epididymis.
- Ductus deferens.
- Seminal vesicles.
- Ejaculatory ducts.

The Sertoli cells also secrete müllerian inhibiting substance (MIS)—a hormone that causes the müllerian ducts to regress (see Fig. 11.3).

The prostate develops as endodermal outgrowths from the urethra surrounded by mesenchyme.

External genitalia

Testosterone secreted by the Leydig cells is also responsible for the development of the male external genitalia shown in Fig. 11.4:
- Phallus enlarges to form the glans (distal end) of the penis.

111

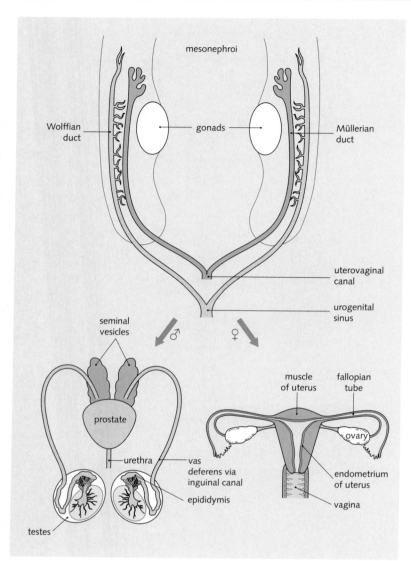

Fig. 11.3 The development of the male and female internal genitalia.

- Urogenital folds fuse ventrally to form the body of the penis.
- Labioscrotal folds fuse to form the scrotum.

All of these structures remain covered in ectoderm that forms the skin covering the penis. A clear ventral line called the scrotal and penile raphe remains from the fusion process. The ectoderm over the glans breaks down to form the foreskin (or prepuce), which remains attached to the glans, preventing retraction of the foreskin until late infancy.

The urethra is an endodermal structure that is enclosed by the urogenital fusion. Failure of this process results in epispadias (see Chapter 13).

 Remember that in the anatomical position the penis is erect and pointing upward. Ventral is underneath and dorsal is on top.

Female development
The ovaries
Female sex is determined by a number of genes on the X chromosome. SRY overrides these genes (e.g., the XXY genotype in Klinefelter syndrome is

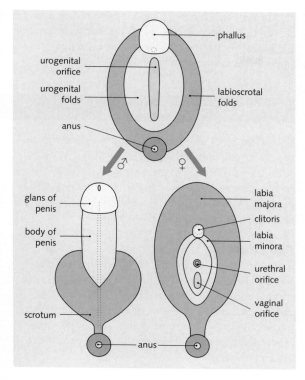

Fig. 11.4 The development of the male and female external genitalia.

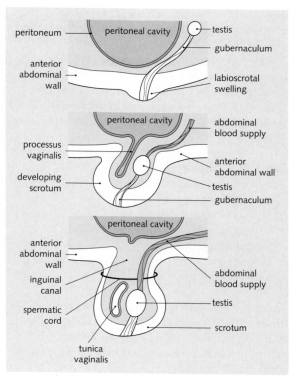

Fig. 11.5 The migration of the testes through the anterior abdominal wall.

phenotypically male). The genes of both X chromosomes are needed for normal female development; therefore, the XO genotype in Turner syndrome usually results in infertility and ovarian degeneration. The signals involved in female development have not been determined.

The mesothelial primary sex cords degenerate and secondary sex cords develop from the mesothelium. The primordial germ cells migrate into these new cords, which then break up to form primordial follicles. The mesenchymal medulla forms the connective tissue stroma that supports these follicles. The primordial germ cells develop into oogonia, which undergo mitotic division to increase the number of germ cells. They enter the first prophase of meiosis before birth, after which further mitosis is not possible; there is no stem cell system equivalent to that found in males. The cells are called oocytes once the meiotic division has begun.

A primordial follicle is composed of:
• A single oocyte from the primordial germ cell.
• A single layer of follicular cells from the mesothelium, which surround the oocyte.

At birth about 750,000 primordial follicles are present; their meiotic division will only be completed many years later (see Fig. 11.2).

The ovaries separate from the mesonephros and become suspended in the pelvis by their mesentery.

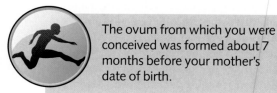

The ovum from which you were conceived was formed about 7 months before your mother's date of birth.

Internal genitalia
The internal genitalia develop due to the absence of testosterone and MIS; the unstimulated wolffian duct regresses, while the müllerian ducts develop. The funnel-shaped end nearest the ovary forms the:
• Fallopian (uterine) tubes.
• Uterine endometrium.

113

The other two layers (including the muscle) of the uterus are formed from surrounding mesenchyme (see Fig. 11.3).

The vaginal epithelium is derived from the endodermal urethra, and the other two layers develop from the surrounding mesenchyme. The hymen is formed from the cloacal membrane covering the urogenital orifice from which the vagina develops.

External genitalia

The external genitalia also develop due to the absence of testosterone (see Fig. 11.4):

- Phallus forms the clitoris.
- Urogenital folds do not fuse completely; they form the labia minora.
- Labioscrotal folds do not fuse completely; they form the labia majora.

The urogenital sinus is formed by the incomplete fusion of these two folds. The vagina and urethra open into this sinus. Skin covers the clitoris, labia majora, and labia minora. There is no breakdown of the skin covering the clitoris (called the prepuce) comparable to the development of the foreskin.

Development of the breast

The mammary glands (breasts) develop from apocrine sweat glands (i.e., those associated with hair follicles) in the mesenchymal layer directly beneath the skin; this accounts for their very superficial nature. Development is identical in males and females until puberty.

At the 4th week of development, a line of thickened ectoderm (skin) develops from the inguinal region to the axilla; this is called the mammary ridge. In humans, this ridge regresses except in the pectoral region; however, failure of regression can cause extra nipples to form.

In the 6th week, single mammary buds develop as downgrowths into the mammary ridge on either side. Under the influence of placental hormones (e.g., human placental lactogen), they branch to form 15–20 lactiferous ducts. The surrounding mesenchyme develops into the fat and connective tissue of the breast. The functional glandular components of the lactiferous ducts in females are called mammary glands; they develop under the influence of estrogen at puberty.

The nipple is formed by depression of the skin before birth. Shortly after birth the skin surrounding the nipple pit begins to grow, raising the nipple to form the usual shape.

Postnatal development

Soon after birth, the anterior pituitary gland begins to secrete gonadotropins (LH and FSH) at roughly adult levels. Within 2 years, secretion declines rapidly to very low levels that are maintained until puberty. Sexual maturation is halted, and the reproductive organs cease to develop.

Adrenarche

At about 8 years of age, the zona reticularis of the adrenal cortex reaches maturity. It begins to secrete adrenal androgens (see Chapter 4). This event is called adrenarche. These weak androgens contribute to the growth of pubic and axillary hair at puberty, especially in females. They do not cause puberty or the growth spurt.

Puberty

Puberty is the reactivation of gonadotropin (LH and FSH) release after the dormancy of childhood. The age of pubertal onset varies widely among individuals (females, 8–13 years; males, 9–14 years). Puberty is characterized by a number of processes:

- Pubertal growth spurt.
- Development of secondary sexual characteristics.
- Achievement of fertility.
- Psychological and social development.

Gonadarche and the initiation of puberty

From an endocrine perspective, puberty is marked by the onset of pulsatile gonadotropin release from the anterior pituitary gland during the night. Gonadotropins stimulate the production of sex steroids (i.e., testosterone and estrogen) from the gonads; the activation of the gonads is called gonadarche.

The onset of puberty is not fully understood; however, the CNS integrates a number of signals. A reduction in hypothalamic sensitivity to the negative feedback of the sex steroids causes the hypothalamus to secrete higher levels of gonadotropin-releasing

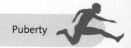

hormone (GnRH) in a pulsatile manner. Secretion of growth hormone (GH), thyroid-stimulating hormone (TSH), and adrenocorticotropic hormone (ACTH) is also increased.

Body weight and puberty

Over the past few decades the onset of puberty has occurred at an increasingly young age. This change is often attributed to improved nutrition and rising body weight. In fact, achieving a body weight of 47 kg (103 lb) is a better predictor of the start of periods than age.

In recent years, a possible mechanism for this effect has been found. The hormone leptin is secreted by adipose tissue, and it is a hormonal indicator of body fat: higher levels of leptin are present with increasing body fat. Puberty cannot begin without leptin, but evidence suggests that it is only one of a number of factors.

The pubertal growth spurt

The earliest developmental event in puberty is an increase in growth velocity called the growth spurt. It occurs about 2 years earlier in females, giving a temporary height advantage. The initial rise in growth velocity is slight; thus growth of the breasts or testes is usually noticed first.

The increase in growth rate is caused by increased GH and sex steroid secretion. Sex steroids also cause bone maturation. As the bones mature, the growing plates (epiphyses) fuse, preventing further growth. This fusion occurs 2 years earlier in females, giving males an extra 2 years of growth. This largely accounts for the increased height of adult males.

Puberty in the male

Puberty usually occurs between 9 and 14 years of age in boys; however, it is considered normal if it occurs between 9 and 16 years of age. Once the testes have developed, male pubertal changes are brought about by the secretion of androgens such as testosterone.

Testes development and early puberty

Growth of the testes is often the first sign of puberty noticed in boys. The increase is mainly due to proliferation of the seminiferous tubules under the influence of FSH. LH stimulates the interstitial Leydig cells to secrete testosterone. The scrotum becomes larger, thicker, and pigmented; pubic hair growth follows.

Spermatogenesis begins once the testes have enlarged and matured. The first ejaculation is often around 13–14 years of age.

Penile development and late puberty

The penis begins to enlarge after the testes at about the same time the growth spurt is noticed. The penis doubles in size during puberty to reach an average size of 9.5 cm (3.7 in.) flaccid or 13.2 cm (5.2 in.) erect.

Facial and axillary hair growth usually starts at about 15 years of age. The sebaceous glands in the skin are also activated, often causing acne.

The breaking of the voice is also a late feature. The larynx, cricothyroid cartilage, and laryngeal muscles enlarge to give an Adam's apple.

Puberty in the female

Puberty usually occurs between 8 and 13 years of age in girls; however, it is considered normal between 8 and 15 years of age. The changes caused by estrogens and progesterone are shown in Fig. 11.6.

Breast development and early puberty

The development of breast buds is often the first sign of puberty noticed in girls. The breast then continues to grow under the influence of estrogen while the ductal system develops (see Fig. 11.6). Pubic hair begins to grow about 6 months later.

The changes caused by estrogen and progesterone during female puberty	
Estrogen-mediated changes	**Progesterone-mediated changes**
Fat deposition and proliferation of the ductal system in the breasts, causing growth	Proliferation of the secretory lobules and acini in the breast
Growth of the vagina and maturation of the epithelium	Contribution to vaginal and uterine growth
Growth of the clitoris	Initiation of cyclical changes in endometrium and ovary

Fig. 11.6 The changes caused by estrogen and progesterone during female puberty.

Menarche and late puberty

The uterus begins to enlarge after the development of pubic hair. The onset of menstruation (periods) is called menarche. The mean age of menarche is 13 years, making it a late feature of puberty. In the ovary, follicular development begins and the first ovulation occurs 10 months after menarche, on average.

The menstrual cycle

The menstrual cycle is regulated by the interactions of a number of hormones. Pituitary FSH stimulates a group of ovarian follicles to develop, and these follicles release estrogen. When estrogen levels reach a threshold, they stimulate a surge of LH from the pituitary gland. This surge causes ovulation and development of the corpus luteum, which secretes progesterone. In the absence of pregnancy, the corpus luteum degenerates resulting in estrogen and progesterone levels falling; this allows FSH secretion to rise restarting the cycle. This sequence of events is described in more detail in Chapter 12. The cycle may take some time to become regular.

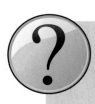

- How is gender determined from a genetic and endocrine perspective?
- Describe the early development of the gonads along with the fate of the three types of cell.
- Describe the two ducts that form the male and female internal genital tracts.
- List the structures formed by these ducts in the male and female.
- Name the five swellings that form the external genitalia.
- What structures do these swellings form in the male and female?
- Describe the development of the breasts, especially the line along which they develop.
- Describe the endocrine changes that characterize puberty.
- What are the changes that occur during male puberty?
- What are the changes that occur during female puberty?

12. The Female Reproductive System

The female reproductive system must perform five main functions:
- Oogenesis and ovulation—production and release of oocytes (female gametes).
- Fertilization—allowing the sperm and oocyte to meet and fuse.
- Pregnancy—providing a suitable environment for the fetus to grow.
- Parturition—expelling the fetus with minimal trauma to the mother and baby.
- Lactation—providing the baby with nutrition.

After menarche (the start of periods) the female body prepares for pregnancy every month until menopause. This process is regulated by four main hormones (Fig. 12.1):
- Follicle-stimulating hormone (FSH).
- Luteinizing hormone (LH).
- Estrogen.
- Progesterone.

These hormones regulate all of the processes described above. In the absence of pregnancy, the hormone levels rise and fall in the same pattern every month. These fluctuations, and the changes they cause, are called the menstrual cycle. Menstrual cycles continue until menopause.

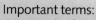

Important terms:
Oocyte: the female gamete that is released at ovulation and fertilized by sperm
Menstruation: vaginal bleeding at the beginning of the menstrual cycle, also called a "period"
Amenorrhea: absence of menstruation
Menorrhagia: excessively heavy periods
Dysplasia: cellular changes that suggest malignancy

After reading this chapter you should be able to:
- Visualize the anatomical structure of the female reproductive system.
- Describe the hormones that regulate the female reproductive system.
- Explain the sequence of events during the menstrual cycle.
- Discuss the common disorders of the female reproductive system.

Organization

The female reproductive system consists of six main components:
- **Ovaries**—produce oocytes and female sex steroids (e.g., estrogens).
- **Fallopian tubes**—connect the ovaries to the uterus; they are the normal site of fertilization.
- **Uterus**—supports the implantation and development of the fetus.
- **Vagina**—normal site for the deposition of sperm.
- **Vulva**—the structures surrounding the introitus (external orifice of the vagina).
- **Breasts**—provide milk for the baby.

The ovaries lie inside the peritoneal cavity while all the other components lie outside; the ovarian ends of the fallopian tubes open into this cavity. The peritoneum covers the uterus and fallopian tubes to form a fold called the broad ligament. Each of these components is discussed individually in the following sections. Their anatomical locations are shown in Fig. 12.2, and their blood supply, lymphatics, and innervation are shown in Fig. 12.3.

Ovaries

The ovaries are two oval organs that produce oocytes (female gametes) and sex steroid hormones in response to pituitary gonadotropins (LH and FSH). The position of the ovaries is variable, but they usually lie lateral to the uterus, fixed to the posterior

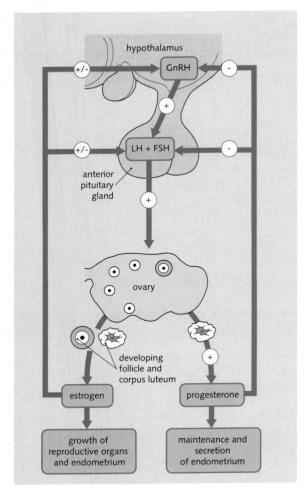

Fig. 12.1 Hormonal regulation of the female reproductive system. (FSH, follicle-stimulating hormone; GnRH, gonadotropin-releasing hormone; LH, luteinizing hormone.)

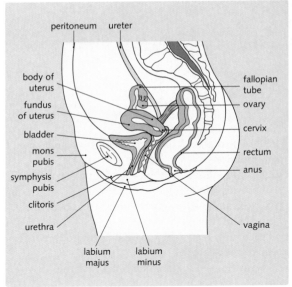

Fig. 12.2 Sagittal section of the female pelvis showing the locations of the reproductive organs.

of the broad ligament. The opening of the fallopian tubes (infundibulum) lies laterally to the ovaries, allowing oocytes to enter the infundibulum at ovulation.

The ovaries are held on the surface of the broad ligament by a fold of peritoneum called the mesovarium, which is continuous with the germinal epithelium that forms their outer surface. Ovarian nerves, arteries, and veins enter the hilum of the ovary from the mesovarium. The relationship of the ovaries to the uterus, fallopian tubes, and ligaments is shown in Fig. 12.4.

Two peritoneal ligaments attach to the ovary:

- Suspensory ligament of the ovary—from the mesovarium to the pelvic wall; it contains the blood vessels and nerves.
- Round ligament of the ovary—from the ovary to the fundus (top) of the uterus; it is a remnant of the upper section of the gubernaculum.

Microstructure

The ovary has three components (Fig. 12.5):

- Surface—simple cuboidal epithelium called the germinal epithelium.
- Cortex—composed of connective tissue stroma supporting thousands of follicles. Every month a group of preovulatory primary follicles begin to enlarge and synthesize steroid hormones. One of these follicles will eventually ovulate and form a postovulatory corpus luteum whilst the others will regress. Therefore, the cortex supports preovulatory, postovulatory, and degenerating follicles.
- Medulla—composed of supporting stroma; it contains a rich network of vessels and nerves that enter the ovary from the mesovarium.

The fallopian (uterine) tubes

The fallopian tubes are two J-shaped tubes lying in the upper border of the broad ligament. The tubes

Blood supply, lymphatics, and innervation of the female reproductive organs				
Organ	Arterial supply	Venous drainage	Innervation	Lymphatic drainage
Ovaries	The ovarian arteries from the aorta via the suspensory ligaments	Forms the pampiniform plexus that drains into the ovarian veins in the suspensory ligaments	Autonomic nerves via the suspensory ligaments	Paraaortic lymph nodes
Fallopian tubes	Uterine and ovarian arteries	Uterine and ovarian veins	From the uterovaginal plexus and suspensory ligaments	Iliac, sacral, and aortic lymph nodes
Uterus	Uterine arteries, branches of the internal iliac arteries	Forms a plexus in the broad ligament that drains into the uterine veins	Uterovaginal plexus in the broad ligament	Iliac, sacral, aortic (and inguinal) lymph nodes
Vagina	Uterine arteries from the internal iliac arteries	Vaginal venous plexus that drains into the internal iliac veins	Uterovaginal plexus in the broad ligament	Iliac and superficial inguinal lymph nodes
External genitalia	Pudendal arteries	Pudendal veins	Pudendal and ilioinguinal nerves, S2–S4	Superficial inguinal lymph nodes
Breasts	Internal thoracic, lateral thoracic, and intercostal arteries	Axillary and internal thoracic veins	Intercostal nerves, mainly T4	Axillary and parasternal lymph nodes and the contralateral breast

Fig. 12.3 Blood supply, lymphatics, and innervation of the female reproductive organs.

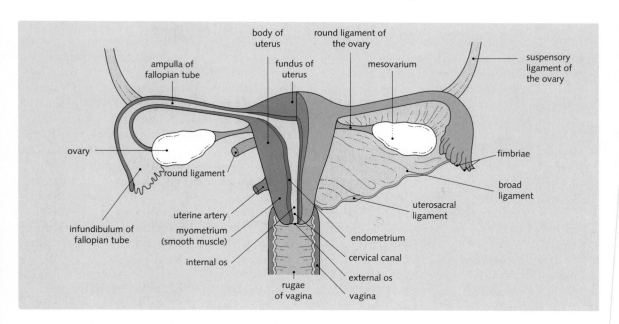

Fig. 12.4 Structure of the ovaries, fallopian tubes, and uterus.

extend from their opening into the peritoneal cavity near the ovaries to the fundus (top) of the uterus, where they open into the uterine cavity. As a result, there is a connection between the peritoneal cavity and the external reproductive tract. Infection can travel up this route, although the cervix acts as a barrier. The fallopian tubes are described in four parts, from lateral to medial:

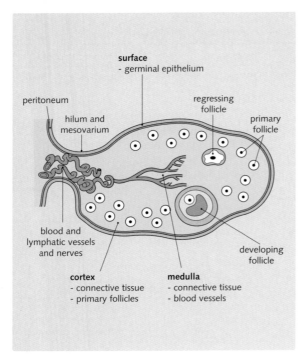

Fig. 12.5 Microstructure of an ovary.

At ovulation the oocyte briefly enters the peritoneal cavity by breaking through the germinal epithelium. The opening of the fallopian tubes is in this cavity, so that there is a direct connection to the outside world via the uterus and vagina.

Uterus and cervix

The uterus is a pear-shaped, muscular organ that can enlarge greatly to accommodate the growing fetus. It is lined by a specialized epithelium called the endometrium. The fallopian tubes join superiorly, and the vagina is inferior. These relationships are shown in Fig. 12.4.

The uterus is described in three sections:
- Fundus—above the entry point of the fallopian tubes.
- Body—the usual site of implantation.
- Cervix—the lower third, which links the uterus and vagina.

The cylindrical cervix is structurally and functionally distinct from the rest of the uterus. The junction of the cervix with the body is called the internal os and that with the vagina, the external os. The passage between these two junctions is called the endocervical canal. The ureters pass 1 cm lateral to the internal os on either side; this relationship is important when considering cervical carcinoma. The external os can be visualized in the conscious patient using a speculum, and the surrounding cells are sampled in a smear test.

The cervix and all structures superior are sterile areas. This sterility is maintained by the frequent shedding of the endometrium, thick cervical mucus, and the narrow external os of the cervix.

Support and ligaments of the uterus

A number of structures hold the uterus in position and prevent prolapse into the vagina. The main support is derived from the pelvic floor formed by the levator ani, coccygeus, and pubococcygeus muscles. The other structures are called "ligaments," although most of them are not actually ligaments. The functions, relations, and locations of these structures are common exam questions:

- Infundibulum—the funnel-shaped opening of the tube that is closely related to the ovary; it collects the oocytes from the surface of the ovary using ciliated, finger-like fimbriae.
- Ampulla—the widest section is where fertilization normally occurs.
- Isthmus—connects the ampulla to the uterus.
- Uterine section—the section as the tube penetrates the uterine muscle.

The fallopian tubes are lined by ciliated and secretory cells that waft the oocyte toward the uterus and supply it with nutrients. Two layers of spiral muscle surround this lining and help move the oocyte and sperm by peristalsis. These muscles are sensitive to sex steroids (e.g., estrogen) so that motility is most rapid when sex steroid levels are highest. The "morning-after pill" uses estrogen to increase this motility so that the oocyte is ejected before the uterus is ready for implantation, thus preventing pregnancy. If motility is slow there is a risk of ectopic pregnancy in which implantation occurs in the fallopian tube. The relationship of the fallopian tubes to the uterus, ovaries, and broad ligament is shown in Fig. 12.4.

- Broad ligament—a double layer of peritoneum that surrounds the uterus with the fallopian tubes, forming its superior border. It does not support the uterus.
- Round ligament—from the uterus body (anteroinferiorly to the insertion point of the fallopian tubes) to the labia majora through the inguinal canal. It is the remnant of the lower sections of the gubernaculum. It holds the uterus in an anteverted position. (The fundus lies superior and anterior to the cervix.)
- Uterosacral ligaments—from the cervix either side of the rectum to the piriformis muscle over the sacrum; these structures support the uterus.
- Transverse cervical (cardinal) ligaments—from the cervix and superior vagina to the lateral pelvic walls; these structures support the uterus.
- Pubocervical ligaments—from the cervix to the pubis bone; they do not support the uterus.

Microstructure of the uterus

The body and fundus are composed of three tissue layers (Fig. 12.6):

- Serosa—the peritoneal covering.
- Myometrium—the thick smooth muscle layer; it is sensitive to hormones (e.g., oxytocin).
- Endometrium—the inner lining of the uterus that varies through the menstrual cycle; it is sensitive to hormones (e.g., estrogen and progesterone).

The endometrium is further divided into two layers:
- Deep basal layer—this changes little through the menstrual cycle and is not shed at menstruation.
- Superficial functional layer—a hormone-sensitive layer that proliferates in response to estrogen and becomes secretory in response to progesterone; it is shed at the end of the menstrual cycle and regenerates from cells in the basal layer.

The arterioles of the superficial endometrial layer lie alongside the glands of the endometrium. They have a characteristic spiral appearance. As progesterone levels fall at the end of the menstrual cycle they respond by constriction. The superficial layer becomes ischemic and undergoes necrosis; this causes the shedding and hemorrhage of menstruation.

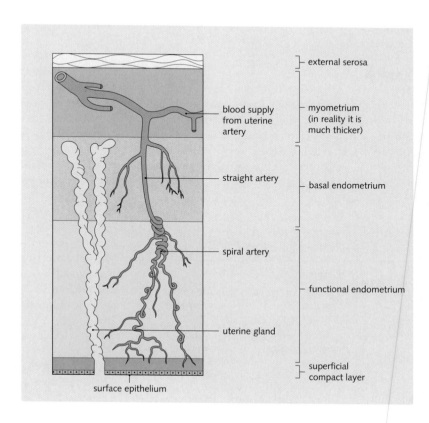

Fig. 12.6 Microstructure of the uterus.

external serosa

myometrium (in reality it is much thicker)

blood supply from uterine artery

straight artery

basal endometrium

spiral artery

functional endometrium

uterine gland

superficial compact layer

surface epithelium

Microstructure of the cervix

The cervix consists mainly of collagen and small amounts of smooth muscle. The columnar epithelium lining the endocervical canal secretes mucus that changes in consistency during the menstrual cycle. Estrogen promotes a watery mucus that allows sperm to pass. Progesterone causes the production of a viscous mucus that is hostile to sperm.

The cervix is divided into two sections:
- Endocervix—superior, related to the uterus body.
- Ectocervix—inferior, related to the vagina.

The anatomical definition of this division is different from the histological definition (Fig. 12.7). The anatomical division is generally located superiorly to the histological division.

During puberty, high estrogen levels cause the columnar epithelium of the cervix to extend beyond the external os into the vagina; this is called cervical ectopy. The acidic vaginal pH induces squamous metaplasia (changing to squamous epithelium) of the columnar epithelium. The cells that change are within an area called the transformation zone, and they are susceptible to dysplasia (precancerous changes). Cervical smears take samples of these cells to detect early signs of dysplasia allowing curative treatment.

Vagina

The vagina is a 9 cm long muscular tube that runs upward and backward from the external genitalia (vulva) to the cervix. The urethra and bladder are anterior and the rectum posterior. In most women the cervix is inserted into the anterior wall of the vagina at an angle of 90°; this is called the anteverted position of the uterus.

Comparison of the endocervix and ectocervix		
	Endocervix	**Ectocervix**
Anatomy	Above the internal os; covered by peritoneum anteriorly	Below the internal os; not covered by peritoneum anteriorly
Histology	Columnar endometrial epithelium; does not menstruate	Stratified squamous vaginal epithelium; does not menstruate

Fig. 12.7 Comparison of the endocervix and ectocervix.

The cervix projects into the vagina creating a small dome with the external os at the center. The vaginal lumen around the cervix is divided into anterior, posterior, and two lateral fornices. The posterior fornix is the deepest and is covered by peritoneum on its internal surface. This is an important relationship since an object that penetrates this area (e.g., during a "backstreet" abortion) will enter the abdominal cavity, potentially causing an infection.

The word *vagina* is Latin for "scabbard."

Microstructure

The structure of the vaginal wall allows expansion during intercourse and childbirth. The wall of the vagina is composed of four layers:
- Stratified squamous epithelial lining for protection.
- Elastic lamina propria.
- Fibromuscular layer (two layers of smooth muscle).
- Fibroelastic adventitia.

The wall contains few sensory fibres and no glands; the lining epithelium is lubricated by cervical mucus. During sexual arousal the vagina is further lubricated by the secretions from Bartholin's glands next to the introitus (external vaginal orifice) and the transudation of fluid across the vaginal epithelium.

Unlike the cervix, uterus, and fallopian tubes, the vagina is a nonsterile area; the main organisms present are the commensal *Lactobacillus vaginalis*. After puberty, estrogen stimulates the cells of the vaginal epithelium to secrete glycogen. The lactobacilli digest this glycogen to release lactic acid and thus lower the pH of the vagina below 4.5; this prevents infection by other organisms. Other commensal organisms present include *Candida* and *Escherichia coli*. As in the gastrointestinal tract, antibiotics can disrupt the flora to cause overgrowth and infections such as candidiasis (thrush). Low estrogen levels can also result in infection.

External genitalia (vulva)

The appearance of the vulva is shown in Fig. 12.8. The introitus or external vaginal orifice opens into

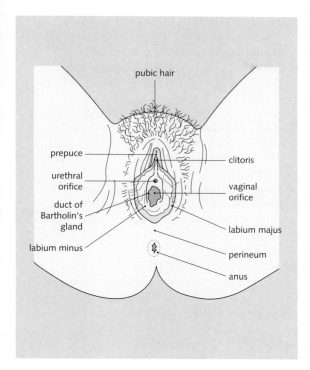

Fig. 12.8 Structure of the vulva.

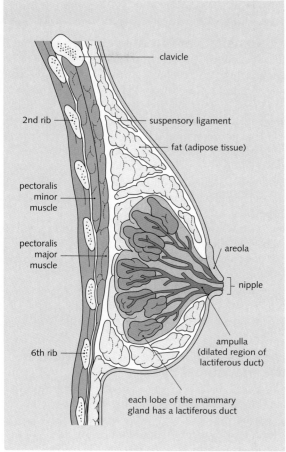

Fig. 12.9 Internal structure of the breast.

the vestibule, which is the area between the labia. The short urethra opens anterior to the introitus within the vestibule. The labia minora are two hairless folds of skin that surround the vestibule; they fuse anterior to the urethral opening to form the prepuce (hood) of the clitoris. Beneath the prepuce lies the clitoris; this is composed of two erectile corpora cavernosa that become engorged with blood upon sexual stimulation.

The labia minora lie within two larger, hair-bearing skin folds called the labia majora; the labia majora fuse posteriorly and extend anteriorly to the mons pubis. The mons pubis is a fat pad covered in pubic hair at the anterior of the vulva.

Two pairs of small glands are located either side of the introitus called the vestibular and Bartholin's glands. During sexual arousal they secrete a lubricating mucus into the vestibule via small ducts.

Female breasts (mammary glands)

The breasts lie in the superficial fascia over the pectoral muscles on the anterior of the chest. They are very superficial structures composed largely of fat; the size and shape varies between individuals. They extend toward the axilla and this axillary tail

must be checked on examination. The pigmented skin around the nipple is called the areola. In white-skinned women it permanently changes from pink to brown during pregnancy.

Microstructure

Embedded in the fatty tissue of the breast there are 15–20 independent glandular lobules with openings on the nipple. Each opening is a lactiferous duct that forms a lactiferous sinus beneath the areola. Within the breast, the lactiferous ducts branch extensively to end in secretory acini potentially capable of secreting milk. The ducts and lobules are surrounded by myoepithelial cells that contract in response to oxytocin and expel the milk on stimulation of the nipple. The internal structure of the breast is shown in Fig. 12.9.

Oogenesis

Meiosis in the female fetus

Oogenesis is the process by which haploid (23-chromosome) oocytes are formed from diploid (46-chromosome) stem cells called oogonia. This process requires a meiotic division that is begun before birth and ends when the oocyte is fertilized.

Oogonia are ovarian stem cells derived from the primordial germ cells in the yolk sac (see Chapter 11); initially they divide by mitosis to increase their numbers. In the second trimester of pregnancy all the oogonia develop into primary oocytes and enter the prophase of the first meiotic division. The meiotic division is arrested at this stage until menarche. Since no oogonia remain, further mitotic divisions to increase the number of oocytes are not possible.

A single layer of flat granulosa cells surrounds each primary oocyte to form a primordial follicle. The follicles are located within the ovarian cortex.

Meiosis and follicle development in the menstrual cycle

The primordial follicles and primary oocytes remain unchanged until puberty and menarche. Once the menstrual cycle has become established, FSH secretion stimulates the development of a selection of primordial follicles each month. The chosen follicles go through the following stages (see Fig. 12.13):

- Unilaminar primary follicle—the primary oocyte and a single layer of granulosa cells enlarge in size.
- Multilaminar primary follicle—the granulosa cells divide to form layers, and the zona pellucida (glycoprotein shell) forms around the primary oocyte.
- Secondary follicle—the surrounding ovarian cortex forms the secretory theca interna and theca externa.
- Graafian (tertiary) follicle—a fluid-filled cavity called the antrum develops within the granulosa cell layer.

Once the Graafian follicle has matured, the primary oocyte completes the first meiotic division under the influence of LH. Unlike most cell divisions this process produces two cells of differing size and function:

- Secondary oocyte—the mature haploid oocyte that is capable of fertilization; it has the majority of the cytoplasm and organelles.
- First polar body—a small haploid cell that degenerates; it has virtually no cytoplasm.

The secondary oocyte begins the second meiotic division immediately; however, it is arrested at metaphase II until fertilization.

The secondary oocyte is released at ovulation surrounded by two layers:
- Zona pellucida—the glycoprotein layer.
- Corona radiata (also called the cumulus oophorus)—a covering of granulosa cells from the follicle.

Meiosis at fertilization

The second meiotic division is not completed unless the secondary oocyte is fertilized. The calcium influx caused by the fusion of the sperm and secondary oocyte stimulates the completion of this division. Two haploid cells are produced:

- Female pronucleus—the functional gamete; it has the majority of the cytoplasm and fuses with the male pronucleus (see Chapter 14).
- Second polar body—another small haploid cell that degenerates; it has virtually no cytoplasm.

Hormones

Ovarian sex steroids

The ovaries produce a number of steroid hormones in response to gonadotropins from the anterior pituitary. The main hormones produced are:
- Estrogens (e.g., estradiol).
- Progestogens (e.g., progesterone).
- Androgens (e.g., androstenedione).

Estrogens

Estrogens are secreted at the start of the menstrual cycle in response to LH and FSH. Their synthesis takes place in the developing ovarian follicle, requiring both the thecal and granulosa cells. The theca interna secretes androgens in response to LH. LH activates the enzyme that converts cholesterol to pregnenolone (i.e., the first step in steroid production); however, the thecal cells lack the aromatase enzyme necessary to convert androgens to estrogens.

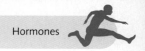

Fig. 12.10 Synthesis of estrogens by the developing follicle. (FSH, follicle-stimulating hormone; LH, luteinizing hormone.)

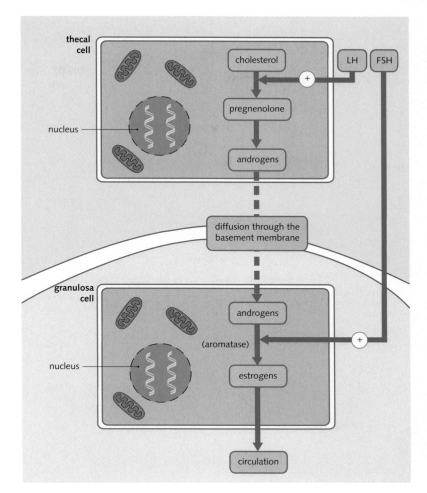

The majority of androgens cross the basement membrane into the granulosa cells. FSH activates the aromatase enzyme produced by the granulosa cells allowing the thecal androgens to be converted to estrogens (mainly estradiol-17β). The process of estrogen synthesis is shown in Fig. 12.10. After ovulation, estrogens are produced by the corpus luteum formed from the follicle.

Estrogens are transported in the blood bound to sex hormone-binding globulin (SHBG) and albumin. They act via intracellular receptors in the target cells. Estrogens act on the anterior pituitary and hypothalamus to provide feedback (usually inhibition), which regulates the system. The actions of estrogens are shown in Fig. 12.11. The main actions are:

- Development of the reproductive organs and secondary sexual characteristics.
- Proliferation of the functional layer of uterus endometrium.

Progestogens

Progesterone is secreted in the second half of the menstrual cycle by the corpus luteum. This structure is formed by the transformation of the granulosa cells in the follicle after ovulation; LH maintains the secretory activity of these cells. The main progestogen is progesterone, which is synthesized from cholesterol in just two steps. During pregnancy, progesterone production is taken over by the placenta.

Progesterone is transported in the blood bound to corticosteroid-binding globulin (CBG) and albumin. It acts via intracellular receptors in the target cells. Progesterone acts on the anterior pituitary and the hypothalamus to provide negative feedback. The

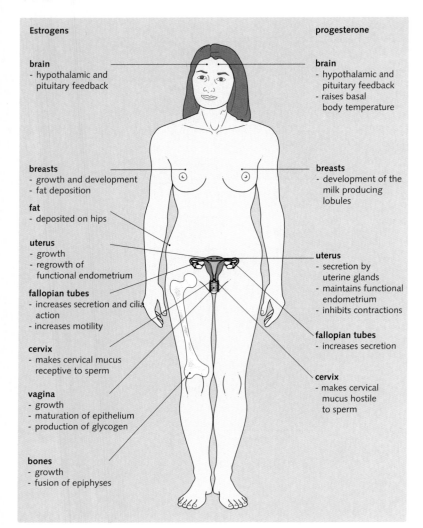

Fig. 12.11 Actions of estrogens and progesterone.

Estrogens

brain
- hypothalamic and pituitary feedback

breasts
- growth and development
- fat deposition

fat
- deposited on hips

uterus
- growth
- regrowth of functional endometrium

fallopian tubes
- increases secretion and cilia action
- increases motility

cervix
- makes cervical mucus receptive to sperm

vagina
- growth
- maturation of epithelium
- production of glycogen

bones
- growth
- fusion of epiphyses

progesterone

brain
- hypothalamic and pituitary feedback
- raises basal body temperature

breasts
- development of the milk producing lobules

uterus
- secretion by uterine glands
- maintains functional endometrium
- inhibits contractions

fallopian tubes
- increases secretion

cervix
- makes cervical mucus hostile to sperm

actions of progesterone are shown in Fig. 12.11. Its main actions are:
- Maintenance of the uterine endometrium.
- Stimulation of uterine secretions.

Androgens
The androgens are precursors of estrogens; however, small quantities are released systemically. They act with adrenal androgen to promote pubic and axillary hair growth during puberty.

Control of ovarian steroid production
Ovarian steroids are regulated in a similar manner to many other major hormones (as shown in Fig. 12.1). Gonadotropin-releasing hormone (GnRH) is

synthesized by the hypothalamus and transported to the anterior pituitary gland in the portal veins. Here, it acts on gonadotroph cells to stimulate the release of gonadotropins (i.e., LH and FSH). This process is described in more detail in Chapter 2.

Gonadotropins in the blood reach the ovaries and stimulate the release of the ovarian sex steroids. Both LH and FSH stimulate enzymes involved in estrogen synthesis. LH also allows the formation and maintenance of the corpus luteum which synthesizes progesterone.

Estrogens and progesterone feed back to the anterior hypothalamus to regulate their release. This feedback is usually inhibitory and it prevents excess secretion. Before ovulation the feedback becomes positive triggering the surge in LH and FSH release that causes ovulation.

Other ovarian hormones

Inhibin and activin

Inhibin and activin are polypeptide hormones secreted by the granulosa cells of the ovarian follicles. Inhibin stimulates androgen synthesis but inhibits conversion to estrogens while activin inhibits androgen production but stimulates conversion to estrogens. Together they regulate local sex steroid levels and the balance between estrogens and androgens.

Relaxin

This is a polypeptide hormone secreted by the corpus luteum and placenta. It prepares the body for childbirth by causing cervical softening and relaxation of pelvic ligaments.

The menstrual cycle

The menstrual cycle is the process by which the female prepares for possible fertilization of the oocyte. The cycle lasts 28–32 days and begins on the first day of menstruation (also called a "period"). A number of changes occur in the ovaries and endometrium; these are regulated by hormones. The hormonal, ovarian, and endometrial changes are shown in Fig. 12.12.

The cycle is divided into two stages, each lasting about 14 days. Between these stages (about the 14th day) ovulation occurs.

The first half of the cycle

The first half of the cycle begins on the first day of menstruation and lasts until ovulation. The length of 14 days is variable; if a woman has a long cycle it is the first stage that is prolonged.

Ovarian changes

This stage of the cycle is called the follicular stage in the ovary.

During menstruation LH and FSH levels rise. As its name implies, FSH stimulates several primary follicles to mature into secondary follicles. This involves proliferation of the granulosa cells while stromal cells surrounding the follicle line up to form thecal cells. These two components allow estrogen production to begin and for the next 12 days estrogen levels rise exponentially.

A few days later, fluid begins to collect between the granulosa cells forming a cavity called the antrum. The follicle is now called a tertiary or antral follicle. The estrogens stimulate synthesis of FSH and LH receptors in the granulosa cells and growth accelerates. The estrogens also have a negative feedback effect on the pituitary gland to cause a drop in FSH and LH levels. Usually only one follicle will maintain growth as the levels of FSH fall. The other follicles regress (a process called atresia).

Further growth results in the formation of a mature Graafian follicle with a diameter of about 2.5 cm just before ovulation. The development of a follicle is shown in Fig. 12.13. Follicles are composed of seven layers; from the inside out they are as follows:

- Oocyte—the female gamete, arrested in first meiotic prophase.
- Zona pellucida—a glycoprotein layer that surrounds the oocyte like an eggshell.
- Granulosa cells—cuboidal cells surrounding the oocyte; they secrete estrogens.
- Antrum—fluid-filled cavity within the granulosa cells.
- Basement membrane/lamina.
- Theca interna—a layer of stromal cells that secrete androgens.
- Theca externa—a nonsecretory stromal cell layer.

Oral contraceptives: Administration of synthetic estrogen and/or progesterone through the first half of the menstrual cycle prevents FSH secretion. This prevents follicular growth so that ovulation cannot occur.

Endometrial changes

The first half of the cycle is separated into two phases:

- Menstrual phase.
- Proliferative phase.

During the menstrual phase (days 1–4) the ischemic and necrotic functional layer of the endometrium is lost. This dead tissue passes out of the vagina, along with blood from the degenerating spiral arteries.

The proliferative phase (days 4–13) is caused by the rising estrogen levels. These stimulate cells in the

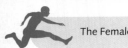

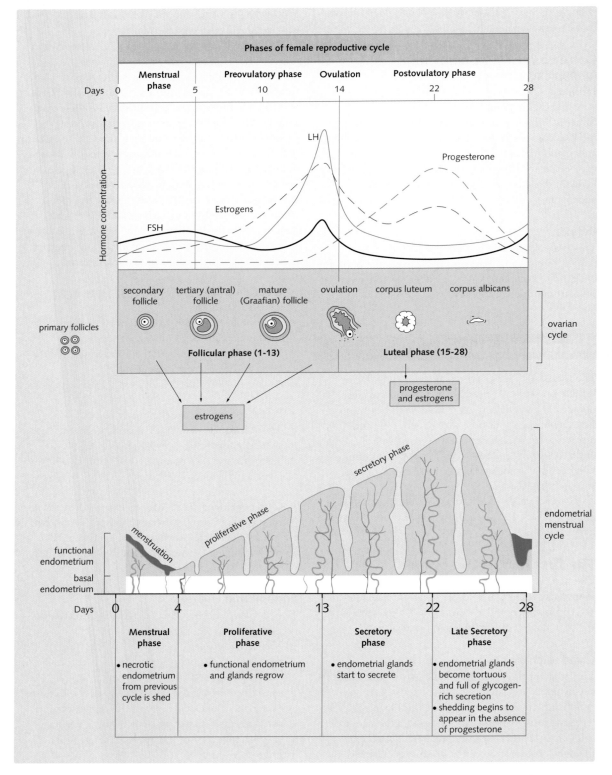

Fig. 12.12 The hormonal, ovarian, and endometrial changes during the menstrual cycle. (FSH, follicle-stimulating hormone; LH, luteinizing hormone.)

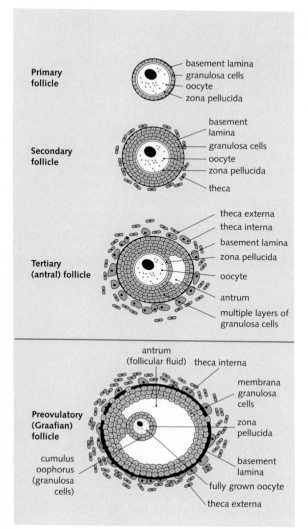

Primary follicle
- basement lamina
- granulosa cells
- oocyte
- zona pellucida

Secondary follicle
- basement lamina
- granulosa cells
- oocyte
- zona pellucida
- theca

Tertiary (antral) follicle
- theca externa
- theca interna
- basement lamina
- zona pellucida
- oocyte
- antrum
- multiple layers of granulosa cells

Preovulatory (Graafian) follicle
- antrum (follicular fluid)
- theca interna
- membrana granulosa cells
- zona pellucida
- basement lamina
- fully grown oocyte
- theca externa
- cumulus oophorus (granulosa cells)

Fig. 12.13 Development of an ovarian follicle through the follicular phase of the menstrual cycle.

basal layer of the endometrium to proliferate and form a new functional layer. Glands are formed in this layer but they are not yet active.

The rising estrogen also stimulates secretion of a clear, watery cervical mucus that facilitates sperm transport across the cervix. At other times the mucus is scant and thick.

Oral contraceptives: Administration of progesterone through the first half of the cycle causes the cervical mucus to remain thick. This forms a barrier that prevents the passage of sperm.

Ovulation
At the end of the follicular stage, the mature Graafian follicle secretes such large quantities of estrogen that the feedback on the pituitary gland changes. The feedback turns from negative to positive and the very high estrogen levels cause a dramatic surge in the release of LH and FSH. LH causes the Graafian follicle to rupture through the germinal epithelium—a process called ovulation. The oocyte and its first polar body are released into the peritoneal cavity; they are surrounded by the zona pellucida and a few granulosa cells. The ovulated oocyte is swept into the fallopian tubes by the wafting action of the cilia of the fimbriae.

Oral contraceptives: Administration of estrogen and/or progesterone through the first half of the menstrual cycle can prevent the preovulatory surge of LH that stimulates ovulation.

The second half of the cycle
The second half of the cycle is the time between ovulation and menstruation; the average length is 14 days and this remains constant despite changes in cycle length. The length is determined by the lifespan of the corpus luteum (about 10 days).

Ovarian changes
This stage of the cycle is called the luteal stage in the ovary.

The LH surge continues to act on the granulosa and theca cells in the empty follicle once ovulation has occurred. The cells divide and become yellow. They are now called lutein cells (*luteus* means yellow, hence the name luteinizing hormone), and the ruptured follicle is called the corpus luteum.

Over the next 10 days these cells secrete high levels of progesterone and estrogens, but they then spontaneously involute (shrink) and lose their secretory ability.

The progesterone and estrogen secreted by the corpus luteum inhibit LH and FSH release from the pituitary gland. The falling LH levels fail to maintain the corpus luteum so it undergoes involution. As a result progesterone and estrogen levels fall dramatically so their negative feedback to the pituitary gland is lost. FSH and LH secretion rise causing ovarian follicles to grow, thus starting the next cycle.

Oral contraceptives: The use of estrogen and/or progesterone in oral contraceptives aims to mimic the early stages of the second half of the menstrual cycle.

Endometrial changes

After ovulation the progesterone secretion by the corpus luteum activates the endometrium. A number of changes occur:

- Nutrients are stored in the cells.
- Glands become tortuous (irregular-shaped) in preparation for secretion.

About 5 days after ovulation, the glands begin to secrete a glycogen-rich "milk" in preparation for a potential embryo; as a result, the changes to the endometrium during the second half of the menstrual cycle are called the secretory phase.

As progesterone and estrogen levels fall, the spiral arteries supplying the functional endometrium begin to coil and constrict causing ischemia and necrosis. Blood leaks from the damaged vessels into the endometrium before the whole functional endometrium is shed. Menstruation occurs and this marks the first day of the next cycle.

Disorders of the ovaries and fallopian tubes

Pelvic inflammatory disease

Inflammation of the ovaries, fallopian tubes, or uterus is called pelvic inflammatory disease (PID), whereas inflammation specific to the fallopian tubes is called salpingitis. PID can run an acute or chronic course and it is usually caused by the following organisms:

- Sexually transmitted diseases ascending from the vagina (e.g., *Chlamydia trachomatis* [60% of all PID] and *Neisseria gonorrhoeae* [30%].
- Direct infection following childbirth, surgery, or the insertion of a coil.
- Infection from adjacent organs (e.g., from appendicitis).
- Blood-borne infection (e.g., tuberculosis).

These last three infections are usually caused by staphylococci, streptococci, *E. coli*, or anaerobes. Together they account for only 10% of PID.

Acute pelvic inflammatory disease

In acute PID the lining of the internal genital tract becomes inflamed and swollen; excess mucus is secreted along with a fibrinous exudate (pus). Acute PID can be asymptomatic, but moderate infection causes the following symptoms:

- Severely painful and tender lower abdomen.
- Fever, often with rigors.
- Vaginal discharge.
- Painful intercourse (dyspareunia).

On examination there is often abdominal guarding and vaginal examination will cause extreme pain. Acute PID must be treated with antibiotics since failure of treatment causes damage to the fallopian tubes in 10% of cases. Recurrent asymptomatic infection with *Chlamydia trachomatis* can also cause damage and potential infertility.

Chronic pelvic inflammatory disease

A failure to treat acute PID can also result in chronic PID. The fallopian tubes can become sealed by the pus resulting in the following complications:

- Hydrosalpinx—severe swelling due to outflow obstruction.
- Pyosalpinx—an abscess develops in the fallopian tube and adhesions form to surrounding structures, especially the ovaries.
- Infertility.

The patient may complain of menorrhagia and intermittent pelvic pain, often worse before menstruation. On vaginal examination, a tender swelling may be felt and further investigation by laparoscopy may be needed. It is usually treated by surgical removal of the affected organs, especially the fallopian tubes.

Polycystic ovarian syndrome

Polycystic ovarian syndrome (PCOS) is a common but very complicated disease characterized by several endocrine abnormalities and multiple cysts in the ovaries. The "cysts" are actually multiple immature follicles that develop in the ovaries and are visible on ultrasound examination. Twenty per cent of women have polycystic ovaries (PCO); however, only a fraction develop symptoms. The symptoms are caused by endocrine abnormalities, of which the most important are:

- Excess of LH and deficiency of FSH secretion from the anterior pituitary.
- High insulin levels and insulin resistance, though this is linked to weight gain.
- Excess testosterone.

These endocrine abnormalities cause the following symptoms:

- Amenorrhea or oligomenorrhea (no or infrequent periods) with infertility.
- Hirsutism (male pattern hair growth).
- Acne.
- Weight gain.

PCOS is diagnosed from the history, ultrasound examination, and raised LH:FSH ratio. The syndrome is linked to obesity and the best treatment is weight loss. Further treatment is aimed at treating the symptoms:

- Infertility is treated by raising pituitary FSH secretion, often by using the antiestrogen clomiphene.
- Insulin resistance can be treated by the diabetic medication metformin, and this may also help reduce infertility.
- Antiandrogen drugs are given with a combined oral contraceptive pill to improve the hirsutism, though cosmetic treatment is often better.
- In severe cases, destruction of the follicles by laparoscopic ovarian "drilling" will relieve symptoms for about a year.

Benign ovarian tumors and cysts

Benign ovarian masses are common during the reproductive years; however, it is often impossible to distinguish them from malignant ovarian masses from the history and examination alone. Cysts develop in the ovary during the normal menstrual cycle (i.e., the follicle and corpus luteum). These cysts reach 2–2.5 cm in diameter, at which stage they are visible on transvaginal ultrasound examination but usually impalpable on pelvic examination. They should regress within 1 month. Persistent, large, or abnormal cysts merit further investigation.

There are many types of ovarian masses, which can make this topic difficult to remember. The masses described in the next section are arranged according to the part of the ovary from which they derive (Fig. 12.14). These masses are usually benign; however, many have the potential to become malignant.

Benign masses derived from the follicles

Abnormal development of the ovarian follicles can result in functional ovarian cysts that secrete hormones; they are not neoplastic. They are larger than normal follicles but normally shrink without treatment. They are the most common cause of ovarian masses during the reproductive years. There are two types:

- Follicular cysts—an unruptured and persistent follicle that secretes estrogen often causing menorrhagia (heavy periods).
- Luteal cysts—a persistent corpus luteum secreting progesterone causing irregular bleeding and severe premenstual syndrome (PMS).

Benign masses derived from the epithelium
Cystadenomas

These are benign tumors of the ovarian epithelium that secrete fluid to form a cyst; they can grow to

Common types of ovarian neoplasia			
Tumor origin	Name	Frequency	Description
Epithelial cell	Serous cystadenoma	30%	Benign, clear–fluid-filled cyst
	Serous cystadenocarcinoma	5%	Malignant, clear-fluid-filled cyst
	Mucinous cystadenoma	10%	Benign, mucin-filled cyst
	Mucinous cystadenocarcinoma	0.5%	Malignant, mucin-filled cyst
	Endometrioid	8%	Benign, solid and brown
Germ cell	Benign teratomas	20%	Benign cyst with several tissue types
	Immature teratomas	0.1%	Malignant cyst with several tissue types

Fig. 12.14 Common types of ovarian neoplasia.

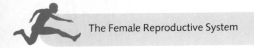
massive sizes. They are the most common cause of neoplasia during the reproductive years. There are two types:

- Serous—secretes a thin, watery substance.
- Mucinous—secretes protein-rich fluid called mucin.

Endometriotic cysts

Endometriosis (see p. 134) can result in functional endometrial tissue being deposited on the ovaries. This tissue is stimulated by the hormonal changes of the menstrual cycle, which results in periodic bleeding. With time the blood becomes dark brown and thick; these cysts are therefore called chocolate cysts.

Brenner tumors

These are very rare, benign, and solid tumors that resemble the transitional epithelium of the urinary tract. They are a type of fibroma.

Benign masses derived from the germ cells
Benign cystic teratomas

These tumors (also called dermoid cysts) are a common type of ovarian tumor. The tumor is composed of cells from at least two germ layers (i.e., ectoderm, mesoderm, and endoderm); they are often lined by skin with hairs and sebaceous glands. Other recognizable structures and tissues may be present (e.g., teeth, bone, muscle, and neural tissue). The teratoma is benign if the tissues are mature.

Struma ovarii

These are very rare types of benign cystic teratoma composed mainly of thyroid tissue; they may present with hyperthyroidism.

Benign masses derived from the stroma

Malignant tumors in the ovarian stroma are exceedingly rare; however, the stromal mesenchyme of the ovarian cortex and medulla can become neoplastic. These rare benign tumors are often associated with hormone production:

- Thecomas—develop from the thecal cells; they often secrete estrogens causing endometrial hyperplasia and a higher risk of endometrial carcinoma.
- Granulosa cell tumors—develop from the granulosa cells; like thecoma, they often secrete estrogens with similar effects.
- Androblastoma—the tumor resembles testicular cells (e.g., Sertoli and Leydig cells); they secrete androgens.

- Fibromas—solid, white tumor made of fibrous tissue.

Malignant ovarian disease

Ovarian carcinoma is a relatively rare form of carcinoma, but the 5-year survival is poor because of late detection. It usually affects postmenopausal women. Risk is increased by the BRCA1 gene and low parity (i.e., few children); the contraceptive pill has a protective effect. All large, abnormal, or persistent ovarian masses should be considered malignant until proven otherwise.

As with benign ovarian masses there are many types, and they are described according to their tissue of origin (see Fig. 12.14).

Malignant masses derived from the epithelium
Cystadenocarcinomas

Benign cystadenomas may undergo malignant change to form malignant cystadenocarcinomas. The two types remain:

- Serous—the most common type of ovarian malignancy (about 50%).
- Mucinous—accounts for 10% of ovarian malignancy.

Endometrioid tumors

These are primary tumors that resemble adenocarcinoma of the endometrium. They usually arise spontaneously, though rarely they develop from endometrioid cysts. Uterine adenocarcinoma is sometimes present.

Clear cell tumors

These are a less common type of endometrioid tumor with pale, glycogen-rich cytoplasm that resembles the secretory phase endometrium.

Malignant masses derived from the germ cells
Dysgerminomas

These are the most common malignant germ cell tumor; the cells resemble seminomas found in the male testes. They occur mainly in adolescents and young women; they are highly malignant.

Yolk sac tumors

Derived from the endoderm of the yolk sac, these are highly malignant tumors that secrete α-fetoprotein (AFP), which can be detected in the blood. They occur mainly in adolescents and young women.

Solid teratoma
Teratomas that contain embryonal tissues are highly malignant. They occur mainly in adolescents.

Choriocarcinoma
These are highly malignant tumors that secrete human chorionic gonadotropin (hCG); they are derived from trophoblastic tissue found in teratomas.

Metastatic ovarian tumors
Tumors may metastasize to the ovaries, especially from:
- Endometrium.
- Breast.
- Stomach (Krukenberg tumor).
- Colon.

Diagnosis and treatment of ovarian masses
Symptoms
Ovarian masses are frequently asymptomatic. Pelvic or abdominal pain may occur; large masses can cause noticeable increases in abdominal girth. Advanced malignancy may cause appetite and weight loss, tiredness, and general malaise. Ovarian masses are most commonly detected through pelvic examination or ultrasound scans.

Investigations
The definitive diagnosis of an ovarian mass can only be made from a biopsy taken during laparotomy. Initial investigations aim to determine which masses require surgical exploration. These investigations include:
- Pregnancy test—to eliminate the risk of ectopic pregnancy.
- CA-125—a blood-borne tumor marker.
- Ultrasound scan—determines the location, size, and nature of the mass.

If a malignancy is suspected, further investigations and imaging aim to determine the stage of the carcinoma to allow appropriate treatment.

Unsuspicious (benign) ovarian masses can be followed up using repeated pelvic examinations and ultrasound scans. They usually do not require treatment.

Staging
The staging of ovarian carcinoma is shown in Fig. 12.15.

Staging and prognosis of ovarian carcinoma		
Stage	**Description**	**Five-year survival (%)**
I	Limited to one or both ovaries	80–100
II	Other pelvic sites involved	80–100
III	Sites involved above the pelvic brim within the peritoneal cavity	15–20
IV	Distant metastases	5

Fig. 12.15 Staging and prognosis of ovarian carcinoma.

Treatment
Ovarian carcinoma is usually treated at the initial investigative laparotomy. Suspicious masses are removed along with both ovaries, the uterus, and the omentum. These tissues are sent for histological analysis and diagnosis. The surgeon will also explore the abdomen and pelvis for signs of metastases. Surgery is followed by chemotherapy unless the carcinoma is stage I.

Tumors of the fallopian tubes
Tumors of the fallopian tubes are extremely rare. Benign adenomatoid tumors can form in the superior border of the broad ligament (mesosalpinx). Primary adenocarcinoma of the epithelium rarely occurs in postmenopausal women, and it has an extremely poor prognosis due to late presentation.

Disorders of the endometrium and myometrium

Inflammation of the endometrium (endometritis)
Inflammation of the endometrium is called endometritis; it can follow an acute or chronic course. Acute endometritis is a bacterial infection, often following trauma (e.g., childbirth, surgical termination, cervical surgery, or insertion of the coil). The endometrium usually avoids infection by frequent shedding (menstruation) and the thick cervical mucus. The main causative organisms are staphylococci, streptococci, clostridia, and anaerobes.

Endometritis presents in a similar manner to PID with lower abdominal pain, tenderness, and fever. In severe cases, cervical obstruction can occur so that the uterus fills with pus (pyometra). This is treated with antibiotics following cervical swabs to determine the organism and its antibiotic sensitivity.

Untreated acute endometritis or PID can cause chronic endometritis. Women develop menstrual irregularities, particularly heavy periods, and the infection may spread to affect other reproductive organs.

Adenomyosis

Adenomyosis is when the basal endometrium penetrates the myometrium (muscular layer of the uterus). Cells from the basal layer of the endometrium form small deposits within the smooth muscle that grow and stimulate proliferation of the muscle. The uterus develops a tumor-like mass or enlarges diffusely often causing menstrual pain and heavy periods. Symptomatic adenomyosis is usually treated by hysterectomy since the basal cell layer is insensitive to hormones.

Endometriosis

Endometriosis is the presence of functioning endometrial tissue outside the uterus. It is a very common gynecological disorder, occurring in about 5% of women; however, many are undetected. The main locations of the ectopic endometrial cells are shown in Fig. 12.16. The two most common sites are the:

- Ovaries.
- Ligaments of the uterus.

The ectopic tissue still responds to hormonal stimuli, so cyclic proliferation and bleeding occurs. The bleeding often forms a cyst that enlarges every month. The size of the cyst is limited by rupture; this may cause adhesions.

The exact cause of endometriosis is still under debate; however, there are three theories:
- Retrograde menstruation—menstrual debris enters the peritoneal cavity via the fallopian tube in most women. A lack of immune activity could cause implantation and disease.
- Metaplasia of peritoneal epithelium—an unknown stimulus causes the epithelium to transform into endometrial tissue.
- Metastatic spread—emboli of endometrial tissue may travel via blood and lymph vessels to reach ectopic sites.

In 25% of women endometriosis is asymptomatic. Women who do have symptoms may have:
- Lower abdominal pain during menstruation (75%).
- Constant pain if adhesions are present.
- Menstrual irregularities (60%).
- Deep dyspareunia (pain on intercourse; 30%).
- Infertility (30%).

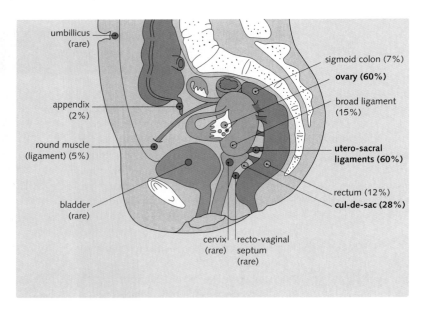

Fig. 12.16 Locations of endometriosis with the relative frequencies (multiple sites are common).

Endometriosis is diagnosed from the history and by laparoscopy, which shows red spots. Since endometriosis is common, it is important to know if it is causing the presenting symptoms. This can be achieved by a short course (up to 6 months) of continuous GnRH analogs that stop cyclical sex steroid changes and endometrial symptoms (they downregulate the GnRH receptors). This investigation also acts as a treatment that persists after the GnRH analog is discontinued.

Endometriosis can be further treated by:

- Continuous use of combined oral contraceptives.
- Medroxyprogesterone acetate (a synthetic progesterone).
- Laparoscopic ablation of the endometrial deposits and adhesions, often used if fertility is desired.
- Danazol—an antiestrogen and antiprogesterone with androgenic activity (up to 6 months).

Severe endometriosis may require hysterectomy and bilateral salpingo-oophorectomy (removal of the uterus, fallopian tubes, and both ovaries).

Endometrial hyperplasia

Endometrial hyperplasia is caused by an excess of estrogens (e.g., from medication, estrogen-secreting tumors, or anovulatory cycles). The proliferation of the functional endometrium during the first half of the menstrual cycle is enhanced, causing irregular and heavy menstruation. Endometrial hyperplasia is important because it carries a higher risk of developing into endometrial carcinoma. A spectrum of malignant change is seen:

- Simple hyperplasia—diffuse enlargement, dilated glands; low risk of carcinoma.
- Complex hyperplasia—focal areas of severe hyperplasia with irregular glands.
- Complex atypical hyperplasia—like complex hyperplasia but cells show atypical malignant changes; there is a high risk of carcinoma.

Endometrial hyperplasia is investigated by biopsy of the endometrium. If there is simple hyperplasia in patients who wish to remain fertile, conservative treatment with cyclical progesterone may be sufficient. In severe and atypical cases hysterectomy is recommended.

Functional endometrial disorders
Anovulatory cycles

At the extremes of reproductive age (i.e., around menarche and menopause) menstruation is frequently irregular. This is due to a failure of ovulation followed by excessive estrogen secretion. The endometrial glands proliferate as a result.

Inadequate luteal phase

A failure in progesterone secretion from the corpus luteum causes inadequate endometrial secretion resulting in infertility.

Oral contraceptives

Starting or changing the "pill" can cause breakthrough bleeding (bleeding in the middle of the cycle). It usually settles down within a few months, and it can be reduced by taking the pill at the same time every day. Higher doses of estrogen may be needed if it does not settle. Prolonged use of oral contraceptives reduces the thickness of the endometrium and inactivates the glands, which reduces the amount of menstrual discharge. There is also a 50% lower risk of endometrial and ovarian cancer.

Menopausal changes

At menopause, ovulation and menstruation become irregular followed by complete cessation of the cycles and menstruation within a few months or years. The endometrium reverts to the prepubertal state and the columnar epithelium may undergo metaplasia to form squamous epithelium; cysts can also develop.

Neoplastic disorders

The most common types of uterine neoplasia are shown in Fig. 12.17.

Benign endometrial polyps

Endometrial polyps are very common around menopause. They are benign tumors caused by the overproliferation of endometrial glands in response to estrogen. The polyps are usually 1–3 cm in size, and they form smooth, firm nodules within the endometrium. They cause menstrual pain and irregularities and can be removed using forceps and a speculum.

Benign leiomyomas (fibroids)

Fibroids are benign tumors of the myometrium (muscle layer of the uterus); they are the most common tumors in the genital tract and affect 20% of menopausal women. The tumors are round, well-defined growths of the smooth muscle cells that

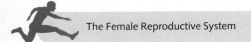

Types of uterine neoplasia			
Uterine layer	Name	Frequency	Description
Endometrium	Endometrial hyperplasia	Common	Benign overgrowth of endometrium
	Estrogen-sensitive endometrial carcinoma	Less common	Malignant tumor derived from endometrial hyperplasia
	Estrogen-insensitive endometrial carcinoma	Less common	Malignant tumor that originates spontaneously
	Endometrial polyps	Common	Benign enlargement of endometrial glands
Myometrium	Leiomyoma	Very common	Benign smooth muscle tumor
	Leiomyosarcoma	Very rare	Malignant smooth muscle tumor

Fig. 12.17 Types of uterine neoplasia.

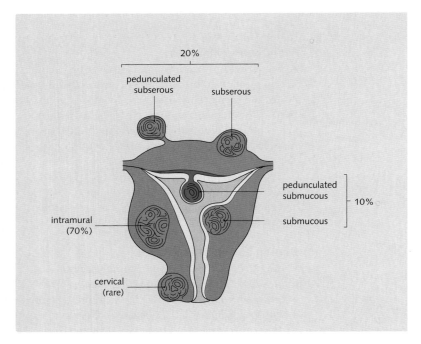

Fig. 12.18 Locations of fibroids with relative frequencies.

often occur in several locations at the same time (Fig. 12.18). Fibroids are estrogen-dependent so they enlarge during pregnancy and with the use of oral contraceptive, but regress after menopause.

The majority of fibroids are asymptomatic. In the remainder, symptoms are caused by the presence of a uterine mass and the extra endometrium required to cover it. Symptoms include:

- Menorrhagia—periods are heavy and prolonged.
- Pelvic pain—torsion of the fibroid can cause ischemia and pain.
- Pelvic mass—large fibroids can be felt in the abdomen and compress surrounding structures.
- Infertility—interference with embryo implantation or recurrent spontaneous abortion.

Treatment is only needed if the fibroids are symptomatic and troublesome. Continuous GnRH agonists may cause the fibroid to regress; however, women who have completed their families often choose hysterectomy. The fibroids can be removed sparing the unaffected uterus (myomectomy), but adhesions are a common complication.

Endometrial carcinoma

Endometrial carcinoma is the most common malignancy of the female genital tract. It is usually found during or after menopause; two patterns are seen:

- Following endometrial hyperplasia—this affects menopausal women; the tumor is an estrogen-dependent adenocarcinoma with a good prognosis.
- Independent of estrogen—this affects postmenopausal women; it can follow endometrial squamous metaplasia and has a poor prognosis.

Endometrial carcinoma spreads mainly by local invasion. Initially, this affects the myometrium but the bladder and rectum may become involved with time. It presents with postmenopausal bleeding that becomes progressively more severe. This symptom must be investigated by hysteroscopy (viewing the endometrium through an endoscope inserted through the cervix) and endometrial biopsy.

The staging of endometrial carcinoma is shown in Fig. 12.19. Early-stage carcinoma can be cured by hysterectomy and bilateral salpingo-oophorectomy (removal of the uterus, fallopian tubes, and both

ovaries) followed by radiotherapy. Patients with inoperable carcinoma may benefit from high doses of progesterone and/or radiotherapy.

Other uterine carcinomas

Rarely, malignancy may develop from the stroma of the endometrium, usually with a poor prognosis. They present in a similar manner to endometrial carcinoma but an epithelial component is often present. There are three main types:

- Endometrial stromal sarcoma—consisting of stromal spindle cells.
- Adenosarcoma—malignant stromal and benign epithelial components.
- Carcinosarcoma—malignant stromal and epithelial components; may contain nonuterine tissues.

Leiomyosarcomas are extremely rare, malignant tumors of the myometrium that tend to occur after menopause. They often metastasize by vascular spread to the lungs.

Menstrual disorders and menopause

Abnormal frequency, duration, and volume of menstruation are common presentations of many gynecological diseases. Normal menstruation:

- Occurs once every 22–35 days.
- Lasts less than 7 days.
- Less than 80 mL of fluid is discharged.

Amenorrhea

If menstruation has not occurred within 35 days of the start of the last cycle, it is called oligomenorrhea. An absence of menstruation for 70 days or more is called amenorrhea; this is normal before puberty, during pregnancy, and after menopause. Pathological amenorrhea is divided into primary and secondary causes.

Primary amenorrhea

This is the failure to start menstruating by the age of 16. It is a relatively rare condition. The most common cause is delayed puberty which will resolve spontaneously; however, a number of diseases and conditions can cause primary amenorrhea:

- Low body fat (e.g., anorexia nervosa, malnutrition).

Staging and prognosis of endometrial carcinoma		
Stage	Description	Five-year survival (%)
I	Limited to the endometrium and myometrium, but not serosa	75–100
II	Limited to the uterus and cervix, but not serosa	60
III	Involvement of serosa and/or metastases to other pelvic organs	50
IV	Distant metastases	20

Fig. 12.19 Staging and prognosis of endometrial carcinoma.

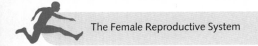

Common causes of secondary amenorrhea		
Cause	**Etiology**	**Frequency (%)**
Weight loss	Deficiency of leptin from fat prevents GnRH release	35
Polycystic ovaries	FSH deficiency and multiple endocrine abnormalities prevent follicle development	25
Pituitary insensitivity	Following the "pill," stress, or illness	15
Hyperprolactinemia	Microadenoma of the pituitary gland (see Chapter 2)	15
Primary ovarian failure	Premature menopause, possibly with autoimmune involvement	5

Fig. 12.20 Common causes of secondary amenorrhea.

- Congenital malformations of the vagina, uterus, or ovaries.
- Imperforate hymen.
- Turner syndrome—lack of an X chromosome (i.e., XO).
- Testicular feminization syndrome—XY but insensitive to testosterone.

Secondary amenorrhea

This is when a woman who has begun to menstruate fails to have a period for 70 days or more. It is a relatively common disorder that affects about 1% of women of reproductive age. The most common causes of secondary amenorrhea are shown in Fig. 12.20.

Investigation and treatment

Amenorrhea is investigated with hormone tests (prolactin, FSH, LH, and thyroid function tests) and an ultrasound scan of the pelvis. Treatment depends on the cause of the amenorrhea.

Menorrhagia

Menorrhagia is excessive (>80 mL) menstrual bleeding; it may also be prolonged. Severe menorrhagia may result in iron deficiency anemia. The main causes are:

- Dysfunctional uterine bleeding (80%).
- Endometrial tumors and polyps that distort the endometrium.
- Adenomyosis.
- Chronic pelvic inflammatory disease.
- Hypothyroidism.

Menorrhagia should be investigated if the woman is over 40 years of age or has intermenstrual bleeding or postcoital bleeding. Hysteroscopy, endometrial biopsy, transvaginal ultrasound, thyroid function tests, and clotting studies are used to exclude pathology. In the majority of patients with menorrhagia no underlying pathology is found, and the disease is termed **dysfunctional uterine bleeding**. This condition can also cause irregular bleeding. It is more common at the extremes of reproductive age and is due to an excess of endometrial prostaglandin synthesis, which may cause excessive uterine contractions and abnormal blood clotting.

If an underlying cause is found, it should be treated; otherwise dysfunctional uterine bleeding can be assumed. Menorrhagia can be treated with:

- Oral contraceptives.
- Mirena® (progesterone-releasing intrauterine system).
- Mefenamic acid (a nonsteroidal anti-inflammatory drug).
- Tranexamic acid (fibrinolysis inhibitor).
- Endometrial ablation or hysterectomy if the bleeding is severe.

Dysmenorrhea

Dysmenorrhea means painful menstrual periods; it has either primary or secondary causes.

Primary dysmenorrhea

This is caused by an imbalance in prostaglandin synthesis that results in ischemia and hyperexcitability of the myometrium. Uterine spasms result, causing cramping pains before and at the start of menstruation. This disorder is very common soon after menarche, when it affects about 75% of girls. It decreases with age, but NSAIDs or oral contraceptives usually help.

Secondary dysmenorrhea

This affects older women and is usually due to endometriosis or PID. Cramping pains are felt before menstruation; however, they persist and worsen through the period. The underlying pathology should be treated.

Premenstrual syndrome

Premenstrual syndrome (PMS) describes a negative mood and several physical symptoms that can occur in the luteal phase (days 14–28) of the menstrual cycle. Mild PMS is very common, but 5–15% of women suffer from life-disrupting symptoms regularly. The symptoms are shown in Fig. 12.21.

The cause remains unknown; however, fluctuating estrogen levels may be responsible, possibly mediated via decreased levels of serotonin (5-hydroxytryptamine; 5-HT) in the CNS. Diagnosis is made from the history and can be confirmed by keeping a diary of symptoms; these must correspond to the menstrual cycle. Treatment can be symptomatic (e.g., analgesia) or aimed at preventing estrogen fluctuations (e.g., oral contraceptives or estrogen patches).

> Extensive research among female medical students at Nottingham University (UK) has revealed the following "treatments" for PMS: bananas, chocolate, vitamin B_6, sage, fennel, chocolate, low fat diet, evening primrose oil, and chocolate.

Menopause

Menopause is the cessation of menstruation and ovulation that usually occurs between the ages of 45 and 55 years (average 51). The term "climacteric" includes the time before and after menopause during which "menopausal" symptoms are noticed.

The ovaries gradually become less sensitive to FSH and LH from about the age of 40 years because of the loss of follicles and receptors. This causes anovulatory cycles and a progressive decrease in estrogen production. As estrogen levels fall, FSH and LH secretion increases because of the lack of negative feedback. The ovaries resist this increase and the woman enters a period of oligomenorrhea followed by amenorrhea. After 6 months of amenorrhea the woman is said to have reached menopause. With time, the FSH and LH levels begin to decline along with estrogen levels.

Other tissues are capable of secreting estrogens independently (e.g., adipose tissue and the adrenal cortex). The estrogens produced do not equal the premenopausal levels so that women become estrogen-deficient. The lack of estrogen predisposes women to three main complications (Fig. 12.22):
- Osteoporosis.
- Heart disease.
- Collagen breakdown.

The climacteric period is symptomatic in 75% of women and severe in 40%. The climacteric symptoms are listed below (those caused by low estrogen levels are in bold):
- **Hot flashes**: usually at night, often with sweating.
- **Dry, burning vagina** with dyspareunia (pain on intercourse).
- Painful joints.

Symptoms of premenstrual syndrome		
Psychological	**Behavioral**	**Physical**
Anxiety	Anger	Acne
Depression	Impulsiveness and accident-prone behavior	Weight gain
Increased appetite		Breast tenderness and swelling
Irritability	Poor concentration	Abdominal bloating
Loss of libido	Poor tolerance to stress	Change in bowel habit
Sleep disturbance		Headache
Tension		Pelvic pain

Fig. 12.21 Symptoms of premenstrual syndrome.

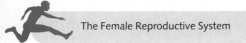

Long-term complications of menopause		
Symptoms/disease	**Cause**	**Consequence**
Osteoporosis	Accelerated bone loss	Increased risk of bone fractures, especially the femoral neck at the hip and crush fractures of the vertebrae
Cardiovascular disease	Estrogens have a beneficial effect on the type of lipid in the blood and in doing so protect against cardiovascular disease	Increased risk of coronary artery disease, myocardial infarction, and strokes
Loss of collagen	Weakening in the pelvic ligaments, joints, and muscles, and loss of elasticity in the skin	Predisposes to uterovaginal prolapse, immobility, muscle weakness, and causes skin wrinkling

Fig. 12.22 Long-term complications of estrogen deficiency following menopause.

- Headaches.
- Depression, anxiety, irritability, and dizziness.
- Palpitations.
- Urinary incontinence and infection.

Menopause is often said to reduce sexual desire. This is true in 20% of women, but 20% report an increase in sexual desire.

Hormone replacement therapy (HRT) is the replacement of estrogens via a tablet, implant, or skin patch. It is often used to treat climacteric symptoms and prevent the long-term complications of estrogen deficiency. There are three types of HRT:

- Cyclical combined HRT—continuous estrogens, 12/28 days of progesterone; they cause regular withdrawal bleeds.
- Continuous combined HRT—continuous estrogens and progesterones; they can only be used 12 months after the last menstrual period.
- Estrogen only—continuous estrogens; they can only be used if the woman has had a hysterectomy.

Progesterone must be included if the woman has not had a hysterectomy to prevent endometrial hyperplasia and carcinoma. Cyclical progesterone causes withdrawal bleeding (similar to using the "pill"); after one year the woman may use a continuous combined preparation in which progesterone is taken constantly to prevent withdrawal bleeds.

Long-term use of HRT has a life-saving effect by reducing cardiovascular disease and osteoporosis;

there is a slight increase in the risk of breast cancer and deep vein thrombosis.

The contraindications of HRT are common exam questions; they include:
- Estrogen-dependent cancer (including breast cancer).
- Thromboembolic disorders.
- Liver disease with abnormal liver function tests (LFTs).
- Undiagnosed vaginal bleeding.
- Pregnancy or breastfeeding.

There is no male equivalent of menopause. Men continue to produce testosterone and spermatozoa well into their 80s, but the amount and quality decline with age. The evolutionary basis for this difference is not fully understood.

Disorders of the cervix

Cervical ectopy
Cervical ectopy is a normal physiological finding that has been called cervical ectropion or erosion in the past. It describes the extension of the columnar epithelium of the endocervix beyond the external os under the influence of estrogen. Any process that raises estrogen levels can temporarily result in a cervical ectopy, including puberty, pregnancy, and the first months of using the "pill." In ectopy, the columnar epithelium appears as a red ring around the external os compared with the pink squamous

epithelium. With time, metaplasia occurs and the columnar epithelium converts to stratified squamous epithelium. The presence of cervical ectopy may account for small amounts of postcoital or intermenstrual bleeding; it may raise susceptibility to sexually transmitted infection.

Inflammation of the cervix

Cervicitis

Cervicitis is inflammation and infection of the cervix. It is usually asymptomatic, although vaginal discharge, postcoital bleeding, dyspareunia, and pelvic pain may be present; on examination it may be inflamed and tender. The infection is often caused by:

- *Chlamydia trachomatis* (very common, see below).
- *Neisseria gonorrhoeae* (common, see below).
- *Trichomonas vaginalis* (see p. 144).
- Herpes simplex (see p. 144).

The infection is diagnosed using swabs (cervical, *Chlamydia* cervical, and high vaginal) along with a wet-mounted cervical smear for *Trichomonas*. Asymptomatic infection should be treated aggressively because of the risk of PID and infertility. The partner often requires treatment to prevent reinfection.

Chlamydia trachomatis   This intracellular bacterium is sexually transmitted. It is thought to cause asymptomatic infection in about 5% of young, sexually active women. Infection is usually asymptomatic; however, it can cause urethritis (infection of the urethra), cervicitis, and pelvic inflammatory disease (PID). It is usually diagnosed by direct fluorescent antibody tests (DFA) that require a special culture medium; it is treated using the antibiotics doxycycline or erythromycin.

Neisseria gonorrhoeae   This Gram-negative diplococcus is an intracellular bacterium that is often called gonococcus; it is a sexually transmitted infection. Like *Chlamydia*, it usually causes asymptomatic urethritis, cervicitis, and pelvic inflammatory disease. It is diagnosed by Gram stain and culture of the swab sample; it is treated with the antibiotics cefixime and ceftriaxone. *Chlamydia* is also present in 50% of gonococcus infections, so doxycycline is often given as well.

Neoplasia of the cervix

During puberty the vagina becomes more acidic owing to the presence of glycogen in the vaginal walls and the action of lactobacilli that colonize the vagina. The columnar epithelium of the endocervix reacts to the acid environment by transforming into stratified squamous epithelium—a process called metaplasia. This results in a transformation zone between the ectocervix and endocervix, which is susceptible to dysplasia (precancerous changes) in a similar manner to the squamocolumnar transformation zone found in Barrett's esophagus. The smear test is used to identify and treat these dysplastic changes before they progress to cervical carcinoma.

Cervical intraepithelial neoplasia

The dysplastic changes leading to cervical carcinoma are called cervical intraepithelial neoplasia (CIN); they are graded from I to III according to the severity and depth of the changes. The risk and rate of progression to cervical carcinoma increases with each grade; however, all stages are treatable. All stages are asymptomatic and undetectable by simply looking at the cervix.

Risk factors

CIN is strongly associated with certain strains of human papilloma virus (HPV); CIN is therefore a sexually transmitted disease. Any factor associated with exposure to HPV increases the risk of CIN, including multiple sexual partners and early age of first intercourse. Cigarette smoking is also a risk factor.

The smear test

Women between the ages of 20 and 64 years are offered free Pap smears (smear tests) every 3 years by their doctor. The test involves scraping cells from the cervix using a speculum to open the vagina and a wooden spatula to take the sample. Between 2% and 5% of smears are reported as abnormal and 10% have an insufficient sample for estimation (a repeat smear is required).

Since the sample is taken from the surface layer, the depth of epithelial involvement cannot be measured directly. The number and severity of dysplastic cells are used to estimate the grade of CIN (Fig. 12.23). This estimate is not entirely accurate; about 30% of normal smears are false negatives and 4% of abnormal smears are false positives. Estimation of borderline smears can be improved by testing for the presence of oncogenic HPV strains.

Management of positive smears

Receiving a diagnosis of a positive (abnormal) smear test is commonly misinterpreted as a diagnosis of

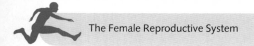

Fig. 12.23 Classification, natural history, and treatment of cervical intraepithelial neoplasia (CIN).

Classification, natural history, and treatment of cervical intraepithelial neoplasia			
Grade	CIN I	CIN II	CIN III
Pap smear classification	Mild dysplasia	Moderate dysplasia	Severe dysplasia/ carcinoma in situ
Extent of epithelium involved on biopsy	Third nearest the basement membrane	Two thirds nearest the basement membrane	Full thickness
Percentage who progress to carcinoma if untreated	1%	8%	20%
Treatment	Follow up in 6 months or refer to colposcopy	Refer to colposcopy	Refer to colposcopy

cervical cancer; the patient will often be afraid and anxious. It is important to explain that it is not a diagnosis of cancer, but that follow-up smears and treatment are very important. The management is shown in Fig. 12.23.

Colposcopy

Abnormal smears are often followed up using colposcopy, which is usually performed at a hospital outpatient clinic. A colposcope looks like a pair of binoculars; it magnifies the cervix by 5–20 times. Acetic acid is applied to the cervix so that abnormal areas of cervical epithelium turn white. These areas are inspected and biopsied so that the depth of involvement can be assessed to accurately diagnose the grade of CIN. It is often treated immediately.

Treatment

Moderate to severe (II and III) CIN is treated by removal or destruction of the abnormal epithelium; this is usually performed in colposcopy using local anesthetic. There are a number of methods of treatment:

- Large loop excision of the transformation zone (LLETZ).
- Laser therapy.
- Cryotherapy.
- Cone biopsy (grade III, may raise miscarriage risk).

Vaginal bleeding and discharge is common for about 2 weeks after treatment; sexual intercourse and the use of tampons should be avoided for 4 weeks after treatment. The treatment is followed up with a Pap smear test 6 months later and yearly smear tests for 5 years. Ninety per cent of women are cured; 10% require repeated treatment.

Cervical carcinoma

Cervical carcinoma is usually a squamous cell carcinoma arising in the transformation zone between the ectocervix and endocervix. There is a clear progression from CIN to carcinoma, and both diseases have the same risk factors, including HPV infection.

Cervical carcinoma usually affects women after menopause, but the incidence in younger women is high enough to warrant population screening from the age of 20 years. The early stages are frequently asymptomatic; by the time of presentation, advanced disease with poor 5-year survival rates is often present. Symptoms include abnormal vaginal bleeding (classically postcoital), vaginal discharge, or renal failure in advanced stages; it can be detected through abnormal smear tests. The staging and 5-year survival figures are shown in Fig. 12.24. Invasion of the ureters (which pass 1 cm lateral to the internal os) in stage IIb is a poor prognostic feature.

Suspected cervical carcinoma is investigated by colposcopy with biopsy; if advanced disease is suspected, then imaging techniques are used to identify the extent of invasion and metastases:

- Stage Ia—cone biopsy or simple hysterectomy.
- Stage Ib/IIa—radical hysterectomy (includes parametrium and pelvic lymph nodes) or pelvic radiotherapy.

Fig. 12.24 Staging and prognosis of cervical carcinoma.

Staging and prognosis of cervical carcinoma		
Stage	**Description**	**Five-year survival (%)**
Ia	Carcinoma only in cervix, <5 mm	95
Ib	Carcinoma only in cervix, >5 mm	85
IIa	Invasion outside the cervix but not the parametrium (surrounding tissue, including ureters)	75
IIb	Invasion outside the cervix including the parametrium (± ureters)	55
III	Invasion of ureters, lower third of the vagina, or pelvic walls	30
IV	Invasion of bladder, rectum, or outside the pelvis	10

- Stage IIb—combination of radical surgery, chemotherapy, and radiotherapy.

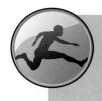

A smear test should be performed once every 3 years on sexually active women aged 20–64 years to detect cervical intraepithelial neoplasia.

Cervical polyps and benign cervical tumors

Cervical polyps are small, round, benign growths of the cervix that often protrude through the external os. They are very common, affecting about 5% of women; they may cause irregular vaginal bleeding or vaginal discharge. They are treated by surgical excision that is often performed in outpatient clinics.

Other benign tumors of the cervix are uncommon, although leiomyomas (smooth muscle tumors) can occur.

Disorders of the vagina and vulva

Infections

The female genital tract is susceptible to many infections, including a number that are sexually transmitted. A summary of the most common female sexually transmitted infections is shown in Fig. 12.25.

Infections of the vagina

Vaginal discharge is a common symptom that can be caused by infections of the cervix (e.g., *Chlamydia*) and vagina (e.g., thrush). The most common causes of vaginal discharge are not sexually transmitted; instead they are caused by overgrowth of normal vaginal flora. This is caused by a rise in vaginal pH (as occurs in pregnancy and diabetes) or loss of the lactobacilli (as occurs when taking antibiotics). These diseases are:
- Bacterial vaginosis.
- Candidiasis (thrush).

Nonetheless, women presenting with vaginal discharge are investigated for a number of sexually transmitted diseases (STDs) owing to the high prevalence of sexually transmitted infection. The main vaginal infections are described below.

Bacterial vaginosis

This disease is usually caused by the overgrowth of the anaerobic bacteria *Gardnerella vaginalis*, although other anaerobes may be responsible. It is classically associated with a smooth, white vaginal discharge with a distinctive "fishy" smell. It is diagnosed if the discharge has:
- pH > 5.5.
- Ammonia smell when mixed with potassium hydroxide.
- Clue cells on microscopic examination.

It is treated using the antibiotic metronidazole.

Candidiasis

Overgrowth of the yeast (a type of fungus) *Candida albicans* is responsible for thrush. Infection causes the following symptoms:

Common sexually transmitted infections in women				
Infection	Site of infection	Organism	Symptoms	Treatment
Pelvic inflammatory disease	Upper genital tract	*Chlamydia trachomatis* (atypical bacteria) or *Neisseria gonorrhoeae*	Abdominal pain and tenderness, dyspareunia, pus discharge	Doxycycline or ceftriaxone
Gonorrhea	Cervix	*Neisseria gonorrhoeae*	Urinary frequency, dysuria, pus discharge	Penicillin or ceftriaxone
Trichomoniasis	Vagina	*Trichomonas vaginalis* (parasite)	Itching, discharge	Metronidazole
Thrush	Vagina	*Candida albicans* (fungus)	Itching, white discharge	Clotrimazole (vaginal pessary)
Herpes	Vulva	Herpes simplex virus	Buming red blisters that may recur	Aciclovir if recurrent
Warts	Vulva	Human papilloma virus	Growths on the vulval skin	Podophyllotoxin cream
HIV and AIDS	Systemic	Human immunodeficiency virus	Chronic, progressive immunodeficiency	Combination antiretroviral therapy
Hepatitis	Systemic (liver)	Hepatitis virus B, C, and E	Chronic liver disease	(Interferon-α)
Syphilis	Systemic (vulval lesion)	*Treponema pallidum*	Ulcerated nodules, but may become systemic	Penicillin

Fig. 12.25 Common sexually transmitted infections in women.

- Vulval itching and soreness.
- Redness of the vulva and vagina.
- Thick, white vaginal discharge.

It is diagnosed by microscopy of the vaginal discharge that reveals dark-purple yeast spores or filaments when stained with potassium hydroxide. A vaginal tablet (pessary) of clotrimazole is used to treat the infection; the partner(s) may also need to be treated to prevent recurrence.

Trichomoniasis

This is an infection with the sexually transmitted flagellated parasite *Trichomonas vaginalis*. It is often asymptomatic, but an accompanying rise in vaginal pH may cause symptoms including:

- Thin, watery (may be green or foamy) vaginal discharge.
- Some itching and redness.

It is diagnosed by viewing the vaginal discharge mounted on saline under a microscope; the organism can be identified by the movement seen. Oral metronidazole cures 90% of infections, but a second vaginal swab should be performed 2 months later. The partner(s) should also be treated.

Infections of the vulva

The vulva is susceptible to sexually transmitted viral infections similar to those that affect skin on other areas of the body:

Herpes simplex

This is caused by the herpes simplex virus (usually HSV type II, though HSV type I can also cause vulval disease). About 25% of patients experience acute symptoms, including:

- Localized itching and burning.
- Multiple painful red vesicles.
- Ulceration of vesicles causing more pain.
- Dysuria if the area round the urethra is involved.
- Fever and malaise.

The vesicles appear about 3 days after infection and take up to 2 weeks to heal, during which the virus is shed and can be transmitted. The virus cannot be transmitted if vesicles are not present, but some vesicles may be hidden. The virus enters the dorsal root ganglion of sensory nerves supplying the infected area. It usually lies dormant, but it may cause recurrent attacks in 5% of patients.

Herpes simplex can be diagnosed from viral culture of fluid in the vesicles and antibody screening. It is treated symptomatically (e.g., anesthetic cream), although the antiviral agent aciclovir can reduce the frequency and duration of recurrent attacks. The virus can be transmitted to other body parts via the hands; the eyes are particularly susceptible. The presence of herpes vesicles in late pregnancy is an indication for cesarean section.

Genital warts

These are benign growths of the epithelium caused by human papilloma viruses (HPV), of which there are many types. Some HPV strains infect the vulval skin, causing small, cauliflower-shaped warts that may cause itching and burning. The infection can spread to the vagina and cervix, and it is readily passed onto sexual contacts. Certain strains of HPV can predispose to dysplastic changes in the cervix, vulva, and anus that may lead to carcinoma; these strains rarely cause obvious growths.

Vulval warts are treated with podophyllotoxin cream, cryotherapy, or minor surgery if they cause the patient distress. Smear tests should be repeated annually.

Bartholin's cyst

This disease is caused by bacterial infection of Bartholin's gland and duct, found on either side of the introitus (vaginal orifice); it is a common vulval disorder. If the duct becomes obstructed, a cyst can form that presents as a vulval swelling. The main causative bacteria are staphylococci, *E. coli*, and gonococci.

Cysts require surgical treatment and antibiotics to prevent abscess formation.

Systemic sexually transmitted infections

Other sexually transmitted diseases cause systemic illness and often have a chronic course. They are briefly described in Fig. 12.25; recent infection with syphilis can result in a genital lesion at the site of infection.

Neoplasia of the vagina

Tumors very rarely develop in the vagina, although they may spread to the vagina from the cervix and endometrium. Of the tumors that do develop in the vagina, the majority are squamous cell carcinomas found in the upper third of the vagina in elderly women. Adenocarcinoma, melanoma, and sarcoma are even rarer but tend to affect younger women.

Vaginal carcinoma presents with abnormal vaginal bleeding, pelvic pain, and the detection of a lump. It is investigated by smear test and ultrasound scan to determine the origins of the carcinoma. The treatment of cervical and endometrial carcinoma is described on p. 142 and p. 137, respectively. Squamous cell carcinoma is mainly treated with radiotherapy, although surgery and chemotherapy may also be required.

Vulval dystrophies

The vulval dystrophies are nonneoplastic, chronic disorders of the vulval skin; they mainly affect menopausal or postmenopausal women, but they may affect prepubescents. They are distinct from the physiological vulval atrophy caused by estrogen deficiency after menopause. There are two patterns of vulvar dystrophy:
- Lichen sclerosus.
- Squamous cell hyperplasia (also called hypertrophic dysplasia or leukoplakia).

These diseases are compared in Fig. 12.26. Both conditions present with vulval itching and pain on contact, leading to superficial dyspareunia; they can undergo malignant change. They are investigated using a colposcope (p. 142) and biopsy of suspicious areas under local anesthetic. Treatment is shown in Fig. 12.26.

Neoplasia of the vulva
Malignant tumors
Vulval intraepithelial neoplasia (VIN)

Precancerous changes can be detected in the vulva (VIN) in a similar manner to the cervix (CIN; see p. 141). These changes are associated with HPV (wart virus) infection, smoking, and the vulval dystrophies described above. The affected vulva may feel itchy and sore, and there may be a lump or ulcer. It is investigated using a colposcope and biopsy to determine the extent of cellular dysplasia; it is graded in a similar manner to CIN to determine treatment (Fig. 12.27). Appropriate treatment ensures a 5-year survival of 100%; untreated VIN may progress to vulval cancer. The risk is significantly higher for VIN III.

Vulval carcinoma

Vulval carcinoma is an uncommon malignancy that mainly affects elderly women. It is usually a squamous cell carcinoma predisposed by HPV infection and smoking; 30% occur as a progression from VIN. They present with similar symptoms to

145

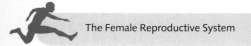
Comparison of lichen sclerosus and squamous cell hyperplasia		
Feature	**Lichen sclerosus**	**Squamous cell hyperplasia**
Epidermis	Thin	Thick
Dermis	Hyalinized (degeneration and replacement with collagen) and edematous	Edematous
Inflammatory cells present	Lymphocytes	Plasma cells
Appearance	Shiny, white, and crinkly plaques	Thick, white/gray areas with deep skin-folds
Treatment	Vaseline or topical steroids	Topical steroids

Fig. 12.26 Comparison of lichen sclerosus and squamous cell hyperplasia.

Classification and treatment of vulval intraepithelial neoplasia			
Grade	**VIN I**	**VIN II**	**VIN III**
Classification	Mild dysplasia	Moderate dysplasia	Severe dysplasia/ carcinoma in situ
Treatment	Topical steroids and regular follow-up	Topical steroids and regular follow-up	Surgical excision or destruction

Fig. 12.27 Classification and treatment of vulval intraepithelial neoplasia (VIN).

Staging and prognosis of vulval carcinoma		
Stage	**Description**	**Five-year survival (%)**
I	Tumor confined to vulva and perineum, <2 cm	>90
II	Tumor confined to vulva and perineum, >2 cm	80–90
III	Tumor involves lower urethra/vagina/anus and/or unilateral lymph nodes	50–80
IV	Distant metastases, involvement of upper urethra/bladder/rectum/pubic bone and/or bilateral metastases	5–30

Fig. 12.28 Staging and prognosis of vulval carcinoma.

VIN and are investigated with colposcope examination and biopsy. The staging system and 5-year survival rates are shown in Fig. 12.28. Vulval carcinoma is treated surgically (radical vulvectomy and lymph node dissection to various extents) and with radiotherapy in stages III and IV.

Other malignancies

Since the vulva is covered with skin, it can develop similar malignant tumors to other areas of skin. The melanocytes can give rise to malignant melanoma, and the vulval ducts can develop cancerous Paget's disease.

Benign tumors

The vulva is prone to the same benign tumors as other areas of skin. One of the most frequent tumors is papillary hidradenoma. This is a benign growth of the sweat (eccrine) glands.

Disorders of the female breast

The most common presenting complaint involving the breast is a lump. Figure 12.29 shows the most common causes and their associated features.

Fig. 12.29 Types of breast lump with associated features.

Types of breast lump and associated features			
Disease	Most common age group	Frequency	Features of lump
Fat necrosis	Any	Rare	Single, hard, and irregular
Mammary duct ectasia	Older women before the menopause	Common	Tender; near the areola
Nodular fibrocystic change	Older women before the menopause	Very common	Single or multiple firm nodules
Cystic fibrocystic change	Just before the menopause	Very common	Rapidly growing smooth, rounded cysts
Fibroadenoma	Younger women (25–35 years)	Common	Single firm, highly mobile, nontender lump
Phyllodes tumor	Older women	Less common	Single, large, rubbery lump
Duct papilloma	Middle-aged women	Common	Lump near the nipple with bloody discharge
Carcinoma	Middle-aged to elderly women	Common	Single hard lump with stromal interference

Congenital abnormalities

Supernumerary nipples

Failure of the fetal mammary ridge to regress can cause extra nipples (polythelia) to develop. The extra nipple is usually just below a normal breast; however, they can be found anywhere along the line of the mammary ridge (axilla to inguinal rings) and very rarely in other locations. It is a common disorder affecting about 1% of people, although the extra nipple is often mistaken for a mole.

Accessory breast tissue

In females, accessory breast tissue (polymastia) can also develop, although it is usually not noticed until puberty. The extra tissue is usually in the axilla, but it can form in the same locations as extra nipples. The accessory breast tissue may be associated with a nipple to form an extra breast.

Congenital nipple inversion

The nipple is usually inverted at birth; development of the areola should cause it to rise. If this process fails, the nipple may be permanently inverted, causing difficulty in breastfeeding. It is important to differentiate between congenital inversion and a recent inversion that may suggest a malignancy.

Inflammatory disorders and infections

Acute mastitis and breast abscess

When the woman is lactating, the breast is prone to bacterial infection through cracks in the nipple and areola. The usual organisms responsible are staphylococci and streptococci.

The initial infection causes an acute inflammation of the breast called mastitis, in which the breast becomes tender and enlarged. It should be treated with antibiotics to prevent breast abscesses that must be drained surgically. Chronic mastitis can also develop, but it is very rare.

Mammary duct ectasia

Mammary duct ectasia is a chronic inflammatory condition of unknown origin that causes the lactiferous ducts near the nipple to dilate. It is most common just before menopause in women who have had children. The dilated duct fills with a creamy, protein-rich fluid that causes a green discharge from the nipple and tender lumps near the areola. The possibility of carcinoma must be excluded by biopsy or surgical excision. The dilated ducts are prone to infection, which requires antibiotic treatment to prevent abscess formation.

Fat necrosis

Relatively minor trauma to the breast can result in necrosis of the adipose tissue (fat cells). This necrosis prompts an inflammatory reaction that can cause fibrous scarring, producing a hard, irregular lump in the breast. These lesions can mimic carcinomas including characteristic interference with the normal breast connective tissue such as skin dimpling. This condition is relatively rare, and it can only be differentiated from a malignancy by excision biopsy.

Fibrocystic change/fibroadenosis

Fibrocystic change is caused by benign growth of the breast tissue resulting in tender lumps. It is a very common disease that affects 50% of women, though only 10% are symptomatic. It is most common in older women before menopause.

The overgrowth occurs in two tissues:
- Epithelial lining of the ducts and lobules.
- Fibrous stroma.

A variation in hormonal response results in a growth imbalance between the fibrous and epithelial tissues causing solid nodules and fluid-filled cysts to develop. The nature of this imbalance can vary, resulting in three patterns of change (described below); these may coexist.

Simple fibrocystic change

Overgrowth of both tissues is seen in simple fibrocystic change, producing a mixture of fibrous nodules and epithelial cysts. The imbalance in tissue overgrowth is a local effect, and many microscopic areas display these changes. Larger growth imbalances can cause symptomatic fibrocystic change.

Single or multiple fibrous nodules can develop, and these frequently become tender toward the end of the menstrual cycle (i.e., premenstrually). It is difficult to differentiate the single lumps from a carcinoma except by biopsy or excision.

Palpable epithelial cysts are most frequent close to the start of the menopause. They can be distinguished from lumps by palpation (smooth, rounded, and flocculent) and their appearance on x-ray mammograms and ultrasound scans. Cysts contain a watery fluid that can be aspirated and examined for evidence of malignancy; this aspiration also treats the cyst. Simple fibrocystic change is entirely benign.

Epithelial hyperplasia

If the epithelial overgrowth predominates, the condition is called epithelial hyperplasia. It is a benign change, but it has an increased risk of breast carcinoma (two times normal risk). The risk of carcinoma is higher if the epithelial cells show signs of dysplasia, called atypical hyperplasia (five times normal risk).

Sclerosing adenosis

If the fibrous overgrowth predominates, the condition is called sclerosing adenosis. This rare variation is entirely benign. It can compress the surrounding glands and cause a histological appearance of solid cords that can be confused with invasive carcinoma on histological and x-ray (mammogram) examination.

Benign neoplasia
Fibroadenoma

Fibroadenomas are common, solitary, benign lumps that occur mostly in young women (below 35 years of age). Lumps develop from the mammary ducts and stroma in response to hormonal stimuli. They contain glandular epithelial components from the duct and fibrous components from the stroma, so they may be caused by a type of fibrocystic change instead of being true benign tumors. The lumps are usually firm, rubbery, and nontender; they are highly mobile and can slip away during palpation (hence the name "breast mice").

Phyllodes tumor

Phyllodes tumors resemble fibroadenomas, but they are often much larger. They can occur at any age after puberty but usually affect older women. These lesions are usually benign, but a spectrum of dysplasia is seen: 10% are malignant.

Duct papilloma

Duct papillomas are benign growths of the mammary duct epithelia. These solitary tumors usually develop in the lactiferous duct just below the nipple in middle-aged women. In younger women they usually develop in the smaller ducts. They cause a lump and bloody nipple discharge. The tumor is surgically excised and the breast is examined by mammography to reveal any underlying carcinoma.

Multiple duct papillomas are rare and have an increased risk of breast carcinoma.

Malignant neoplasia

Breast carcinoma is the most common cancer in women, affecting about 1 in 12 at some point in their life. The risk of breast cancer increases with age, being very rare before 25 years but moderately common by 40 years of age. There are a number of risk factors for breast cancer:

- Family history—including the recently discovered autosomal dominant *BRAC 1* and *BRAC 2* mutations.
- Geographical—there is a higher risk in developed countries.
- Excess estrogen exposure—this can be caused by many factors (e.g., early menarche, late menopause, HRT, no pregnancies) but probably not the "pill."
- Epithelial hyperplasia—see the section on fibrocystic change.

Classification of breast carcinoma

The vast majority of breast cancers are adenocarcinomas. These can develop in three patterns according to their location in the breast:

- Invasive ductal carcinoma (50%).
- Invasive lobular carcinoma (30%).
- Mixed ductal and lobular carcinoma (10%).

The other 10% are rarer forms of breast cancer (see below).

All three patterns of adenocarcinoma can be preceded by noninvasive carcinoma in situ. With time, roughly 25% of these will develop into invasive carcinoma, but early mastectomy usually prevents this. Two forms are seen, identified by location:

- Intraductal carcinoma.
- Intralobular carcinoma.

Three other types of carcinoma occur more rarely. They have a better prognosis than invasive adenocarcinoma. They are:

- Tubular carcinoma.
- Mucoid carcinoma.
- Medullary carcinoma.

Presentation

The majority of breast cancers present as lumps or from mammogram screening. All lumps should be investigated as if they were malignant. This includes:

- Ultrasound or attempted aspiration to differentiate cysts and lumps.
- Fine-needle aspiration or excision biopsy of lumps.

Excision biopsy is carried out only on lumps or cysts with a history or appearance suggestive of malignancy. There are a number of signs of carcinoma that suggest that excision biopsy is needed or that prompt investigation should be done in the absence of a lump. These are mostly caused by interference with the breast stroma or lymphatic drainage:

- Skin dimpling.
- Recent nipple inversion.
- Bloody nipple discharge.
- Peau d'orange (skin with the appearance of orange peel).
- Surface erythema or ulceration.
- Paget's disease of the nipple.

Paget's disease is an eczema-like rash around the nipple caused by local spread of invasive ductal carcinoma.

The features of a lump or cyst that suggest malignancy are:

- Large, hard, or growing masses.
- Fixing of mass to underlying structures.
- Enlargement of the affected breast.
- Blood-stained cystic fluid.
- Recurrence.
- Enlarged axillary lymph nodes.

Spread, prognosis, and staging

Invasive breast carcinoma can spread by three routes:

- Local spread—within the breast or into surrounding structures (e.g., skin, nipple, pectoral muscles, and chest wall).
- Lymphatic spread—to the axillary, internal thoracic lymph nodes, and the other breast.
- Blood-borne spread—especially to the bone (especially vertebral bodies), lungs, and ovaries (called a Krukenberg tumor).

The prognosis of breast cancer is predicted by the stage of the tumor. This is determined from the TNM system, which assigns scores according to three measures (Fig. 12.30): tumor size, nodal involvement, and metastases.

In general, low scores have a better prognosis (e.g., 80% 5-year survival if no nodes are involved). The presence of metastases is a particularly poor prognostic sign, reducing the 5-year survival to 10%.

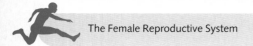

TNM staging system of breast cancer				
Stage	**0**	**1**	**2**	**3**
Tumor (T)	None	<2 cm	2–5 cm	>5 cm
Nodes (N)	None	Nodes involved but mobile	Nodes involved but immobile	
Metastases (M)	None	Metastases		

Fig. 12.30 TNM staging system of breast cancer.

Treatment

The options for treating breast cancer are the same three for most cancers:

- Surgery.
- Radiotherapy.
- Chemotherapy.

Surgical removal of the tumor is necessary if a cure is to be achieved. There are two options, depending on the size of the tumor:

- Simple mastectomy (removal of the affected breast).
- Lumpectomy (removal of the lump) along with a large area of surrounding tissue.

Radiotherapy is used to prevent local and lymphatic spread. The breast, chest wall, and surrounding lymph nodes are often irradiated.

Chemotherapy is aimed at preventing metastatic spread. The standard cytotoxic drugs are used along with tamoxifen, which is an estrogen receptor blocker. This drug causes symptoms of an early menopause in younger women.

- Describe the structure and location of the ovaries.
- Describe the development of an ovarian follicle in the first half of the cycle. How is the oocyte transported from the ovary to the uterus?
- Describe the structure and location of the uterus and cervix. How does the cervix differ from the body of the uterus?
- Describe the structure and location of the vagina and vulva.
- Describe the structure and location of the adult female breast.
- Describe the synthesis and regulation of the three types of ovarian sex steroid.
- List the major effects of estrogens and progesterone.
- Describe the hormonal changes during the menstrual cycle.
- Describe the ovarian changes during the menstrual cycle.
- Describe the endometrial changes during the menstrual cycle.
- Discuss the presentation, diagnosis, and treatment of pelvic inflammatory disease. Which organisms are usually responsible?
- Describe the hormonal changes and symptoms of polycystic ovarian syndrome.
- List the common types of ovarian cysts and tumors along with a brief description of each. How are they treated?
- Describe the presentation, diagnosis, and treatment of endometriosis. How does it differ from adenomyosis?
- List the conditions that can be caused by excess estrogen.
- Describe the presentation, diagnosis, and treatment of fibroids and endometrial carcinoma.
- List the common causes of amenorrhea, menorrhagia, and dysmenorrhea.
- Describe the diagnosis, treatment, and natural progression of cervical intraepithelial neoplasia.
- Discuss common infections of the vagina and vulva.
- List the common causes of lumps in the breast. How are they investigated in clinic?

13. The Male Reproductive System

The male reproductive system must perform two main functions:
- Spermatogenesis—production of sperm (male gamete).
- Ejaculation—expulsion of sperm into the vagina.

The testes begin to produce sperm after puberty and continue to do so until death. This process is regulated by three main hormones (Fig. 13.1):
- Follicle-stimulating hormone (FSH).
- Luteinizing hormone (LH).
- Testosterone.

The ejaculation of sperm is controlled by neural stimuli from the sympathetic system. The sperm are ejected along with seminal fluid that protects them and provides nutrients.

After reading this chapter you should be able to:
- Visualize the anatomy of the male reproductive system.
- Describe the hormones that regulate the male reproductive system.
- Understand the process of sperm production.
- Discuss the common disorders of the male reproductive system.

Important terms:
Inguinal canal: a canal allowing passage of the testes and associated vessels from the abdominal cavity to the scrotum
Androgen: male sex steroids (e.g., testosterone)
Spermatozoa: the medical term for sperm
Spermatid: final stage in the development of a spermatozoon
Spermatogenesis: the process of sperm production

Organization

The male reproductive system consists of five main components:
- Testes—produce the sperm.
- Epididymis—stores and matures the sperm.
- Ductus deferens—transmits the sperm from the epididymis to the penis.
- Prostate and seminal vesicles—secrete seminal fluid to support and protect the ejaculated sperm.
- Penis—becomes erect to penetrate the vagina and deposit the sperm at the cervix.

All of these components lie outside the peritoneal cavity; however, there is no opening into this cavity comparable to the infundibulum of the fallopian tubes in the female. Each of these components is discussed individually in the following sections. Their locations are shown in Fig. 13.2, and their blood supply, lymphatics, and innervation are shown in Fig. 13.3.

Testes
The testes are two oval-shaped organs that produce sperm (the male gametes) in response to gonadotropins (LH + FSH) from the pituitary gland and testosterone from the Leydig cells of the testes. They are suspended in the saclike scrotum by the spermatic cord; this keeps their temperature 2–3°C lower than body temperature. If their temperature rises, sperm production ceases. Each testis is surrounded by a capsule of three layers (starting nearest the testis):
- Tunica vasculosa—loose connective tissue with blood vessels.
- Tunica albuginea—fibrous connective tissue.
- Tunica vaginalis—derived from peritoneum, it also surrounds the epididymis.

Microstructure
Fibrous septa divide each testis into about 300 lobules, each containing 1–4 seminiferous tubules

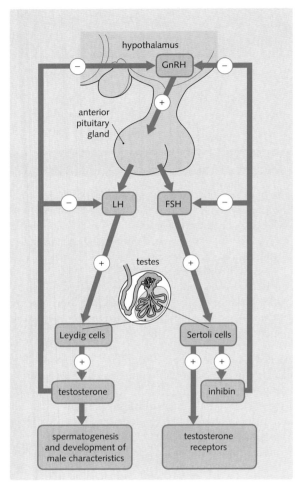

Fig. 13.1 Hormonal regulation of the male reproductive system. (FSH, follicle-stimulating hormone; GnRH, gonadotropin-releasing hormone; LH, luteinizing hormone.)

that produce sperm. The seminiferous tubules are closed loops lined with a specialized epithelium that contains two types of cells:
• Germinal epithelium containing spermatogonia that undergo meiosis to give rise to haploid sperm.
• Sertoli cells that support the developing sperm and secrete testicular fluid into the tubules.

The process of sperm production (spermatogenesis) is discussed on p. 156. Between the seminiferous tubules there are vessels and clusters of testosterone-secreting interstitial (Leydig) cells. The microstructure of the seminiferous tubules is shown in Fig. 13.4.

Inside the testis, the loops of the seminiferous tubules drain into the rete testis. These are convoluted networks of ducts that are lined by simple cuboidal epithelial cells with microvilli and a single flagella. All the vessels that support the testis enter the testis capsule at the location of the rete testis. The sperm pass from the rete testis to the epididymis via about 15 efferent ductules lined by ciliated epithelium.

The prefix *orch-* is used to describe processes relating to the testes and is derived from the Greek word for the testes (*orchis*). This prefix is also used for a group of plants (orchids), perhaps because their roots resemble testes or owing to potential aphrodisiac properties.

Epididymis

The epididymis is a firm, comma-shaped structure attached posteriorly to the top of the testis within the scrotum. Normally it can be distinguished from the testis by palpation. It is described in three sections:
• Head—superior section where the efferent ductules enter.
• Body—between the head and tail.
• Tail—inferior section, continuous with the ductus deferens.

The epididymis contains a single, 5 m long, tightly coiled tube formed by the fusion of the efferent ductules from the rete testis. Testicular fluid is partially reabsorbed by the tall columnar epithelium with long microvilli (stereocilia). The sperm pass slowly through this tube to reach the ductus deferens at the tail of the epididymis. The epididymis is surrounded by a fibrous capsule that is separated from the testis by the tunica vasculosa and tunica albuginea, except at the head where the testis and epididymis join. The tunica vaginalis surrounds the testis and the fibrous capsule of the epididymis.

Scrotum

The scrotum is a saclike structure that contains both testes, the epididymis, and the start of the ductus

Fig. 13.2 Arrangement of the male reproductive system. This diagram is not to scale.

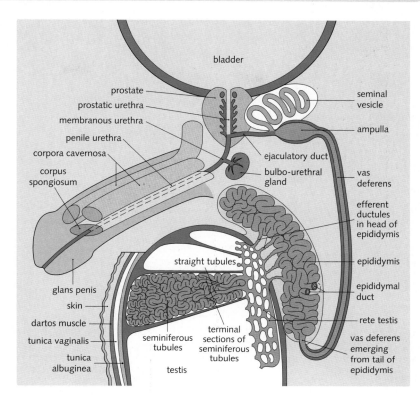

Fig. 13.3 The blood supply, lymphatics, and innervation of the male reproductive organs.

Blood supply, lymphatics, and innervation of the male reproductive organs				
Organ	**Arterial supply**	**Venous drainage**	**Innervation**	**Lymphatic drainage**
Testis	Testicular arteries from the aorta via the spermatic cord	Pampiniform plexus, which forms the testicular veins. Left drains into the left renal vein, right into the inferior vena cava	Sympathetic innervation via the splanchnic nerves	Paraaortic lymph nodes
Scrotum	Pudendal arteries	Scrotal veins	Branches of the genitofemoral, ilioinguinal, and pudendal nerves	Superficial inguinal lymph nodes
Prostate	Vesicular and rectal branches of the internal iliac artery	Prostatic venous plexus drains into the internal iliac veins	Parasympathetic via splanchnic nerves; sympathetic from inferior hypogastric plexus	Internal iliac and sacral lymph nodes
Penis	Internal pudendal arteries	Venous plexus, which joins the prostatic venous plexus	Branches of the pudendal nerve	Superficial inguinal lymph nodes

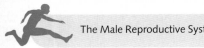
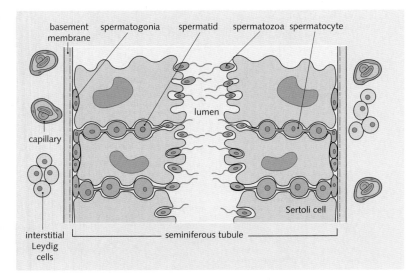

Fig. 13.4 Microstructure of the seminiferous tubule.

Layers of the abdominal wall, spermatic cord, and scrotum		
Abdominal layer	**Spermatic cord layer**	**Scrotal layer**
Skin	None	Skin
Superficial fascia	None	Dartos muscle
External oblique aponeurosis	External spermatic fascia	External spermatic fascia
Internal oblique muscle and fascia	Cremasteric muscle and fascia	Cremasteric muscle and fascia
Transversalis fascia (not the muscle)	Internal spermatic fascia	Internal spermatic fascia

Fig. 13.5 Layers of the abdominal wall, spermatic cord, and scrotum.

deferens. The skin is usually pigmented and wrinkled with a line down the midline called the scrotal raphe.

Microstructure

The wall of the scrotum is formed by five layers; three of these continue as the covering of the spermatic cord. All five are continuous with the abdominal wall, from which they are derived. They are described in Fig. 13.5 and their development is shown in Fig. 11.5. Two muscles are found in the scrotum:

- Dartos muscle—contracts the scrotal skin in response to cold.
- Cremasteric muscle—retracts the testis toward the abdomen.

Ductus (vas) deferens

The ductus deferens is the continuation of the epididymis on each side of the scrotum. It transports sperm from the epididymis to the ejaculatory ducts during the emission phase of an ejaculation (see Chapter 14). It has three muscular layers to propel the spermatozoa along its 40 cm length and a lining epithelium similar to that found in the epididymis. The ductus deferens is palpable in the scrotum; this allows male sterilization with only minimal incisions.

Once the ductus deferens enters the abdomen in the spermatic cord, it passes along the lateral wall of the pelvis, external to the peritoneum. It crosses the ureter and descends to the base of the bladder. The duct widens into the ampulla before the junction with the duct of the seminal vesicle.

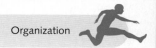

Spermatic cord

The spermatic cord is formed at the deep inguinal ring of the abdominal wall and passes along the inguinal canal and then inferiorly in the scrotum to the testis. It contains five structures:

- Ductus deferens.
- Testicular artery.
- Pampiniform plexus of veins.
- Autonomic nerves (including the sensory nerves that transmit pain from the testis).
- Lymph vessels.

These structures are surrounded by three layers (see Fig. 13.5).

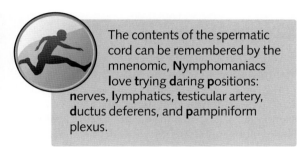

The contents of the spermatic cord can be remembered by the mnemonic, **N**ymphomaniacs **l**ove **t**rying **d**aring **p**ositions: **n**erves, **l**ymphatics, **t**esticular artery, **d**uctus deferens, and **p**ampiniform plexus.

Seminal vesicles and ejaculatory ducts

The seminal vesicles are two 6 cm long, pear-shaped structures found above the prostate between the bladder and rectum. They were originally believed to store sperm (hence their name), but in fact they secrete a fructose-rich, alkaline fluid that forms 70% of ejaculated semen. The duct of the seminal vesicles joins the ductus deferens at the ampulla behind the prostate. Together they form the 1 cm long ejaculatory ducts that pass forward into the prostate gland. The ejaculatory ducts open into the prostatic urethra just before it leaves the prostate (see Fig. 13.2).

Microstructure

Each seminal vesicle is formed from a slightly coiled tube that is 15 cm long. It is covered by two layers of smooth muscle and an external fibroelastic layer. The tube is lined by tall, secretory columnar epithelium.

The ejaculatory ducts have no muscular coverings. They are lined by tall, columnar cells and smaller, rounded cells.

Prostate

The prostate is a walnut-sized gland that surrounds the prostatic urethra at the base of the bladder. The posterior surface is palpable by rectal examination; it should feel regular and firm with a midline groove. The prostate secretes seminal fluid into the urethra during ejaculation. This fluid is rich in acid phosphatase and citric acid.

Inferior to the prostate, the two small bulbourethral glands secrete sugar-rich mucus into the membranous urethra. This fluid may lubricate the urethra prior to ejaculation.

Microstructure

The prostate gland is composed of three concentric rings of glands surrounded by smooth muscle and a fibrous capsule. The smooth muscle contracts during ejaculation to squeeze the prostatic secretions into the urethra. The three types of gland are:

- Inner periurethral (mucosal) glands—these secrete directly into the urethra, which they surround; they can undergo benign prostatic hypertrophy.
- Outer periurethral (submucosal) glands—these secrete into the urethra via short ducts; they can undergo benign prostatic hypertrophy.
- Peripheral zone glands—this ring of glands is incomplete anteriorly; they secrete via long ducts and can give rise to prostatic cancer.

The glands are lined by tall columnar epithelium with a few flat basal cells. Their secretory activity is dependent on testosterone.

Penis

The penis is the outlet for urine and semen. The internal structure of the penis is shown in Fig. 13.6. It is described in three sections:

- Root—the section that is attached to the perineum.
- Body—the free portion, also called the shaft; it is suspended from the pubic symphysis.
- Glans—the sensitive, distal end of the body that includes the external opening of the urethra.

The edge of the glans that joins the body of the penis is called the corona. The penis is composed of three cylinders of erectile tissue, each surrounded by a fibrous capsule called the tunica albuginea. Surrounding these structures is a layer of thin,

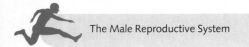

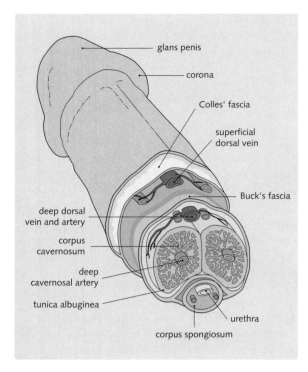

Fig. 13.6 Internal structure of the penis.

pigmented skin; over the glans this skin is called the foreskin or prepuce. The three cylinders of erectile tissue are:

- Two corpora cavernosa—these large cylinders form the dorsum (upper surface) and sides of the penis; they form the crura that support the erect penis in the root.
- One corpus spongiosum—this smaller ventral (lower surface) cylinder surrounds the spongy urethra; it forms the whole of the glans and is called the bulb at the root.

The majority of vessels and nerves supplying the penis are found on the dorsal (upper surface) side. The arteries within the corpora cavernosa are called the deep arteries.

Microstructure and mechanism of erection
The erectile tissues consist of interconnecting vascular spaces that fill with blood during an erection. Erection is normally prevented by shunts between the helicine arteries (branches of the deep arteries) and the deep veins. Stimulation by the parasympathetic nervous system constricts these

shunts so that blood fills sinuses of the cavernosa. The increase in pressure collapses the thin veins, preventing blood from leaving, and erection occurs. Ejaculation requires sympathetic stimulation, which inhibits the parasympathetic system, causing a loss of erection.

Remember "**p**oint and **s**hoot" to recall the function of the **p**arasympathetic and **s**ympathetic innervation of the penis.

Spermatogenesis

Early spermatogenesis
Spermatogenesis is the process by which haploid (23-chromosome) spermatozoa are formed from diploid (46-chromosome) stem cells called spermatogonia. Spermatogonia are found close to the basement membrane of the seminiferous tubules. There are three types:

- Dark A cells (Ad)—these are the true stem cells; they divide by mitosis to produce more Ad cells and a few Ap cells.
- Pale A cells (Ap)—these represent the first step toward differentiation into spermatocytes; they divide by mitosis to produce more Ap cells and a few B cells.
- B cells—these divide by mitosis to produce more B cells and a few primary spermatocytes.

The mitotic cell divisions of spermatogonia are incomplete, so that the daughter cells remain connected by thin cytoplasmic bridges. These bridges remain throughout the development of the spermatocytes and spermatids until the spermatozoa are released into the lumen of the seminiferous tubule.

Meiosis
The primary spermatocytes undergo meiosis, which is the special form of cell division that produces haploid gametes. The first division forms two haploid secondary spermatocytes. The second meiotic division occurs soon afterward to form four haploid spermatids.

> Meiosis in the male gives rise to four functional, haploid sperm. Meiosis in the female produces only one functional haploid oocyte; the other haploid cells are nonfunctional polar bodies.

As meiosis progresses, the germinal cells migrate from the basal membrane to the apex of the Sertoli cells (toward the lumen of the seminiferous tubule). The Sertoli cells perform a number of functions that are essential for spermatogenesis:

- They provide nutrients and remove waste.
- They phagocytose excess cytoplasm or poorly developing spermatids.
- Tight junctions between cells prevent antibodies reaching the haploid cells; they form a blood–testes barrier.
- They produce androgen-binding protein to raise the local androgen concentration.

Spermiogenesis

Having completed the meiotic division, the haploid spermatids are small, spherical cells that must still develop the structure of a mature spermatozoon. This process is called spermiogenesis and takes place on the surface of Sertoli cells in four stages:

- Golgi phase—the Golgi apparatus begins to form an acrosomal vesicle over the nucleus while the centrioles migrate to the other end of the cell. One of the centrioles begins to form the tail.
- Cap phase—the acrosomal vesicle surrounds the front of the nucleus while the nucleus condenses.
- Acrosome phase—the nucleus becomes smaller and lengthens, squeezing the acrosome and cell membrane together. Mitochondria migrate toward the tail to form the "middle piece," while microtubules condense behind the nucleus to form the neck or "manchette."
- Maturation phase—excess cytoplasm is "pinched off" and phagocytosed by the Sertoli cell. The completed spermatozoon is then released into the lumen of the seminiferous tubule by breaking off the cytoplasmic bridges.

Final maturation

The maturation from Ad cells to released spermatozoa in the seminiferous tubule lumen takes about 64 days. Further maturation occurs as they pass through the epididymis to make the spermatozoa motile and capable of fertilization. The spermatozoa are pushed through the rete testis and efferent ductules by the movement of testicular fluid, caused by the action of the cilia, to reach the epididymis.

The epithelium of the epididymis secretes glycoproteins that bind to the surface of the spermatozoa causing the phospholipid membrane to be remodeled. The epididymis is also capable of removing degenerate or poorly formed spermatozoa by phagocytosis. Spermatozoa pass through the epididymis by the movement of testicular fluid and peristalsis.

The fully mature spermatozoa are stored in the epididymis until they are ejaculated or broken down. The epididymis contracts during orgasm to transport the spermatozoa into the ductus deferens. The ductus deferens has a thick muscular layer that propels the sperm along the duct at ejaculation.

Continuous fertility

After puberty males are always fertile, although their fertility may decline with age. Continuous fertility is achieved because there is a population of stem cells in the testes (cf. ovaries):

- A new cycle of spermatogenesis starts every 16 days (and lasts 64 days) at each point in the tubule.
- Sertoli cells are arranged in bands in which cycles of spermatogenesis begin at different times.
- Cycles are at different stages in different segments of the seminiferous tubules.

Mature spermatozoon

Mature spermatozoa have a distinct head and tail (Fig. 13.7). The head is composed largely of condensed chromatin in the pointed nucleus; the front is surrounded by a giant lysosome called the acrosome that allows the spermatozoa to penetrate the oocyte.

The tail is a long and specialized flagellum derived from one of the centrioles. It has the usual pattern of microtubules with nine outer pairs around a central pair; this structure is called the axoneme. There are four sections of the tail:

- Neck—this narrowing contains the centrioles connected to the axoneme.
- Middle piece—the axoneme is surrounded by elongated spiral mitochondria. These release

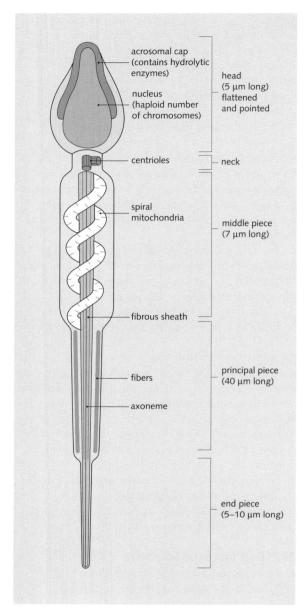

Fig. 13.7 Microstructure of a mature spermatozoon. This diagram is not to scale.

acrosomal cap (contains hydrolytic enzymes)

nucleus (haploid number of chromosomes)

head (5 μm long) flattened and pointed

centrioles

neck

spiral mitochondria

middle piece (7 μm long)

fibrous sheath

fibers

axoneme

principal piece (40 μm long)

end piece (5–10 μm long)

energy to drive the axoneme by the anaerobic respiration of fructose.
- Principal piece—this forms the majority of the tail. It contains fibers, which are not present in the smaller end piece.
- End piece.

Hormones

Testicular sex steroids

The testes secrete 95% of the male sex steroids called androgens; the adrenal cortex is responsible for the remaining 5%. The main androgen is testosterone.

Testicular androgens are secreted by the interstitial Leydig cells found between the seminiferous tubules. They convert cholesterol into the steroid testosterone by a series of reactions. The Leydig cells also secrete small quantities of estrogens and progestins as byproducts of testosterone synthesis.

Testosterone is a strong androgen. However, some target tissues can convert it to the more potent form called dihydrotestosterone (DHT). The conversion requires the 5-reductase enzyme and occurs in:
- Seminiferous tubules.
- Prostate gland.
- Skin.

Testosterone is transported in the plasma by sex hormone-binding globulin (SHBG) or albumin. It acts via intracellular receptors to regulate protein synthesis producing the actions shown in Fig. 13.8. The main actions are:
- Growth and development of the male reproductive tract.
- Development of male secondary sexual characteristics (e.g., male hair pattern, muscle growth).
- Stimulation of spermatogenesis.
- Stimulation of growth and the fusion of the growth plates of the long bones (see Chapter 9).

Control of testicular steroid production

Testosterone synthesis and release are controlled by the same hormones in the male as estrogen synthesis in the female. Gonadotropin-releasing hormone (GnRH) from the hypothalamus is transported to the anterior pituitary gland by the portal veins. It stimulates the gonadotroph cells to secrete gonadotropins (LH and FSH). This process is described in more detail in Chapter 2.

LH acts on the Leydig cells to stimulate the first step in testosterone production. Testosterone feeds back to the hypothalamus and pituitary gland to inhibit LH release, but it has little effect on FSH.

Fig. 13.8 Actions of testosterone.

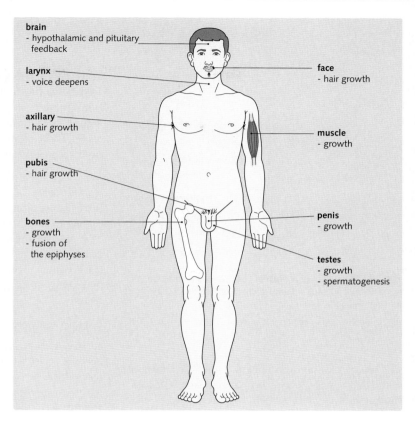

brain
- hypothalamic and pituitary feedback

larynx
- voice deepens

axillary
- hair growth

pubis
- hair growth

bones
- growth
- fusion of the epiphyses

face
- hair growth

muscle
- growth

penis
- growth

testes
- growth
- spermatogenesis

FSH acts on the Sertoli cells; it increases the number of testosterone receptors to stimulate spermatogenesis. It also causes inhibin release from the Sertoli cells, which feeds back to the hypothalamus and pituitary gland to inhibit further FSH release. It has little effect on LH.

Other testicular hormones

The fetal Sertoli cells produce the müllerian inhibiting substance (MIS; described in Chapter 11). This hormone prevents development of the female internal genitalia by causing the müllerian ducts to regress.

Disorders of the testes and epididymis

Congenital abnormalities and regression

Cryptorchidism

Cryptorchidism is the medical term for testes that have failed to descend into the scrotum. It is a common finding in newborns (3–4%), especially premature babies, and it can affect one or both testes. An undescended testis must be distinguished from a testis retracted due to cold (by the cremasteric muscle). It is undescended only if it cannot be massaged into the scrotum or cannot be felt at all. An impalpable testis usually lies in the inguinal canal or at its abdominal entrance (deep inguinal ring). The descent of the testis and formation of the scrotum are described in Chapter 11.

In the majority of babies, this condition resolves with no treatment. However, if the testes still have not descended after a year, their development can be affected. Failure to treat the condition at this stage causes a high risk of infertility because the spermatogonia (stem cells) need cooler temperatures to survive. Testosterone production is not affected because the Leydig cells are not as sensitive. Cryptorchidism also carries a higher risk of germ-cell testicular cancer in later life. It is corrected by surgically fixing the testes in the scrotum—an operation called orchidopexy.

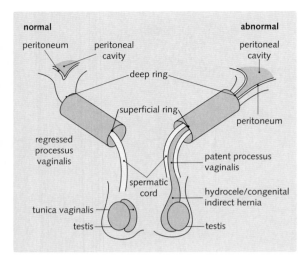

Fig. 13.9 Diagram of a normal testis and one with a persistent processus vaginalis, causing a hydrocele or indirect hernia.

The cause of cryptorchidism is unknown, but both testosterone deficiency and estrogen excess (from the environment) have been suggested.

Abnormalities of the tunica vaginalis
Congenital hernia
The processus vaginalis is a tube of peritoneum that connects the tunica vaginalis to the abdominal cavity through the inguinal canal in the fetus. This structure is shown in Fig. 11.5; a persistent processus vaginalis is shown in Fig. 13.9. If it fails to close, intestines may pass into the scrotum, causing an indirect inguinal hernia (through the inguinal canal). This condition is more common in the presence of undescended testes. It must be corrected surgically to prevent the risk of bowel obstruction and ischemia due to the narrow inguinal ring. Femoral and direct inguinal hernias are very rare in neonates.

Congenital hydrocele
If the processus vaginalis persists but is too small for a hernia to form, peritoneal fluid may enter the tunica vaginalis, causing a hydrocele. This presents as a transluminable swelling within the scrotum that cannot be distinguished from the testis. It often regresses without treatment; if not, it should be drained. Recurring or large hydroceles require surgical correction. Throughout life hydroceles are the most common cause of intrascrotal swelling; the

fluid may be a sign of inflammation or neoplasia of the testis.

Trauma and vascular disturbances
Testicular hemorrhage
Hematoma
Trauma to the groin can cause bleeding within the testes. If the bleeding remains within the intact tunica albuginea, it is called a testicular hematoma. It is extremely painful.

Hematocele
If the tunica albuginea splits, blood can collect in the tunica vaginalis, forming a hematocele. This can also be caused by a testicular tumor in the absence of trauma. If the hemorrhage is not drained, the blood can coagulate and constrict around the testis, potentially causing ischemia and necrosis of the testis.

Torsion of the testis
Torsion of the testis occurs when the spermatic cord becomes twisted, blocking the blood vessels from a testis. It can occur only if the testes are free to rotate within the scrotum owing to a congenital abnormality. Normally the tunica vaginalis attaches to the spermatic cord close to its origin from the epididymis to prevent rotation. In the abnormal state the tunica vaginalis attaches further along the spermatic cord. If the testis rotates excessively, the pampiniform venous plexus within the spermatic cord can become twisted and occluded. Arterial blood continues to enter the affected testis but cannot leave, so the testis swells and undergoes venous infarction, leading to hemorrhagic necrosis.

Testicular torsion is most common in children and adolescents following mild trauma, especially sporting injuries. It presents with the sudden onset of pain and tenderness in one testicle. On palpation the affected testis is high in the scrotum, and the spermatic cord may be thickened. With time, the pain becomes severe with vomiting and dull abdominal pain as the affected testicle swells.

It can be difficult to distinguish the later stages of torsion from acute orchitis. Since testicular torsion is an acute surgical emergency, an unclear diagnosis needs surgical exploration. Without treatment the testis will undergo necrosis and need to be removed. Early surgery (before about 6 hours) can untwist and save the testicle; both testes should be secured to the scrotum to prevent recurrence.

Varicocele

When the pampiniform plexus in the spermatic cord becomes varicose (dilated and tortuous), it is called a varicocele. It is found in about 10% of young men, and in 90% of these the spermatic cord on the left is affected. This may be due to the higher pressure in the renal vein compared with the inferior vena cava (see Fig. 13.3). The underlying cause is not known, although rapidly developing varicoceles may very rarely be caused by carcinoma of the left kidney obstructing the left testicular vein.

The testes should be examined with the patient standing up because the blood often drains out of the plexus when the patient lies down. This response is inhibited if there is an underlying obstruction (e.g., renal carcinoma). The full varicocele feels like a "bag of worms" above the testes.

Occasionally varicoceles present with discomfort, but the vast majority are asymptomatic. The excess blood can warm the testes, reducing the fertility of the patient. Varicoceles can be treated surgically, but this is considered only if discomfort or infertility is present.

Inflammation and infection
Acute orchitis and epididymitis

Inflammation of the testis is called orchitis, while inflammation of the epididymis is called epididymitis. These two conditions often occur together and are managed in a similar manner. The following acute bacterial infections are the most common causes of epididymo-orchitis:

- *Escherichia coli* and other coliforms (from a urinary tract infection [UTI]).
- *Chlamydia trachomatis* (a sexually transmitted disease [STD]).
- *Neisseria gonorrhoeae* (STD).

Patients complain of either one or two painful, tender, and enlarged testes, which may be accompanied by a secondary hydrocele, general malaise, fever, or headache. It is diagnosed from the history and examination of the urine, but surgical exploration is often performed to exclude testicular torsion. Antibiotics are used to treat the infection; otherwise scarring and infertility can develop.

Other infections
Mumps

The mumps virus often causes viral orchitis if it infects postpubertal males. It tends to cause a single tender and enlarged testis. Rarely it can cause infertility if the disease is bilateral.

Tuberculosis

Tuberculosis (TB) can infect the epididymis and testis from the blood or urinary tract. It causes chronic granuloma with caseous necrosis that can persist long after infections at other sites have been successfully treated.

Syphilis

The rare tertiary stage of *Treponema pallidum* infection (i.e., syphilis) can produce the characteristic chronic syphilitic granuloma (called gumma) in the testes.

Autoimmune granulomatous orchitis

Granulomatous orchitis is a rare autoimmune disease that causes chronic inflammation of the testis and destruction of the seminiferous tubules. The tight junctions between the Sertoli cells normally prevent an immune reaction against the developing haploid sperm, but this barrier appears to break down.

It presents in a similar manner to a testicular tumor; the affected testis becomes firm and enlarged, sometimes with a secondary hydrocele.

Epididymal cysts

Epididymal cysts often develop in adult life and are found in the head of the epididymis. The cysts contain either a watery fluid or a milky, fluid-containing sperm (this can be called a spermatocele). They usually present as painless swellings that can be distinguished from the testis and transluminated. If they cause symptoms they can be removed surgically.

Neoplastic disorders

Tumors of the testes are important because they are the most common type of cancer in young adult males. They are often highly malignant but frequently curable with early detection. If undetected, they can spread to the paraaortic lymph nodes or, by blood, to the lungs and liver. Patients often present with:

- A painless, enlarged, hard testis or testicular lump.
- Secondary hydrocele.
- Gynecomastia (due to human chorionic gonadotropin [hCG] or estrogen secretion).
- Metastases to the lungs or liver.

Testicular ultrasound is used to distinguish cystic swellings from testicular tumors. Two tumor markers can be detected in the blood; these are used in diagnosis and monitoring treatment:

- α-Fetoprotein (AFP).
- Human chorionic gonadotropin (hCG).

Other tests are aimed at detecting any tumor spread:
- Chest x-ray to check the lungs.
- Abdominal computed tomography (CT) for liver and lymph nodes.

Testicular carcinoma is treated by orchidectomy (removal of testis), using an inguinal incision. The spermatic cord should be clamped before the testis is removed to help prevent venous spread. If the testis appears normal and on-the-spot biopsy analysis does not reveal malignancy, the testis can be returned to the scrotum. Confirmed carcinoma is followed up with radiotherapy or chemotherapy, depending on the type of testicular tumor. The prognosis also depends on the type of tumor, but it is generally very good. If the lymph nodes are not involved, there is almost a 100% 5-year survival rate.

There are two groups of testicular tumor:
- Germ-cell tumors (97%).
- Sex-cord stromal tumors (3%).

The different types within these groups are shown in Fig. 13.10.

Germ-cell tumors

Germ-cell tumors develop from the gamete-producing spermatogonia in the seminiferous tubules. They are predisposed by undescended testes. There are three types of germ-cell tumors, described below.

Seminoma

This tumor accounts for 50% of germ-cell tumors, and it is most common in 40- to 50-year-old men. It presents as a painless enlargement of one testis, and histology reveals a creamy-white tumor. Ten per cent of tumors secrete hCG as an ectopic hormone. They usually spread via the lymphatics. They are very sensitive to radiotherapy, so the prognosis is good.

Teratoma

These tumors are most common in 20- to 30-year-old men. Teratomas are composed of a number of tissue types derived from endoderm, mesoderm, and ectoderm. Well-differentiated tumors are usually benign; more commonly, the tissues are undifferentiated and immature, causing a highly malignant tumor (cf. ovarian teratomas). There are a number of categories of teratoma according to their histological appearance. They often secrete α-fetoprotein and hCG because they develop from yolk sac and trophoblast tissues. They metastasize early to the lungs and have a poorer prognosis than seminomas, but they are very sensitive to chemotherapy.

Mixed tumors

Some tumors contain different types of teratomas or a combination of seminoma and teratoma tissues. Their behavior and prognosis depend largely on the types of teratoma involved.

Sex-cord stromal tumors

Tumors that develop from the other tissues in the testes are called sex-cord stromal tumors. They account for only 3% of testicular tumors. There are three types, described below.

Types of testicular tumor and the age group they commonly affect			
Tumor type	Tumor	Main age group (years)	Testicular malignancy (%)
Germ-cell tumors	Seminoma	40–50	50
	Teratoma	20–30	35
	Mixed tumor	20–40	12
Sex-cord stromal tumors	Leydig cell tumor	Any	<1
	Sertoli cell tumor	40–50	<1
	Primary lymphoma	65+	2

Fig. 13.10 Frequency of types of testicular tumors and the age group that they commonly affect.

Leydig cell tumors

These are also called interstitial or stromal cell tumors. They can occur at any age and are usually benign. They frequently secrete testosterone or estrogens, which can affect the reproductive system.

Sertoli cell tumors

These are also called androblastomas or sex-cord tumors. They can occur at any age, but they are most common between 40 and 50 years of age. They are often benign, but they may secrete ectopic estrogens.

Primary lymphoma

In the elderly, lymphomas can develop in the testes; aggressively malignant non-Hodgkin's lymphomas are the most common type of testicular tumor in those aged 65 years or over.

Disorders of the prostate

Inflammation and infection
Bacterial prostatitis

The prostate can become inflamed owing to bacterial infection, which can follow an acute or chronic course.

Acute

Bacteria reach the prostate from the urethra; thus the common causative organisms are those that cause urinary tract infections or are sexually transmitted:
- *E. coli* and other coliforms (UTI).
- *Neisseria gonorrhoeae* (also called gonococcus; an STD).
- *Chlamydia trachomatis* (STD).

Patients present with increased urinary frequency, penile and testicular pain, and systemic illness (e.g., fever). The prostate gland becomes enlarged and acutely tender on rectal examination. Severe inflammation can obstruct the urethra, causing urinary retention, and abscesses may develop, leading to a urethral discharge of pus.

It is diagnosed from urine culture and treated with appropriate antibiotics (e.g., trimethoprim or erythromycin).

Chronic

Failure to cure acute prostatitis can lead to chronic prostatitis. It can also be caused by tuberculosis infection, often from the kidney or epididymis. The symptoms are similar to acute prostatitis but ill-defined and less severe. It is managed in the same manner as an acute infection or with treatment for TB.

Abacterial prostatitis

Chronic prostatitis can also be caused by noninfective disease in which anti-inflammatory drugs may ease symptoms. The exact etiology is unknown, but theories include:
- Allergy, since it is associated with asthma.
- Autoimmune disease.
- Urine reflux.

Benign prostatic hypertrophy

The prostate gland begins to enlarge from the age of 45 years. By the age of 70 years, the vast majority of men have some benign enlargement, making it the most common disease of the prostate gland. It is caused by nodular hyperplasia (increased cell division forming nodules) of the inner and outer periurethral glands of the prostate. The underlying fault is believed to be an imbalance between estrogen and androgen secretion. It does not develop into prostate carcinoma.

The enlarged prostate gland can compress the urethra, causing difficulty urinating called "prostatism." This occurs only in more severely affected men and is characterized by the following symptoms:
- Increased frequency of urination.
- Increased urgency.
- Reduced size and force of urinary stream.
- Hesitancy and interruption.
- Dribbling at the end of urination.

If the hypertrophy is very severe, urinary obstruction may result due to compression of the internal urethral sphincter. Chronic urine retention follows, leading to recurrent urinary tract infections or renal impairment.

Benign prostatic hypertrophy is diagnosed by the history and rectal examination in the absence of evidence for renal failure or carcinoma of the prostate. Mild disease can be treated medically with α-blockers to lower prostate tone. More progressive disease may be treated by transurethral resection of the prostate (TURP); however, this procedure can often cause retrograde ejaculation and occasionally impotence. The histology of the resected prostate tissue should be examined under a microscope to exclude malignancy.

Neoplastic disorders

Prostatic carcinoma is the second most common male carcinoma after lung cancer. It usually affects the elderly, but the incidence is currently increasing in younger men. It is an adenocarcinoma that develops in the glands of the peripheral zone of the prostate. It is not preceded by the benign hyperplasia discussed above, since the two conditions affect different zones of the gland.

The risk factors for prostate cancer are not known. They are often sensitive to testosterone, but an endocrine imbalance does not appear to be the underlying cause.

Adenocarcinomas of the prostate show a wide variation in behavior. Some remain confined to the prostate for many years, whereas others metastasize early and are highly invasive.

Presentation

Since prostate carcinoma develops in the external glands of the prostate, away from the urethra, it is initially asymptomatic. As the tumor grows, it begins to compress the urethra, causing symptoms similar to those of benign prostatic hyperplasia, although they tend to progress more rapidly. This is a relatively late feature. Systemic and metastatic symptoms can be the first signs in advanced disease, including:

- Weight loss.
- General malaise.
- Anemia.
- Back pain.

Rectal examination can reveal a hard nodule on the posterior surface of the prostate gland. As the tumor grows, the median groove of the gland is obliterated. The staging system of prostate tumors is shown in Fig. 13.11.

Diagnosis and investigation

The possibility of prostate cancer should be excluded in all patients with symptoms of prostatism. Raised levels of the blood-borne tumor marker called prostate-specific antigen (PSA) suggest carcinoma. This marker can also be used to monitor treatment. Blood specimens for PSA measurement should be taken prior to rectal examination, since this can raise the levels. Further investigation includes:

- Transrectal ultrasound.
- Rectal or transurethral needle biopsy.
- Bone x-rays to locate metastases.

Treatment

The prostate can be removed by TURP, though this procedure carries a high risk of retrograde ejaculation (into the bladder, causing infertility) or, less commonly, impotence. Resection is performed in patients with urinary obstruction or late-stage tumors. Early-stage, asymptomatic tumors are often simply observed or treated with radiotherapy, although resection is recommended by some clinicians.

If the patient has incurable metastatic disease, the following medical treatments may help:

- Cyproterone acetate blocks androgen receptors, which can reduce tumor size and invasion.
- Continuous GnRH analogs can inhibit LH secretion from the pituitary gland, reducing testosterone secretion.

Staging and prognosis of prostate carcinoma			
Stage	**Description**	**Symptoms**	**Five-year survival (%)**
A1	Microscopic, focal, and well-differentiated tumors	None	95
A2	Microscopic, diffuse, and/or poorly differentiated tumors	None	80
B	Larger tumors that are palpable rectally	None	75
C	Tumors that involve the entire prostate gland ± local invasion	Prostatism	50
D	Metastatic spread to lymph nodes or organs including bones	Prostatism and systemic/metastatic symptoms	35

Fig. 13.11 Staging and prognosis of prostate carcinoma.

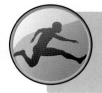

Because prostate cancer develops in the outer part of the prostate gland, it can be missed following transurethral biopsy.

Invasion and metastasis

Prostate carcinoma can spread in the following manners:

- Local spread within the gland and to the bladder and seminal vesicles.
- Lymphatic spread to the pelvic and paraaortic lymph nodes.
- Blood-borne spread to the bones, especially the pelvis, spine, and skull. It causes characteristic osteosclerotic lesions (i.e., bone is formed but not destroyed).

Disorders of the penis

Structural abnormalities
Congenital abnormalities
Hypospadias

The body of the penis is formed by the fusion of the urogenital folds round the urethra, as described in Chapter 11. This fusion can fail to varying degrees, resulting in hypospadias in which a meatus (opening) of the urethra forms along the ventral surface (underneath) of the penis, usually at the base of the glans (Fig. 13.12); it is the most common structural abnormality of the penis.

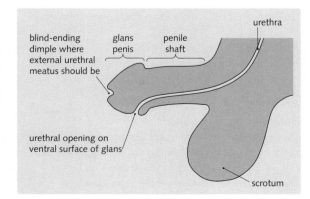

Fig. 13.12 Congenital hypospadias of the penis.

Hypospadias is caused by a deficiency of fetal testosterone production. It is associated with undescended testes, a "hooded" foreskin, and a downward curvature of the penis called congenital chordee. It can be corrected surgically using the foreskin.

Epispadias

This is a much rarer condition than hypospadias. It is a similar abnormality except that the urethral meatus is on the dorsal (top) surface of the penis, usually at the base of the body. It can cause urinary incontinence and recurrent urinary infections; it is corrected surgically. It is often associated with other abnormalities of the genitalia or urinary tract.

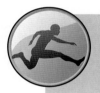

Never circumcise a child without checking for hypospadias because the foreskin is essential for the repair.

Phimosis

When the foreskin is too narrow to retract over the glans of the penis, the condition is called phimosis. It is normal after birth, but the foreskin should become retractable within a few years as the adhesions between the glans and foreskin break down. Phimosis can be congenital, but this is rare. More commonly, inflammation and fibrosis can cause narrowing following chronic or recurrent *Candida* infection. It is treated by topical steroids and exercising (gently stretching) the foreskin. Fibrosis can also be caused by balanitis xerotica obliterans (BXO), a disease of unknown etiology that causes inflammation of the glans and is treated by circumcision.

Phimosis causes dyspareunia (pain on intercourse) and, in severe cases, can obstruct urinary flow. Attempts to retract the fibrosed foreskin during erection can cause paraphimosis, in which the foreskin gets stuck behind the glans. The venous drainage becomes obstructed, restricting blood flow and causing edema. This is treated by squeezing the glans hard to allow the foreskin to return.

Inflammation and infection

The penis, especially the glans and urethra, is very susceptible to the same sexually transmitted infections that affect the female reproductive tract. A summary of these infections is shown in Fig. 13.13.

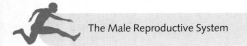

Summary of infections of the male reproductive tract			
Infection	**Organism**	**Symptoms**	**Treatment**
Herpes	Herpes simplex virus	Burning red blisters that may recur	Aciclovir if recurrent
Warts	Human papilloma virus	Growths on the penile skin	Podophyllotoxin cream
Gonorrhea	*Neisseria gonorrhoeae*	Dysuria, white urethral discharge	Penicillin or ceftriaxone
Nongonococcal urethritis	*Chlamydia trachomatis*	Milder dysuria, white urethral discharge	Erythromycin
Syphilis	*Treponema pallidum*	Ulcerated nodules, but may become systemic	Penicillin
Balanitis	*Candida albicans* (fungus)	Itching, white urethral discharge	Nystatin cream

Fig. 13.13 Summary of infections of the male genital tract.

Viral infection

The penis is prone to the same viral infections as the female vulva.

Herpes simplex

This is a sexually transmitted disease caused by herpes simplex virus (HSV, usually type II). It causes a recurrent, acute, and itchy skin infection. This progresses to form vesicles and painful skin erosions on the glans. The inguinal lymph nodes are often enlarged and painful.

The primary infection is often subclinical, but the virus then remains latent in the dorsal root ganglion that supplies that area of skin. The virus can be reactivated, causing recurrent attacks.

HSV can be diagnosed from viral culture of the fluid in the blisters. It is treated symptomatically (e.g., anesthetic cream), but aciclovir is often used for asymptomatic contacts, the initial infection, or immunosuppressed patients. The virus can be transmitted to other body parts on the hands; the eyes are particularly susceptible.

Genital warts

This is a sexually transmitted disease caused by human papilloma virus (HPV), of which there are many types. They cause benign, warty skin lesions called condyloma acuminatum, usually on the glans or inner surface of the foreskin.

The warts are treated with cryotherapy, in which a liquid nitrogen spray freezes and kills infected cells, or with podophyllin cream, which burns the infected cells chemically. The warts often recur despite treatment. Some strains of HPV predispose to malignant change of the penile skin (see below).

Bacterial infection

Gonorrhea

This sexually transmitted disease is caused by the bacterium *Neisseria gonorrhoeae* (often called gonococcus) that infects the distal urethra. Symptoms include dysuria (pain on urinating) and a discharge of a whitish pus. It is diagnosed by microscopy and culture of the pus to identify the organism and its antibiotic sensitivity; many gonococcus bacteria are now resistant to penicillin, in which case ceftriaxone is used.

Untreated gonorrhoea can lead to the following complications:
- Epididymo-orchitis.
- Proctitis (infection of the rectum).
- Infective arthritis.
- Septicemia.

Nongonococcal urethritis

More commonly the urethra can be infected by other bacteria, particularly *Chlamydia trachomatis*. It causes similar but milder symptoms. Epididymo-orchitis can also develop, but nongonococcal urethritis is usually cured by a single dose of erythromycin.

Syphilis

This sexually transmitted disease is caused by the bacterium *Treponema pallidum*, which initially infects the glans or the inner surface of the foreskin. Today syphilis is a rare disease; the complications are almost never seen because of effective treatment. The untreated disease follows four stages:

- Primary syphilis—a solitary, painless ulcerated nodule appears at the infection site. The inguinal lymph nodes become enlarged but not painful.
- Secondary syphilis—two months later a systemic disease may develop, including scaly rashes and mucosal ulcers over much of the body surface. It normally resolves after several months.
- Tertiary syphilis—rarely the disease may enter a chronic stage in which characteristic rubbery granulomas (called gummata) develop throughout the body.
- Quaternary syphilis—with time syphilis may affect the cardiovascular and central nervous system with potentially fatal effects.

Syphilis is diagnosed by serological (antibody) tests and treated with penicillin, which is also given to recent sexual contacts.

Fungal infection

The penis can be infected by *Candida albicans* causing thrush. This fungal infection is often an endogenous infection (from another body part), but it can be sexually transmitted.

Thrush causes inflammation of the foreskin and glans called balanitis producing red, itchy patches and a white urethral discharge. It is diagnosed by microscopy and culture of the discharge. Treatment is with topical antifungals (e.g., nystatin). Chronic balanitis can cause phimosis.

Neoplastic disorders
Benign tumors

Benign tumors of the penis take the form of warts caused by HPV. These are called condyloma acuminatum; they are discussed with the other viral infections of the penis.

Malignant tumors

Carcinoma of the penis is rare, but squamous cell carcinoma can develop in the penile skin. A series of dysplastic changes from carcinoma in situ to invasive carcinoma are grouped together as "penile intraepithelial neoplasia" (PIN). Dysplastic change affects elderly uncircumcised men. It is predisposed by poor hygiene and HPV infection.

The initial neoplasia is called Queyrat's erythroplasia. This is a raised, red plaque that is noninvasive but has the histological appearance of squamous cell carcinoma. It is usually found on the inner surface of the foreskin or the base of the glans.

With time this carcinoma in situ can develop into invasive squamous carcinoma of the penis. This is a slow-growing tumor with a warty appearance. It can spread to the inguinal lymph nodes.

PIN is treated with radiotherapy, partial or complete penile amputation, and lymph node dissection, depending on the extent of the tumor and its spread.

Disorders of the male breast

Gynecomastia

The male breast contains the same tissue components as the female breast in the undeveloped, prepubescent state. If the male breast enlarges, the condition is called gynecomastia. The development of the male breast in gynecomastia resembles the changes that the female breast undergoes during puberty; there is growth and development of the mammary ducts and connective tissues. It is caused by any condition or process that raises estrogen or lowers testosterone levels. It often occurs during puberty but will usually resolve with time. The underlying cause should be treated. Surgical removal of breast tissue may be performed in severe cases for cosmetic reasons.

Carcinoma

Breast carcinoma in men is very rare compared with women; it accounts for <1% of all breast cancer. The carcinoma is usually of the intraductal or infiltrating duct types (described in Chapter 12). It presents in elderly men as a breast lump or nipple discharge. The tumors have often metastasized to the axillary lymph nodes, lungs, brain, bone, or liver by the time of presentation; thus the prognosis is poor.

- Describe the structure and location of the testes.
- Describe the structure and layers of the epididymis and scrotum.
- Describe the course and layers of the spermatic cord. How do these relate to the abdomen and scrotum?
- Draw a diagram to illustrate the structure and location of the prostate.
- Describe the structure of the penis and the mechanism of erection.
- Name three hormones involved in the male reproductive system, along with their origins and actions.
- How is the male reproductive system regulated hormonally?
- Describe the process of spermatogenesis. Explain the roles of the Sertoli and Leydig cells.
- How is continuous fertility achieved?
- Draw a diagram to illustrate the structure of a mature sperm. What are the functions of the different components? Where are mature sperm stored?
- Name and briefly describe three congenital abnormalities of the testes.
- Compare testicular torsion and epididymo-orchitis. How are they treated?
- Describe the differential diagnosis of a scrotal lump.
- Name three types of testicular carcinoma, the cells from which they are derived, and the age groups that they affect.
- Describe the etiology, presentation, and treatment of benign prostatic hypertrophy. Is it premalignant?
- Describe the location, presentation, and treatment of prostatic carcinoma.
- Describe the common congenital malformations of the penis, along with three other conditions with which they are associated.
- Discuss four sexually transmitted diseases, including their presentation and treatment.
- Describe the series of changes seen in penile intraepithelial neoplasia.
- Compare gynecomastia and male breast carcinoma.

14. The Process of Reproduction

The previous two chapters have described the organization of the male and female reproductive systems along with how the gametes are produced. This chapter describes how the gametes meet and the processes that occur from fertilization until the baby is born and breastfed.

During pregnancy many processes and changes take place under hormonal control. The main hormones are:

- Progesterone.
- Estrogens.
- Human chorionic gonadotropin (hCG).
- Human placental lactogen (hPL).
- Prolactin.
- Oxytocin.

After reading this chapter you should be able to:

- Explain the process of sexual intercourse and the common associated disorders.
- Understand the processes involved in fertilization and implantation.
- List the most common methods of contraception and describe their modes of action.
- Give an account of the development and functions of the placenta.
- Appreciate the adaptations required for a successful pregnancy.
- Picture the stages of childbirth.
- Explain the physiology and process of lactation.

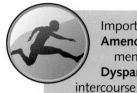

Important terms:
Amenorrhea—when menstruation fails to occur
Dyspareunia—pain on sexual intercourse
Menorrhagia—large volumes of blood lost during menstruation
Contraception—a method of preventing pregnancy
Trimester—the developmental period of the fetus in the uterus, divided into three periods of equal length (about 13 weeks)

Sexual intercourse and dysfunction

Sexual arousal and sensation

In both men and women sexual arousal is derived from two components: physical stimulation and psychological stimulation.

Sexual arousal activates the parasympathetic nerves to the genitalia to cause erection of the penis or clitoris; the mechanism of erection is described in Chapter 13.

Physical stimulation

Physical stimulation of the glans of the penis in the male or the clitoris in the female results in sexual arousal; however, other parts of the body can also have this effect (erogenous zones). These structures contain an abundance of sensory receptors that are stimulated by the massaging action of sexual intercourse. Stimulation of the external and internal genitalia can add to these sensations (e.g., vagina, urethra, and prostate). These signals reach the spinal cord via the pudendal nerves and are transmitted to the central nervous system (CNS). They also initiate reflexes in the lumbar and sacral spinal cord. These reflexes produce the physical signs of sexual arousal to the extent that erection and ejaculation are possible in male patients with severed spinal cords, although there is no accompanying sensation.

Psychological stimulation

Psychological stimuli greatly enhance the response to physical stimuli. Erotic thoughts can activate the limbic system in a similar manner to physical stimuli, causing sexual arousal, including lubrication and erection.

Physiology of sexual intercourse
Stages of sexual intercourse

Sexual intercourse is also called coitus. The changes in sexual arousal during coitus are often described in the four stages of the EPOR model (Fig. 14.1):

- Excitement phase—initial rapid rise in the level of sexual arousal.
- Plateau phase—sexual arousal is maintained at a high level.
- Orgasmic phase—sexual arousal crosses the threshold, resulting in orgasm.
- Resolution phase—the fall in sexual arousal following the cessation of coitus; physical and behavioral changes revert to normal.

Excitement and plateau phases

Sexual arousal causes stimulation of the parasympathetic nerve plexuses supplying the genitalia; this results in the following physical changes in the male:

- Vasocongestion of the penis (leading to erection) and scrotum.
- Secretion of small amounts of preejaculatory fluid that may contain sperm.

Similar changes occur in the female:

- Vasocongestion of the clitoris (leading to erection), vagina, labia minora, and nipples.
- Secretion of lubricating fluid by Bartholin's glands on either side of the vestibule and a fluid exudate from blood vessels in the vaginal wall.

These physical changes increase the level of stimulation, and the increase in stimulation causes further sexual arousal, resulting in a positive feedback system.

Systemic changes occur in both sexes; these changes reach a peak at the point of orgasm:

- Rise in heart rate and blood pressure.
- Rise in respiratory rate.
- Rise in temperature and blood supply to the skin.
- Increase in muscle tone.

The male orgasm and resolution

When sexual arousal reaches the "threshold," a reflex is initiated in the lumbar sympathetic nerves called an orgasm; it is accompanied by intense physical sensations. In the male the orgasm is accompanied by the expulsion of roughly 200 million spermatozoa in

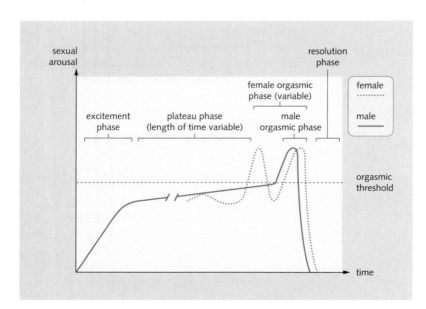

Fig. 14.1 The EPOR model of sexual arousal.

2–4 mL of seminal fluid. The sperm are projected deep into the vagina, close to the external os of the cervix. This expulsion occurs in two phases:

- Emission—the epididymis, ductus deferens, seminal vesicles, and prostate begin to contract, pushing sperm and seminal fluid into the urethra. This urethral sensation heightens stimulation and contraction.
- Ejaculation—the urethra contracts rhythmically, expelling the semen in a series of pulses.

The sympathetic stimulation of male ejaculation inhibits the erection maintained by the parasympathetic input. The male enters a short "absolute refractory" period during which further arousal is not possible; resolution will follow unless there is further stimulation.

The female orgasm and resolution

The female orgasm causes intense physical sensations and muscle contraction throughout the body in a manner similar to the male orgasm. A female orgasm is not necessary for pregnancy to occur, although it may raise fertility. Following the female orgasm sexual arousal returns to the plateau phase without an absolute refractory period. Continued stimulation can result in further orgasms; otherwise resolution will occur.

A single ejaculation contains 200 million spermatozoa, whereas the female produces only 2 million oocytes throughout her entire life, of which only 400 are ovulated. Theoretically, a man could fertilize the entire fertile female population of the world with just 10 ejaculations.

Sexual dysfunction

The term "sexual dysfunction" includes any process that interferes with a normal sex life. This can be caused by stress or physical or mental illness, but the majority of conditions result from ignorance, embarrassment, or poor communication between sexual partners. Any therapy should involve both partners and encourage discussion and intimacy.

Male sexual dysfunction
Reduced libido

This is a lack of sexual desire; it is less common in men than women. It can be caused by psychological reactions to a deteriorating relationship or depression. It can also be caused by physical conditions, including systemic illness, medications, and a decrease in testosterone levels with age.

Impotence

Impotence is the inability to maintain an erection suitable for vaginal penetration despite normal sexual desire. It is the most common presentation of sexual dysfunction in men and can be caused by many conditions (Fig. 14.2). Impotence can be treated by the following methods, according to the cause:

- Sexual counseling.
- Vacuum aids.
- Oral medications (including sildenafil citrate [Viagra®]).
- Medications injected directly into the penis.
- Implants.

Premature ejaculation

The definition of premature ejaculation depends on the expectations and desires of both partners. In severe cases, ejaculation may occur prior to penetration. It is made worse by anxiety and can be treated by relaxation techniques.

Female sexual dysfunction
Reduced libido

A lack of sexual desire can be present from puberty, or it can develop with time, in which case it is often a reaction to a deteriorating relationship or depression. It can be caused by physical illness that prevents the enjoyment of sexual intercourse (e.g., vaginal infection, general illness, or medications).

Anorgasmia

The majority of women require more time and greater stimulation to achieve orgasm than men. Anorgasmia is the complete failure to achieve orgasm; it is not infrequent orgasms. The best treatment involves teaching both partners about the female body; encouraging masturbation may also benefit some women.

Dyspareunia

Dyspareunia is pain on intercourse. There are two kinds:

- Superficial—felt on the external genitalia.
- Deep—felt internally.

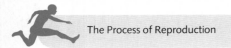

Causes of male sexual dysfunction		
Cause	Examples	Mechanism
Psychological	Performance anxiety, stress	Stress inhibits the parasympathetic nervous system that maintains erection
Alcohol	Brewer's droop	Acutely inhibits sensory nerves, chronically damages liver raising estrogen levels
Medications	Antihypertensives	Reduce blood flow to the penis
	Antidepressants and antipsychotics	Antagonize sexual arousal in the CNS
Endocrine	Diabetes	Long-term complications can damage the nerves and blood vessels of the penis
Vascular disease	Atherosclerosis	Prevents sufficient blood reaching the penis to maintain erection
Neurological	Multiple sclerosis	Inhibits sexual arousal in the CNS

Fig. 14.2 Causes of male sexual dysfunction.

Causes of female dyspareunia		
Type of dyspareunia	Disease process	Symptoms and signs
Superficial	Vulval/vaginal infections	Lesions and discharge
	Previous surgery or trauma	Scars
	Cystitis and UTIs	Urinary frequency, urgency, and pain
	Estrogen deficiency	Lack of lubrication, postmenopausal
Deep	Endometriosis	Recurrent pelvic pain in time with the menstrual cycle
	Pelvic inflammatory disease	Abdominal pain
	Fibroids	Menorrhagia and pelvic pain
	Ovarian cysts/tumors	Pelvic pain and menorrhagia

Fig. 14.3 Causes of female dyspareunia. (UTIs, urinary tract infections.)

Apart from the common vaginismus (see below), dyspareunia tends to have a physical cause (Fig. 14.3).

Vaginismus
This is involuntary contraction of vaginal muscle upon attempted penetration, causing apareunia or dyspareunia. It is a common psychological condition caused by fear of penetration, sometimes resulting from previous dyspareunia. It can be treated by teaching relaxation techniques together with insertion of vaginal dilators of increasing size until penile insertion is possible. The woman should be in control of all insertion until she can relax enough to allow her partner to do so.

Apareunia
This is the inability of the vagina to accept penile penetration. It can be caused by congenital malformations of the vagina or severe vaginal infections, but most commonly it is caused by vaginismus.

Fertilization and contraception

Fertilization
Oocyte
At ovulation the oocyte is released from the mature ovarian follicle onto the surface of the ovary in the

peritoneal cavity. At this stage, it has completed the first division of meiosis and has arrested at metaphase of the second meiotic division. It is surrounded by two layers:

- Zona pellucida—a glycoprotein layer.
- Corona radiata—granulosa cells from the follicle (also called cumulus oophorus).

The oocyte is wafted into the fallopian tube by the action of cilia on the fimbriae. Further ciliary action and peristalsis move the oocyte along the fallopian tube to the ampulla. It is capable of fertilization for less than 24 hours.

Sperm

About 200 million sperm are ejaculated deep into the vagina close to the external cervical os. They are suspended in the fructose-rich, alkaline seminal fluid; this provides the energy required by the sperm and acts as a buffer to the acidic vaginal environment. The motile sperm must cover a significant distance to reach the oocyte in the fallopian tubes. Their passage is obstructed by two narrow openings that act as filters against damaged sperm:

- External os of the cervix.
- Uterine entrance of the fallopian tubes.

Their passage may be assisted by physiological changes brought about by the female orgasm and chemical signals directing them toward the oocyte.

Within the female genital tract, sperm are viable for less than 48 hours. The majority degenerate and are absorbed by the female, with only about 200 sperm reaching the oocyte in the ampulla of the fallopian tube. The quickest sperm can arrive in just 5 minutes.

Capacitation

The ejaculated sperm cannot reach and penetrate the oocyte until they undergo capacitation. The following changes occur in the uterus or fallopian tubes:

- Removal of glycoproteins covering the acrosome.
- Reorganization of membrane phospholipids to alter the membrane potential and charge.
- Influx of calcium that increases flagellar activity and motility.
- Activation of the acrosome allowing the release of enzymes.

Capacitation must be mimicked during in-vitro fertilization (IVF) by incubation in a suitable medium.

Fertilization

Fertilization normally occurs in the ampulla of the fallopian tube. The sperm must penetrate the layers surrounding the oocyte and, in the process, prevent other sperm from fertilizing the oocyte a second time. This process requires several steps:

1. *Penetration of the corona radiata*   The acrosome membrane begins to perforate, releasing the enzyme hyaluronidase, which disrupts the cell matrix allowing sperm to push through the remaining granulosa cells.
2. *Penetration of the zona pellucida*   Receptors on the acrosome bind to ZP3 molecules causing the release of acrosin, an enzyme that digests the glycoprotein chains of the zona pellucida. The sperm can then push through the weakened structure.
3. *Fusion of the plasma membranes*   The membranes of the sperm and oocyte bind via integrin receptors and fuse. The sperm nucleus enters the oocyte cytoplasm leaving its tail and membrane behind. (No sperm mitochondria enter the oocyte.)
4. *Fast block*   The membrane fusion causes the oocyte to depolarize preventing other sperm from binding for about a minute.
5. *Slow block*   The fusion also causes calcium to enter the oocyte resulting in the release of granules containing hydrolytic enzymes. These enzymes break down the ZP3 molecules of the zona pellucida, permanently preventing other sperm from binding.
6. *Second meiotic division*   The calcium influx also causes the oocyte to complete the second meiotic division. This produces two haploid cells:
   - Female pronucleus with the majority of the cytoplasm.
   - Second polar body with almost no cytoplasm.
7. *Formation of the pronuclei*   The nucleus of the sperm enlarges to form a pronucleus that is indistinguishable from the female pronucleus. The DNA within each pronucleus is replicated.
8. *Mixing of the chromosomes*   The nuclear membranes surrounding the pronuclei break down and the maternal and paternal chromosomes mix producing a diploid (46-chromosome) zygote.
9. *First mitotic division*   The zygote immediately begins to divide by mitosis and a copy of the replicated DNA enters each cell. This division takes about 30 hours to complete.

The fast and slow blocks do not always prevent multiple fertilizations. Triploid (three sets of chromosomes) zygotes are formed, but they usually die within the uterus, although the mechanism for this abortion is unknown.

Development and implantation
Early development
The zygote divides into two cells called blastomeres as the embryo is transported along the fallopian tube. The blastomeres continue to divide mitotically, becoming smaller with each division. The cells then reorganize to form a tighter ball, a process called compaction. When the embryo reaches the 12- to 15-cell stage, it is called a morula.

The morula enters the uterus about 3 days after fertilization. Glands in the endometrial lining secrete a glycogen-rich fluid under the influence of progesterone from the corpus luteum. Glycogen can cross the zona pellucida to nourish the morula.

Soon after the morula enters the uterus, a cavity develops, forming an inner and outer layer of cells:
- Trophoblast—the outer cell layer that will form the placenta.
- Embryoblast—the inner cell mass that will form the embryo.

The morula is now called a blastocyst. Over the next 2 days the zona pellucida breaks down allowing the blastocyst to increase in size. It is now ready for implantation. These changes are shown in Fig. 14.4.

Implantation
About 6 days after fertilization the blastocyst binds to the endometrial lining. This usually occurs in the body of the uterus with the embryoblast nearer to the endometrium and the cavity closer to the uterus lumen. The trophoblast layer grows rapidly and differentiates to form two layers:
- Cytotrophoblast—the layer nearest the embryoblast, composed of dividing cells that join the syncytiotrophoblast.
- Syncytiotrophoblast—the layer nearest to the endometrium, composed of cytoplasm containing many nuclei without cell boundaries.

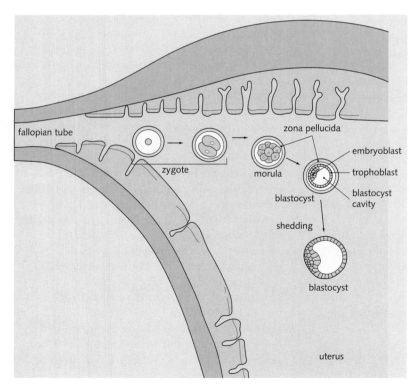

Fig. 14.4 Early development of the zygote, morula, and blastocyst.

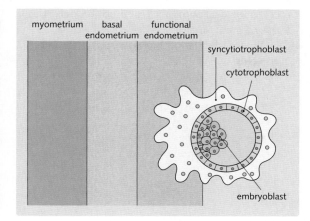

Fig. 14.5 Implantation of the blastocyst.

The syncytiotrophoblast develops fingerlike projections that invade the surrounding endometrium to hold the blastocyst in place. It releases enzymes that break down the glycogen-rich endometrial stroma to release nourishment for the developing embryoblast. This entire process is called implantation (Fig. 14.5).

Contraception

Humans are most unusual animals since neither the female nor the male is aware of the time of ovulation. The majority of female animals display ovulation with dramatic changes in color, smell, and behavior, to which the male responds appropriately. On the good side, this allows humans to engage in sex at any time throughout the year. However, it makes pregnancy very difficult to avoid.

A wide range of reliable contraceptive methods are now available, allowing people to choose a method that suits their lifestyle and beliefs. No method of contraception can prevent pregnancy 100% of the time in 100% of women. The failure rate is measured as the percentage of women who become pregnant during 1 year of use. This percentage varies widely among contraceptive methods and the reliability of the user; the lower the figure, the more effective the contraception. Figure 14.6 shows examples of common contraceptive methods, and Fig. 14.7 shows where their contraceptive actions take place.

Natural contraception
None
The average age of first contraceptive use is 8 months later than the average age of first sexual intercourse. Many adolescents have disproved the myth that you cannot get pregnant the first time you have sex. Without any form of contraception 90% of women become pregnant during 1 year of regular sex.

Examples of methods of contraception						
Method	Rhythm method	Condoms	COCP	IUD	Mirena® (IUS)	Vasectomy
Action	Natural	Barrier	Hormonal	Prevents implantation	Hormonal	Surgical sterilization
Failure rate (%)	2.5–30	1.5–7	1	2	0.1	0.05 per lifetime
Advantages	Free, approved by Catholic church	Cheap, easy, portable, and protects from STDs	Cheap, effective, light periods	Lasts up to 5 years	Very effective, light periods, minimal effort	Very effective, simple operation
Disadvantages	Requires high motivation and control	Reduces spontaneity and may affect sensitivity	Several side effects including risk of cardiovascular disease and breast cancer	Must be fitted by doctor, risk of PID and heavy menstrual bleeding	Must be fitted by doctor, risk of PID	Irreversible

Fig. 14.6 Examples of methods of contraception. (COCP, combined oral contraceptive pill; IUD, intrauterine device; IUS, intrauterine system; PID, pelvic inflammatory disease; STDs, sexually transmitted diseases.)

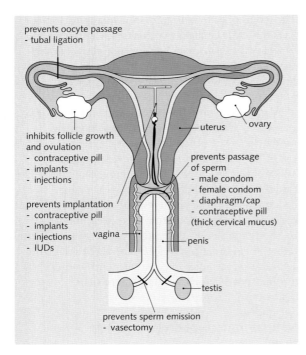

prevents oocyte passage
- tubal ligation

uterus

ovary

inhibits follicle growth
and ovulation
- contraceptive pill
- implants
- injections

prevents passage
of sperm
- male condom
- female condom
- diaphragm/cap
- contraceptive pill
(thick cervical mucus)

prevents implantation
- contraceptive pill
- implants
- injections
- IUDs

vagina

penis

testis

prevents sperm emission
- vasectomy

Fig. 14.7 Locations of contraceptive actions. (IUDs, intrauterine devices.)

Postcoital douche

Since the sperm are deposited in the vagina, washing the vagina out after sex reduces fertility. This method is very ineffective: it has a failure rate of 45% because the sperm are rapidly transported through the cervix.

Coitus interruptus

This is also called the withdrawal method; the man withdraws his penis from the vagina just before ejaculation. While the theory is good, in practice the sympathetic system hijacks the body to propagate the species. Even with successful withdrawal, pregnancy can still result since sperm is also present in the male preejaculatory secretions. The failure rate of 35% speaks for itself.

Rhythm method

The oocyte can only survive for 24 hours without fertilization, whereas the sperm can survive for 48 hours. In theory, fertilization can only occur following sexual intercourse in the 3 days around ovulation. By determining the exact date of ovulation and avoiding sex before and after this date, pregnancy can be avoided. In practice, a wider period of sexual abstinence is used, usually about 9 days per

cycle. There are a number of methods for detecting the date of ovulation:

- Keeping a calendar of the menstrual cycle and changes.
- Changes in cervical mucus; it becomes clear, sticky, and stretchy at ovulation.
- Changes in temperature; there is a rise of about 0.3°C after ovulation.
- Changes in the types of estrogens and luteinizing hormone (LH) levels in the urine using over-the-counter kits.
- Occasionally women may experience "ovulation pain."

The failure rate ranges from 2.5% to 30%, depending on the motivation of both partners and the regularity of the menstrual cycle.

Barrier contraception

The aim of barrier protection is to prevent the sperm from reaching the oocyte, thus preventing fertilization. All barrier methods offer some protection against sexually transmitted diseases, including human immunodeficiency virus (HIV) infection. The failure rate ranges from 1.5% to 7%, depending on the motivation of both partners.

Male condom

Condoms are currently the only method of contraception where the responsibility is entirely on the part of the man. Condoms are sheaths of lubricated latex that fit over the erect penis to prevent sperm from entering the vagina. After intercourse the penis should be withdrawn as soon as possible while holding the condom in place. Modern condoms do not interfere with sensation significantly, but they may reduce spontaneity. They are readily available, cheap, and portable and offer good protection against many sexually transmitted diseases (STDs), including HIV.

Female condom

These are larger versions of male condoms that fit into the vagina. There is a risk of the penis "missing" the condom, but a large ring at the open end aims to prevent this by holding it against the vulva. They do not need to be fitted by a specialist. The main disadvantage is the rustling noise, similar to a plastic bag, that accompanies intercourse.

Diaphragm

Diaphragms are reusable circular latex devices that fit in the vagina (or caps that fit over the cervix); they are used with a covering of spermicidal cream to kill the sperm. They can be inserted a couple of hours before sex, but they must not be removed for at least 6 hours afterward. They must initially be fitted by a medical professional and require teaching and practice for reliable use.

Hormonal contraception

Hormonal contraception is the artificial administration of estrogens and/or progesterone to reduce fertility. They mimic the hormonal changes of pregnancy to prevent further ovulation. Estrogens act in the following ways:

- Strongly suppress follicle-stimulating hormone (FSH) to prevent follicle development.
- Suppress the LH surge to prevent ovulation.
- Weakly inhibit implantation.

Progesterone has slightly different effects:

- Thickens the cervical mucus to inhibit sperm transport.
- Inhibits development of the endometrium to prevent implantation.
- Weakly suppresses FSH to prevent follicle development.
- Weakly suppresses LH release to prevent ovulation.

The use of estrogen-containing contraception has a number of beneficial effects:

- Lighter, shorter periods.
- Regular, controllable periods.
- Reduces symptoms of premenstrual syndrome (PMS).
- Reduces the risk of ovarian and endometrial cancer.
- Controls the symptoms of endometriosis.

Unfortunately estrogens also increase the risk of two serious diseases:

- Thromboembolism—the hormones increase the levels of many clotting factors so that the blood is prone to coagulate causing deep vein thrombosis (DVT) and a risk of pulmonary embolus (PE). There is also a risk of hypertension.
- Cancer—there may be a small and temporary increase in the incidence of breast cancer in young women. This is offset by the reduction in risk of ovarian and endometrial cancer.

Since both these diseases are rare in the younger age groups that use hormonal contraception, the overall risk remains very small. In fact, it is less than the risk of childbirth or abortion. Smoking greatly increases these risks.

A number of less serious side effects are occasionally experienced:

- Breakthrough bleeding—irregular menstrual bleeding is common in the first few months of use.
- Slight weight gain—this is usually temporary.
- Headaches and migraine.
- Acne—caused by estrogen.
- Dry eyes—a concern for contact lens users.
- Loss of libido due to androgen inhibition.

The side effects do result in a number of contraindications for estrogen-containing contraception; in most cases, progesterone-only contraception can be used instead. These are similar to the contraindications for hormone replacement therapy (HRT) and, likewise, are frequently screened in exams:

- Estrogen-dependent cancer (including breast cancer).
- Cardiovascular and thromboembolic disorders.
- Liver disease with abnormal liver function tests (LFTs).
- Undiagnosed vaginal bleeding.
- Pregnancy or breastfeeding.
- Smokers aged over 35 years.
- Severe migraines.

Combined oral contraceptive pill (COCP)

The "pill" is the most common method of contraception used by young women. It contains low doses of both estrogen and progesterone, giving a failure rate of 1%. It is taken for 21 days, followed by a 7-day break, during which withdrawal bleeding occurs; this is not real menstruation. The side effects are described above.

Progesterone-only pill (POP)

As the name suggests, this oral contraceptive contains only progesterone. It has a higher failure rate (2%), especially in younger women, but it can be used in women in whom COCPs are contraindicated or not tolerated. It must be taken continuously at the same time (within 3 hours) every day. The main side effect is the menstrual irregularity, which occurs in 25% of users.

Depot progesterone

Long-acting progesterone can be injected intramuscularly to give 2–3 months of contraception.

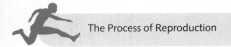

It has similar side effects and failure rate to POPs, but it carries a risk of amenorrhea and temporary infertility for several months after discontinuation.

Subdermal implants

A progesterone-containing tube (Implanon®) can be implanted in the upper arm to give 3 years of contraception. The side effects and failure rate are similar to POPs. It must be removed after 3 years, but it can be removed earlier to rapidly restore fertility. In the past, six rods were implanted, but this method was discontinued because they were difficult to remove.

Intrauterine system (IUS or Mirena®)

This is a type of plastic intrauterine device (IUD) that releases progesterone; it does not contain copper. The progesterone acts locally to give excellent contraception; it reduces menstrual bleeding and prevents side effects. They last 5 years and the failure rate is about 0.1%. There are some cases emerging where bleeding recommences after 2 years, even though the implant is still releasing progesterone. This phenomenon is currently under investigation.

Prevention of implantation
Intrauterine devices

These are small plastic devices surrounded by copper wire that are inserted into the uterine lumen. The copper inactivates sperm to prevent fertilization. The device also inhibits implantation. Threads are attached to the device to allow insertion and removal, which must be performed by a trained medical professional. Insertion can be difficult in young or nulliparous women (i.e., women who have never given birth). The woman can check that the IUD remains in place by feeling for these threads at the cervix os. The IUD can be left in place for 5 years, throughout which the failure rate is about 1%. There are several side effects and risks:
- Expulsion—especially in the first 2 months.
- Cramping and bleeding—usually diminish with time.
- Pelvic inflammatory disease (PID)—caused by bacterial infection at insertion.
- Increased risk of ectopic pregnancy.

An IUD can prevent implantation and, therefore, pregnancy if it is inserted within 5 days of sexual intercourse.

Postcoital medication

Within recent years, the use of emergency contraceptive pills (EPCs; e.g., PC4® or Levonelle®) has become a viable option for prevention of implantation. These are also referred to as "morning-after" pills in lay terms. In the United States, EPCs are available by prescription only, whereas in many other countries they are sold over the counter. These pills contain high levels of estrogen and progesterone which increase the motility of the fallopian tubes so that the embryo reaches the uterus before the endometrium is prepared for implantation. The emergency hormonal contraception is effective if it is taken within 72 hours (3 days) of unprotected sexual intercourse, and the dose must be repeated 12 hours later. PC4 often induces nausea and vomiting so an antiemetic is sometimes prescribed. The side effects of Levonelle are milder, allowing it to be available over the counter. The failure rate of both pills is about 3%.

Irreversible contraception

Sterilization is the most popular form of contraception in older men and women. It involves surgery to prevent the sperm or oocyte from reaching the site of fertilization. Since the male operation is simpler and more effective, it should be considered the preferred technique in stable couples who have completed their family. Both techniques should be considered a permanent form of contraception, although microsurgery can successfully reverse sterilization in about 50% of cases.

Vasectomy

This is a quick operation, performed under local anesthetic, in which a section of each ductus deferens is removed. The cut ends are tied or burnt closed by diathermy to prevent sperm from reaching the urethra. It does not interfere with testosterone production or sensation. The man is potentially fertile for 3 months after the operation owing to sperm within the proximal ductus deferens; during this time other contraception should be employed. There is a risk of postoperative bruising and bleeding. It is the most effective form of contraception with a failure rate of about 0.05% per lifetime.

Tubal ligation

This is the equivalent operation in the female. It is usually performed under general anesthetic using a laparoscope to cut, burn, or clip both fallopian tubes. The woman becomes infertile after her next period,

Fig. 14.8 Causes of male infertility.

Causes of male infertility	
Abnormality	**Cause**
Azoospermia	Blockage of genital tract
Oligospermia	Testosterone deficiency
	Hyperprolactinemia
Asthenozoospermia	Raised scrotal temperature, e.g., varicocele
	Antisperm antibodies
Oligospermia or asthenozoospermia	Genetic disorders, e.g., Klinefelter's
	Genital tract infection (current or previous with scarring)

and the failure rate is low at 0.5% per lifetime. The major complications are due to the general anesthetic.

Infertility

Infertility is defined as the inability to conceive after 1 year of regular unprotected sex. It is a common problem, affecting about 1 in 10 couples. Infertility is caused by:

- Abnormalities in the male (30%).
- Abnormalities in the female (45%).
- Idiopathic (unknown) origin (25%).

Male infertility

Male infertility is usually caused by abnormalities in sperm production. These include:

- Azoospermia—no sperm.
- Oligospermia—also called a low sperm count (less than 20 million/mL; the average is about 60 million/mL).
- Asthenozoospermia—decreased sperm quality due to reduced motility or abnormal morphology (shape).

Some of the conditions that can cause these abnormalities are shown in Fig. 14.8.

Female infertility

The causes of female infertility are more varied:

- Oligomenorrhea or amenorrhea (45%).
- Structural abnormalities of the fallopian tubes (45%).

Causes of female infertility	
Abnormality	**Cause**
Oligomenorrhea or amenorrhea	Weight loss
	Post-COCP pituitary insensitivity
	Polycystic ovaries
	Hyperprolactinemia
Abnormal fallopian tube	Pelvic inflammatory disease (Chlamydia)
	Endometriosis
	Pelvic surgery
Abnormal cervix	Cervical stenosis
Abnormal cervical mucus	Immunological reaction against sperm

Fig. 14.9 Causes of female infertility. (COCP, combined oral contraceptive pill.)

- Structural abnormalities of the uterus and cervix (5%).
- Disorders of the cervical mucus (5%).

The main conditions that cause these abnormalities are shown in Fig. 14.9. Some clinicians believe that an inadequate luteal phase can also cause infertility because the blastocyst does not have time to implant successfully before the corpus luteum regresses. Infertility can also be caused by sexual dysfunction.

179

Investigation

Counseling and reassurance are extremely important in the management of infertility. Many of the questions and procedures can be very embarrassing; the couple must feel that they can trust the practitioner. The investigations should be aimed at diagnosing and treating the cause of infertility, not finding which partner is "at fault."

Infertility is investigated by:
- Examination of sperm under a microscope.
- Hormone investigations—FSH, LH, prolactin, progesterone, estrogen, testosterone, and thyroid hormone.
- Pelvic ultrasound—looks for gross abnormality and can detect the presence of correctly developing ovarian follicles.
- Hysterosalpingography or laparoscopy—contrast media/dye is injected into the uterus to image the fallopian tubes by x-ray or visually (see Fig. 17.9).
- Postcoital test—checks cervical mucus and sexual technique.

Treatment

Infertility is rarely absolute; it is usually caused by the reduced fertility (subfertility) of one or both partners. Where possible, treatment is aimed at the underlying cause. Medical treatment includes:
- Bromocriptine—which treats hyperprolactinemia.
- Clomiphene—an antiestrogen, which stimulates FSH release and follicle development.
- hCG—which can trigger ovulation by acting like LH.
- LH and FSH injections; follicle stimulants, if clomiphene fails.
- GnRH analogs; follicle stimulants, if clomiphene fails.

Medications that stimulate follicle development may induce multiple pregnancies.

If these simpler treatments fail, assisted fertilization techniques can be used. These are both expensive and emotionally draining, although they have a 20–30% success rate (live births per cycle). This is compared with a rate of about 15% in fertile couples without assisted fertilization. Assisted fertilization techniques require hyperstimulation of the ovaries using the medications described above. The ovary responds by producing several eggs that are harvested using a transvaginal needle under ultrasound control. The techniques then differ:

- In-vitro fertilization (IVF)—oocytes are fertilized in vitro and reintroduced into the uterus. This is the only treatment for blocked fallopian tubes.
- Intracytoplasmic sperm injection (ICSI)—used alongside IVF if the sperm are abnormal and incapable of fertilization.
- Gamete intrafallopian transfer (GIFT)—oocytes are reintroduced into the fallopian tubes along with sperm for in-vivo fertilization.

Therapeutic abortion

In the United States, induced abortion is legal until 24 weeks of gestation, although it is rarely performed beyond 20 weeks. It is sometimes recommended to prevent physical illness, although 95% are performed for social or psychiatric reasons. It is a relatively safe procedure with no risk of subsequent reduced fertility if performed without complications before 13 weeks of gestation. An appropriate method of contraception is usually included as part of the treatment.

Surgical termination of pregnancy (STOP) can be performed until the 13th week of gestation. It is an outpatient procedure performed under general anesthetic in which the uterus is evacuated using suction.

Medical termination can be performed until the 24th week of gestation. Two drugs are used:
- Oral mifepristone—this drug is administered first; it raises the sensitivity of the uterus to prostaglandins.
- Prostaglandins—these are given 48 hours after mifepristone; they can be taken orally or applied vaginally and they induce uterine contractions.

The fetus is usually expelled vaginally within 12 hours of the prostaglandin treatment. Medical termination often causes bleeding and pain, but pain relief is available.

The placenta

Development

The placenta develops from the trophoblast surrounding the developing fetus. The development of the trophoblast is described in the section "Implantation" (p. 174). The placenta develops mainly from fetal tissues and partially from the

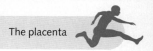

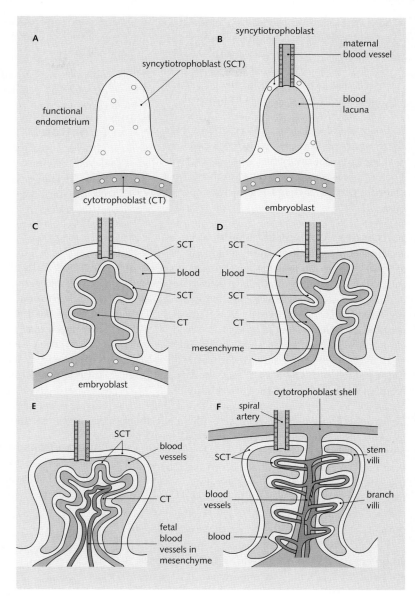

Fig. 14.10 Development of the placenta: (A) Syncytiotrophoblast invasion; (B) Lacunar phase; (C) Primary chorionic villi; (D) Secondary chorionic villi; (E) Tertiary chorionic villi; (F) Mature chorionic villi. See text for details.

maternal endometrium; the development is shown in Fig. 14.10.

Lacunar phase

Eight days after fertilization, the syncytiotrophoblast begins to erode endometrial capillaries. Cavities called lacunae develop within the syncytiotrophoblast; they are continuous with the maternal capillaries and fill with maternal blood. They supply oxygen and nutrition to the blastocyst through diffusion and represent the early maternal circulation in the developing placenta. The lacunae

link together to form a network, while the capillaries enlarge to form sinusoids.

Chorionic villi

The chorionic villi are branching projections from the blastocyst into the syncytiotrophoblast and functional endometrium. They increase the surface area in contact with maternal blood. Development progresses in three stages:

* Primary villi—two weeks after fertilization, swellings in the cytotrophoblast extend into the syncytiotrophoblast and begin to branch.

181

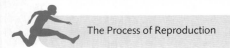

- Secondary villi—at the start of the third week, mesenchyme from the embryo invades the cytotrophoblast of the primary villi.
- Tertiary villi—the mesenchyme forms blood vessels that link up with the newly formed fetal circulation by the end of the third week.

At this stage, the placenta has a blood supply from the mother and fetus, allowing more efficient exchange of nutrients, gases, and waste products. The placenta continues to develop throughout pregnancy, in advance of the growing needs of the fetus.

Further development of the villi

As the tertiary villi form, the cytotrophoblast extends through the syncytiotrophoblast at the tip of each villus. These cells are now in direct contact with endometrial cells, and they form a cytotrophoblast shell that holds the embryo in place. This shell remains directly connected at the top of the chorionic villi that are now called stem villi.

Branching villi at the sides of the stem villi are called branch villi. These are surrounded by maternal blood in the lacunae, and they are the site of exchange between fetal and maternal blood. The cytotrophoblast lining of the branch villi breaks down to reduce the distance molecules must diffuse between the two circulations. As the placenta continues to grow, the lacunae become supplied by the spiral arteries and endometrial veins. Deoxygenated fetal blood reaches the placenta via the two umbilical arteries and oxygenated blood returns to the fetal circulation via the umbilical vein.

Further growth of the placenta occurs at the embryonic pole (the side to which the umbilicus is attached) by widening and lengthening; it does not penetrate further into the endometrium. This forms the familiar platelike shape on one side of the uterus. The endometrium on the same side also changes to form the decidua basalis; this grows into the placenta forming incomplete septa that divide it into sections called cotyledons.

Structure

It is important to remember that maternal and fetal blood do not mix within the placenta. Maternal blood enters large lacunae (cavities) from spiral arteries and is drained by endometrial veins. Fetal circulation in the branch villi is separated from the maternal circulation by two layers:

- Thin syncytiotrophoblast layer.
- Single cell layer of endometrium in the fetal capillary.

This allows rapid diffusion between the two circulations. A diagram of the fully developed placenta is shown in Fig. 14.11.

Functions

The placenta supplies all the requirements of the developing fetus while maintaining an environment in which the fetus can grow. The metabolic rate of the placenta is very high owing to protein synthesis, active transport, and growth. The many actions involved in this task fall into four categories and are described below.

Gaseous transport

Oxygen and carbon dioxide cross the placenta by passive diffusion. The rapid metabolism of the fetus uses up oxygen, so blood in the umbilical arteries has less oxygen than the maternal blood. This forms a concentration gradient that allows oxygen to diffuse across the placenta into the fetal blood. This process is also aided by fetal hemoglobin, which binds oxygen more strongly than adult hemoglobin. High levels of CO_2 are generated, crossing the placenta in the opposite direction.

Nutrient transport

Nutrients cross the placenta by two processes:
- Passive facilitated diffusion.
- Active transport.

Toward the end of pregnancy an excess of nutrients is transported so that the fetus can develop energy stores such as glycogen and fat. This includes brown adipose tissue that is broken down within the first few days after birth to create heat.

Immune protection

The process of meiosis and the presence of paternal DNA cause the maternal immune system to recognize the fetus as foreign. The placenta must act as a barrier to prevent immunological rejection.

A graft from a child to its mother would normally be rejected. However, as a fetus, the same child is protected by the placenta from rejection.

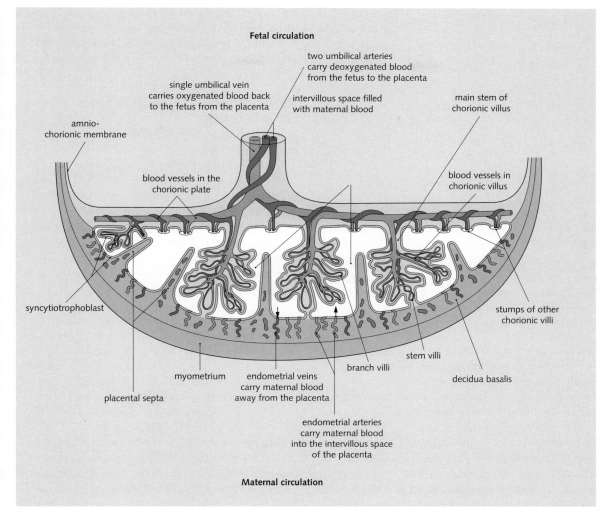

Fetal circulation

two umbilical arteries
carry deoxygenated blood
from the fetus to the placenta

single umbilical vein
carries oxygenated blood back
to the fetus from the placenta

intervillous space filled
with maternal blood

main stem of
chorionic villus

amnio-
chorionic membrane

blood vessels in the
chorionic plate

blood vessels in
chorionic villus

syncytiotrophoblast

stumps of other
chorionic villi

myometrium

stem villi

branch villi

decidua basalis

placental septa

endometrial veins
carry maternal blood
away from the placenta

endometrial arteries
carry maternal blood
into the intervillous space
of the placenta

Maternal circulation

Fig. 14.11 Structure of the mature placenta. (Adapted from Moore KL, Persaud TVN: The Developing Human: Clinically Oriented Embryology, 5th ed. Philadelphia, W.B. Saunders, 1999.)

Secretion of hormones

The placenta secretes high levels of steroid and peptide hormones that regulate and maintain pregnancy. It also allows maternal and fetal hormones to cross. These hormones are described in the next section.

Reproductive hormones in pregnancy

Sources of reproductive hormones

Endocrine signals are essential for implantation and the maintenance of pregnancy. As the pregnancy progresses, the hormone levels change as shown in Fig. 14.12. There are two phases of hormonal secretion during pregnancy:

- Corpus luteum phase—the corpus luteum secretes hormones to maintain the endometrium and the developing placenta.
- Placental phase—the placenta takes over hormonal secretion to allow maternal adaptation to pregnancy, birth, and lactation.

Corpus luteum phase

In the normal menstrual cycle, the corpus luteum secretes progesterone and estrogen for about 10 days following ovulation, after which it regresses. The

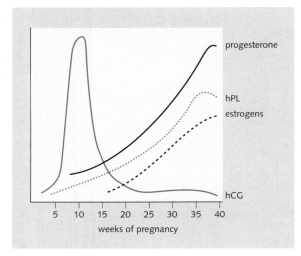

Fig. 14.12 Changes in the maternal blood levels of hormones during pregnancy. (Adapted from Llewellyn-Jones D: Fundamentals of Obstetrics and Gynceology, 6th ed. St. Louis, Mosby, 1994.)

dramatic fall in progesterone levels causes degeneration and shedding of the endometrium, resulting in menstruation. The blastocyst must prevent the next menstruation by maintaining the corpus luteum and its steroid secretion.

Soon after implantation, around day 6, the syncytiotrophoblast (outer layer of cells) secretes human chorionic gonadotropin (hCG). This hormone is equivalent to LH and acts on the corpus luteum to prevent regression. Progesterone levels continue to rise and the functional endometrium is maintained. This demonstrates the power of endocrine signals, since the tiny blastocyst can alter the physiology of the mother who is many millions of times larger.

The corpus luteum continues to be the main source of progesterone and estrogen for the first 6 weeks of development.

Placental phase
The placenta secretes the following hormones:
- Human chorionic gonadotropin (hCG).
- Progesterone.
- Estrogens.
- Human placental lactogen (hPL).
- Relaxin.

By the sixth week the placenta is the main source of progesterone and estrogens, which help the mother's body adapt to pregnancy. hPL helps regulate nutrient levels and metabolism; it also causes the glandular tissue of the breast to develop. Relaxin is secreted toward the end of pregnancy to prepare the body for birth.

Reproductive hormones from the placenta
Human chorionic gonadotropin
hCG is a peptide hormone secreted by the syncytiotrophoblast of the blastocyst from implantation. It has a similar structure and actions to LH. These actions include:
- Maintenance of the corpus luteum.
- Regulation of placental estrogen secretion.
- May be a factor in blocking the maternal immune response to fetus.
- Stimulation of testosterone secretion in the male fetus.

The corpus luteum is initially formed and maintained by the ovulatory LH surge and hCG simply replaces the falling levels of LH to prevent regression. hCG is secreted for the first 10 weeks of pregnancy until the placenta is capable of secreting sufficient sex steroids to maintain the pregnancy. After 10 weeks the corpus luteum is no longer needed for hormone production and hCG levels begin to fall.

The β-subunit of hCG can be detected in the urine just before the first day of a missed period, usually about 10 days after potential fertilization. This allows time for the blastocyst to implant and hCG levels to rise. This principle is used for the urine pregnancy testing available in hospitals and over the counter in pharmacies. Since hCG levels fall after the corpus luteum phase, these tests no longer work after 20 weeks. False positives may rarely indicate underlying disease (see the section on placental disorders).

Progesterone
The structure and synthesis of progesterone are described in Chapter 12. Plasma levels of progesterone rise throughout pregnancy, secreted initially by the corpus luteum, then by the placenta. It is the single most important hormone in the maintenance of pregnancy. Actions include:
- Maintenance and development of the functional endometrium.
- Inhibition of smooth muscle in the uterus to prevent premature expulsion.

- Metabolic changes, including fat storage.
- Physiological adaptation to pregnancy (described in the next section).
- Relaxation of smooth muscle throughout the body, which may cause some side effects (e.g., constipation and esophageal reflux).

Estrogens

The structure and synthesis of estrogens are described in Chapter 12. Plasma levels of estrogens (especially estriol) rise throughout pregnancy, secreted initially by the corpus luteum, then by the placenta. Like the granulosa cells, the placenta lacks several key enzymes for the synthesis of estrogen from cholesterol. These steps must be performed by the fetal adrenal gland, allowing the fetus to regulate placental estrogen secretion. This does not affect progesterone secretion, which is formed from cholesterol in just two steps.

The actions of estrogen prepare the body for birth and lactation. They include:
- Growth of the smooth muscle of the uterus (myometrium).
- Increased blood flow to the uterus.
- Softening of the cervix and pelvic ligaments.
- Stimulation of breast growth and development.
- Stimulation of pituitary prolactin secretion.
- Inhibition of pituitary LH and FSH secretion.
- Stimulation of oxytocin receptor synthesis in the myometrium in late pregnancy.
- Water retention.

Human placental lactogen

hPL is a peptide hormone secreted by the placenta; levels rise throughout pregnancy. It is sometimes called human chorionic somatomammotropin because its actions are similar to growth hormone and prolactin. These actions include:
- Maternal lipolysis (fat breakdown) and fatty acid metabolism, sparing glucose.
- Maternal insulin resistance, sparing glucose for the fetus.
- Enhancing active amino acid transfer across the placenta.
- Stimulating the growth and development of the breasts.

Relaxin

Relaxin is a peptide hormone secreted by the placenta late in pregnancy. It relaxes the myometrium, cervix, and the pelvic ligaments,

allowing the uterus to enlarge and the pelvis to stretch during birth. It acts by stimulating collagenase enzymes, which break down collagen in these tissues.

Reproductive hormones from other sources
Inhibin

Inhibin is a peptide hormone secreted by the ovary in the pregnant and nonpregnant state. It may suppress pituitary FSH secretion and stimulate progesterone production during pregnancy.

Prolactin

The structure, synthesis, and control of prolactin are described in Chapter 2. Prolactin secretion from the pituitary gland rises throughout pregnancy owing to stimulation by estrogens. It has a similar action to hPL in that it stimulates the growth and development of the breasts and regulates fat metabolism.

During pregnancy the high levels of placental estrogens prevent the secretion of milk. After birth the fall in estrogen levels allows prolactin to act on the breast. If the mother breastfeeds the baby, sensory signals from the nipple cause further prolactin secretion after pregnancy. The high prolactin levels have two effects:
- Secretion of milk, though it is oxytocin that causes the milk to be ejected.
- Inhibition of pituitary FSH and LH, which has a contraceptive effect.

Maternal adaptations to pregnancy

Throughout pregnancy the mother's body is undergoing changes that achieve three main purposes:
- Maintenance of a suitable environment for fetal growth.
- Preparation of the mother for childbirth.
- Preparation of the mother for lactation.

A summary of these changes is shown in Fig. 14.13.

Symptoms and signs of pregnancy
Presentation

The diagnosis of pregnancy may be a joyful or disastrous moment, depending on the situation and beliefs of the mother. There is also a wide range of

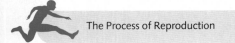

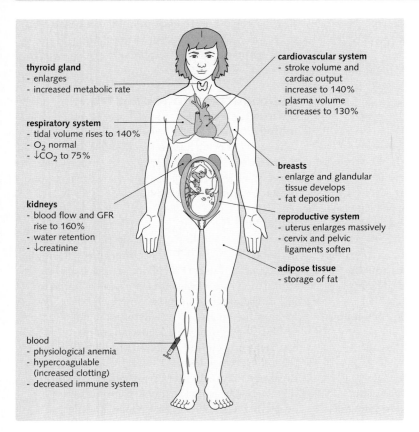

Fig. 14.13 Maternal adaptations to pregnancy.

thyroid gland
- enlarges
- increased metabolic rate

respiratory system
- tidal volume rises to 140%
- O_2 normal
- $\downarrow CO_2$ to 75%

kidneys
- blood flow and GFR rise to 160%
- water retention
- $\downarrow$creatinine

blood
- physiological anemia
- hypercoagulable (increased clotting)
- decreased immune system

cardiovascular system
- stroke volume and cardiac output increase to 140%
- plasma volume increases to 130%

breasts
- enlarge and glandular tissue develops
- fat deposition

reproductive system
- uterus enlarges massively
- cervix and pelvic ligaments soften

adipose tissue
- storage of fat

knowledge and experience among women of different backgrounds and age groups. The earliest signs of pregnancy are:
- A missed period.
- Nausea, possibly with vomiting.
- Temporary increase in frequency of urination.
- Fuller breasts and larger nipples, possibly with tenderness.

A positive urine β-hCG test confirms the diagnosis, and many patients will have done this test at home before presenting to a doctor. Further confirmation can be obtained using ultrasound, but this is not normally necessary.

Side effects

In addition to the early signs mentioned above, the maternal adaptations to pregnancy can cause symptomatic side effects; the common side effects are shown in Fig. 14.14.

Genital tract

Placental hormones cause changes mainly in the lower genital tract:

- Uterus—expands dramatically through pregnancy; the muscle layer hypertrophies massively in preparation for birth.
- Cervix—softens and becomes more readily dilated.
- Vagina—hypertrophy of muscle and becomes more readily dilated.

Cardiovascular system

The effectiveness of the cardiovascular system must increase to cope with:

- Increased oxygen demands of the fetus and placenta—about 130% of normal.
- Extra vascular space created by the expanding uterus and placenta.

The early adaptations are mostly caused by an increase in stroke volume with a slight increase in heart rate. Together these factors raise cardiac output to about 140% of normal by the sixth month. Cardiac output then begins to fall because pressure from the enlarged uterus inhibits venous return. Blood pressure does not increase for the first 7 months

Fig. 14.14 Common symptoms of pregnancy.

Common symptoms of pregnancy		
Symptom	**Cause**	**Stage of pregnancy**
Morning sickness (nausea ± vomiting)	Rising estrogen levels	From 4 weeks but then declines
Increased pigmentation	Raised levels of melanocyte-stimulating hormone (MSH) from the pituitary causing pigmentation of the face (chloasma) and abdominal striae	Gets progressively worse through pregnancy
Breathlessness	Changes in the cardiorespiratory system	
Gestational diabetes	Impaired glucose tolerance due to cortisol and hPL	
Constipation	Relaxation of smooth muscle caused by progesterone	
Heartburn and reflux		
Carpal tunnel syndrome	Water retention caused by estrogen	
Ankle edema		
Goiter	Raised thyroid-stimulating hormone (TSH) acting on the thyroid gland	
Severe abdominal distension	Fetus developing inside the uterus	
Prurigo of pregnancy	Itchy rash over abdomen and limbs	Late
Backache	Softening of ligaments due to estrogen	
Urinary frequency	Fetal head presses on the bladder, increased blood volume	

because of the fall in peripheral resistance caused by the developing placenta. It then begins to rise until birth.

 The increase in cardiac output may cause a systolic flow murmur over the pulmonary valve; it usually disappears after birth.

Blood volume rises in the latter half of pregnancy to about 130% of normal, although there is a slight rise throughout pregnancy. Aldosterone and estrogen cause renal water retention so that plasma volume increases. There is also an increase in red blood cells, but this is less than the fluid retention so the blood becomes diluted, causing a physiological anemia. The excess blood volume fills the placental vasculature and also protects the mother from hemorrhage during birth.

Respiratory system

The increased oxygen demands of the fetus and placenta also require adaptations in the respiratory system. Progesterone makes the chemoreceptors more sensitive to CO_2, causing the tidal volume to increase to 140% of normal while the respiratory rate remains the same. This maintains arterial oxygen saturation at normal levels while arterial CO_2 levels are about 75% of normal. These adaptations often give a sensation of breathlessness during pregnancy.

187

Renal system

Blood flow to the kidney increases during early pregnancy and then remains high. This causes the glomerular filtration rate (GFR) to rise to about 160% of normal. This would normally result in sodium loss, but increased secretion of renin, angiotensin II, and aldosterone counteract these changes.

Progesterone causes the smooth muscle of the collecting ducts and ureters to become dilated. This slows the excretion of urine making urinary tract infections (UTIs) more common. The urethra is also relaxed and the fetus exerts pressure on the bladder, so urinary incontinence is relatively common in late pregnancy.

Endocrine system

The secretion of the anterior pituitary hormones is altered during pregnancy (Fig. 14.15):

- FSH and LH secretion is almost completely stopped.
- Prolactin secretion rises throughout pregnancy.
- Thyroid-stimulating hormone (TSH) secretion initially falls then increases.
- Adrenocorticotropic hormone (ACTH) secretion increases.

- Melanocyte-stimulating hormone (MSH) secretion increases.

The anterior pituitary gland enlarges as a result of these changes.

The rise in secretion of most hormones is caused by direct actions of placental hormones and an increase in plasma binding proteins (caused by the action of estrogens on the liver) that reduces negative feedback.

Thyroid glands

hCG inhibits TSH secretion in the first trimester but, as the hCG levels fall in the second and third trimesters, TSH then rises above normal. The increase in TSH together with a reduction in iodine from the overactive kidneys causes the thyroid gland to enlarge. Thyroid hormone synthesis also increases but so does the synthesis of thyroid hormone binding proteins stimulated by estrogen. Overall active/free thyroid hormone levels remain normal.

Adrenal glands

In contrast, free cortisol levels do rise, despite the increase in plasma binding proteins. This raises amino

Changes that occur in pituitary hormone secretion during pregnancy and the effects caused by these changes		
Secretion of anterior pituitary hormone	Hormone secretion in pregnancy (compared with nonpregnancy)	Effect of altered plasma hormone level in pregnancy
Prolactin ↑↑↑	Enhanced by placental estrogens	Promotes growth and development of the breasts and regulates fat metabolism
FSH ↓ and LH ↓	FSH secretion is suppressed by inhibin and placental estrogens LH secretion is suppressed by the combined effect of progesterone and estrogen	Prevents further follicular development and ovulation during pregnancy
GH ↓	Suppressed by hPL	Unknown (hPL has similar effect to GH)
ACTH ↑	Rises	Stimulates increased cortisol secretion from the adrenal cortex
TSH	Falls in first trimester but then rises in second and third	Changes in thyroid hormone secretion are counteracted by changes in plasma protein synthesis

Fig. 14.15 Changes in secretion of anterior pituitary hormones during pregnancy. (ACTH, adrenocorticotropic hormone; FSH, follicle-stimulating hormone; GH, growth hormone; hPL, human placental lactogen; LH, luteinizing hormone; TSH, thyroid-stimulating hormone.)

acid and glucose levels in the blood to improve fetal growth.

Aldosterone secretion from the adrenal cortex also rises slowly in response to the rising ACTH levels. It helps prevent the sodium loss caused by the raised GFR in the kidney.

Changes in metabolism

The mother usually gains 9–15 kg (20–33 lb) during pregnancy, the majority of which is caused by the fetus, placenta, and fluid retention. Six months after birth, maternal weight is usually just 1 kg higher than before the pregnancy. Women have a larger appetite during pregnancy to supply the developing fetus, placenta, and breasts. The excess of nutrients is regulated by changes in metabolism.

Carbohydrates

The hormone hPL causes insulin resistance to develop, and this effect is enhanced by the raised cortisol. As a result, the maternal metabolism uses a higher proportion of fatty acids and glucose use decreases. This glucose is spared for the growing fetus.

If the mother already has a degree of impaired glucose tolerance (e.g., obesity), diabetes mellitus can result. The glucose levels should be strictly controlled because hyperglycemia predisposes to large babies, difficult births, and other pediatric complications. After birth this gestational diabetes mellitus usually resolves.

Amino acids

Progesterone inhibits the breakdown of amino acids in the liver to increase their availability for the fetus. The raised cortisol also increases the blood levels while hPL aids transport across the placenta.

Fat

Fat stores are initially broken down through the action of hPL to drive maternal metabolism. Toward the end of pregnancy fat is stored in the breasts and subcutaneous tissues. Fat accounts for only a fraction of weight gain through pregnancy.

Other changes

Other minor changes occur during pregnancy:
- Increase of clotting factors so that coagulation occurs more easily. In fact, intravascular coagulation and embolism are a relatively common cause of pregnancy-related mortality.
- Immune system is repressed to prevent rejection of the fetus. This can predispose to infection.
- Pelvic ligaments soften to allow the fetus to pass during birth.
- Venous congestion in lower limbs due to the pressure of the fetus on venous return; it can cause varicose veins.

Parturition and labor

Position of the fetus

It is important to determine the position of the fetus before the onset of labor so that potential problems can be identified and preparations made. The position is assessed through palpation and ultrasound scans. There are three aspects to the fetal position, described below.

Lie

The lie describes the orientation of the baby's long axis; in simple terms, it is the orientation of the back. It can be:
- Longitudinal—this is the normal position with the back lying along the uterus.
- Oblique—the back is at an angle across the uterus.
- Transverse—the back lies across the uterus.

Palpation can also reveal which side the back is on, in a longitudinal lie.

Presentation

This is simply the part of the fetus that is nearest the cervix and, therefore, most likely to come out first. There are three main presentations:
- Cephalic—head first; this is normal.
- Breech—the bottom or feet first.
- Shoulder—associated with a transverse lie.

Cephalic presentations are further divided according to which part of the head is presenting. The term "denominator" is used to describe the foremost part of the head. This is important because it affects the widest part of the head that must be born. The different types of cephalic presentation are shown in Fig. 14.16; occipitoanterior is the normal presentation. Figure 14.17 shows some important points on the fetal skull along with the widest diameters of each presentation.

Clinically the presentation is described along with the extent to which the presenting part is palpable;

Comparison of the four variations of cephalic presentation				
Presentation	Vertex (occipitoanterior)	Deflexed (occipitoposterior)	Brow	Face
Position of the neck	Flexed	Deflexed	Extended	Very extended
Denominator	Occiput	Vertex	Bregma	Chin
Widest diameter	Suboccipitobregmatic	Occipitofrontal	Mentovertical	Submentobregmatic
Width	9.5 cm	11.5 cm	13.5 cm	9.5 cm

Fig. 14.16 Comparison of the four variations of cephalic presentation.

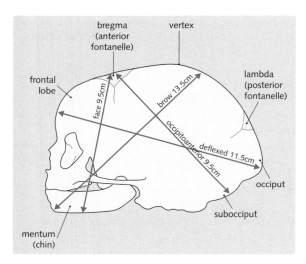

Fig. 14.17 Anatomy of the fetal skull and the widest diameters in the four types of cephalic presentation.

Secondly:
- Anterior (A)—faces the pubis bone.
- Transverse (T)—across the pelvis.
- Posterior (P)—faces the sacrum.

These two sections are combined with the name of the denominator to describe the position (e.g., left occipitoanterior [LOA] or occipitoposterior [OP]). The occipitoposterior position is often associated with a deflexed presentation.

Sequence of labor

Labor is the sequence of actions leading to childbirth (parturition), including the expulsion of the placenta. In normal pregnancies childbirth occurs after 37–42 weeks; the average is 40 weeks (280 days). Labor begins with regular, painful uterine contractions accompanied by cervical dilatation. It is often preceded by several weeks of false labor with irregular, painful contractions (called Braxton Hicks contractions) and no cervical dilatation. True labor is divided into three stages: first, second, and third.

First stage

This is from the onset of true labor until full cervical dilatation (10 cm). The length of the stage varies widely among women; however, the cervix should dilate at a rate of 1 cm/hr:
- 8–10 hours in first labor (nulliparous women).
- 2–6 hours in subsequent labors (multiparous women).

As labor progresses, the uterine contractions become stronger and more frequent. The contractions push the fetal head into the pelvis toward the cervix. The pain experienced is due to hypoxia of the uterus caused by occlusion of the blood vessels during the

this is described in fifths so that a fully palpable head scores 5/5, which decreases as the head descends (e.g., 3/5).

Position

The position of the fetus describes the direction that the denominator is facing compared with the pelvis. This is divided into two sections, which are then subdivided.

Firstly:
- Left (L)—faces the mother's left.
- Right (R)—faces the mother's right.
- Straight—faces the pubic symphysis or sacrum directly.

muscular contractions. The amniotic membrane often ruptures during this stage, resulting in the loss of amniotic fluid (breaking of the waters). The baby performs two actions before or during the first stage:
1. Engagement of the head into the pelvis.
2. Descent of the head through the pelvis, usually in left occipitoanterior (LOA) position.

The first stage is subdivided into two phases:
• Latent phase—the cervix dilates slowly from 0 to 4 cm.
• Active phase—the cervix dilates more rapidly from 4 to 10 cm.

Second stage

This is from full cervical dilatation until the birth of the baby. It usually lasts 40–60 minutes in nulliparous women and 10–15 minutes in multiparous women. The baby must perform eight actions for normal birth to occur:
1. Flexion of the neck so its chin is on its chest and the occiput will be presented.
2. Internal rotation of the head so that it faces the sacrum.
3. Crowning of the occiput (when the baby is visible between contractions).
4. Extension of the neck as the head is born (support the head and check for the umbilical cord at the back of the neck).
5. Restitution as the head rotates back to the normal position outside of the mother.
6. External rotation of the head toward the mother's thigh as the shoulders rotate.
7. Birth of the anterior (top) shoulder (push the baby's head down).
8. Birth of the posterior (bottom) shoulder and body (pull the baby's head up and support the body).

Uterine contractions continue and are assisted by voluntary "pushing" by the mother (contractions of the diaphragm and abdominal muscles). Once the head has crowned, the mother is asked to stop pushing so that the head can pass the vaginal opening smoothly to prevent tearing.

The pain is most severe during the second stage; it is caused by stretching of the cervix, vagina, and perineum. The pain is conducted by normal somatic sensory nerves.

Third stage

This is from birth of the baby until the delivery of the placenta and membranes. Naturally, it lasts between 10 and 45 minutes, although current practice is to actively manage this stage. This involves:
• Intramuscular injection of Syntometrine® (5 units oxytocin and 500 µg ergometrine) during the birth of the body.
• Pulling the umbilical cord once there are signs of placental separation (lengthening of the cord, contraction of the uterus, or a gush of blood).

The uterus shrinks to the 20-week size, and contractions continue. The entire placenta and decidua basalis detach from the uterus and are expelled, causing hemorrhage from the ruptured blood vessels. The hemorrhage is stopped by the muscle fiber arrangements within the uterus; this is more effective using active management. The contractions slowly subside once the afterbirth has been expelled. The placenta is inspected carefully to ensure that no sections remain in the uterus.

Initiation of parturition

The myometrium of the uterus becomes more excitable toward the end of gestation, causing false labor that blends into the coordinated contractions seen in true labor. The exact mechanism that initiates this increase in excitability and onset of labor are not known, although several factors have been identified.

Estrogen:progesterone ratio

Progesterone inhibits contractions during pregnancy, but its secretion stabilizes or drops toward the end. Estrogens stimulate contractions, and secretion continues to increase until birth. The balance of these hormones moves in favor of estrogen, causing increased excitability.

Uterine distension

Stretching the muscle of the uterus increases contractility so that fetal growth and movement may have a stimulatory effect.

Cervical distension

Irritation and stretching of the cervix cause oxytocin release, which stimulates contractions. The fetal head activates this release by pressing against the cervix.

Fetal hypothalamus maturation

At full term the fetal hypothalamus and pituitary secrete more CRH, ACTH, and oxytocin. This oxytocin may cross the placenta to act on the uterus.

Fetal adrenal activity

Cortisol secretion from the fetal adrenal glands increases as fetal ACTH rises. This stimulates placental estrogen secretion and prostaglandin synthesis in the uterine muscle, which raises contractility.

Hormonal control of parturition
Oxytocin

Oxytocin is a peptide hormone synthesized in the hypothalamus and secreted by the posterior pituitary gland (it is described in Chapter 2).

During labor, oxytocin levels rise owing to cervical stimulation by the head. It stimulates uterine contractions that push the fetus against the cervix, stimulating further oxytocin release. A positive feedback mechanism develops called the Ferguson reflex.

Oxytocin receptors in the uterine muscle are increased during late pregnancy by the action of estrogen. Oxytocin binding stimulates prostaglandin production, which causes the increased contractility (especially PGE_2).

Prostaglandins

Prostaglandins are locally acting eicosanoids that regulate many processes throughout the body (see Chapter 1). During labor the prostaglandin PGE_2 is synthesized in the uterine muscle cells in response to oxytocin. It stimulates the release of calcium ions, which cause muscle contractions.

PGE_2 is also synthesized in the cervix, where it stimulates cervical softening and dilatation.

Relaxin

Relaxin promotes the relaxation of the pelvic ligaments and softens the cervix prior to parturition. This allows both structures to stretch so the fetus can pass through the pelvis.

Induction of labor

Labor can be induced by three methods, which can be used in combination or alone:
- Prostaglandins (PGE_2) by vaginal pessary or gel, which acts within a few hours.
- Intravenous oxytocin, which takes about 12 hours to act.
- Rupture of the amniotic membrane (amniotomy), which can be performed only if the cervix is more than 4 cm dilated.

Disorders of labor

Prolonged labor

The progress of labor is plotted on a partogram that records measurements, including the frequency and strength of contractions, dilatation of the cervix, and descent of the fetus. The pattern on the partogram can be used to distinguish between two types of prolonged labor (Fig. 14.18).

Primary dysfunctional labor

Primary dysfunctional labor describes slow dilatation of the cervix or descent of the mature fetus. It is a common condition, especially in first-time mothers. It is usually due to inefficient uterine contractions and can be treated using intravenous oxytocin to improve the strength of contractions. Alternatively, artificial rupture of the membranes (if they have not already ruptured) using an "amnihook" can have a similar effect.

Secondary arrest of labor

Secondary arrest describes a labor that "gets stuck" after progressing normally. The head fails to descend, and the cervix remains at the same dilatation. This is less common than primary dysfunctional labor, although it is often difficult to distinguish the two patterns. Secondary arrest should be suspected when prolonged labor occurs in a multiparous woman; it can also occur in first-time mothers. It is caused by:
- Inefficient uterine contractions.
- Cephalopelvic disproportion (the head is too large for the pelvis).
- Malposition of the fetus (e.g., breech).

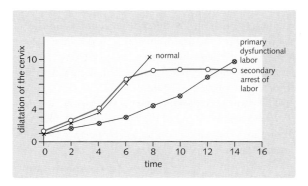

Fig. 14.18 Dilatation of the cervix in normal, primary dysfunctional, and secondary arrested labor.

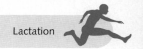

Since inefficient uterine contractions are the most common cause, intravenous oxytocin is used. If the labor still fails to progress, or if fetal distress is detected, then cesarean section is needed.

Assisted delivery

The second stage of labor is a critical period for the fetus and mother. If the second stage progresses slowly (beyond 1 hr in multiparous women or beyond 1.5 hr in nulliparous women) or fetal compromise is suspected, an assisted delivery may be considered. There are four main types of assisted delivery:

- Kjelland's forceps—rotational forceps used to correct a malposition; they are rarely used in developed countries.
- Neville–Barnes forceps—the most common forceps used for midpelvic cavity deliveries.
- Wrigley's forceps—short forceps used for low pelvic cavity deliveries and cesarean sections.
- Ventouse extraction—a suction device that fits onto the fetal vertex.

All assisted deliveries carry the risk of increased trauma to the fetus and mother. A number of criteria must be met before an assisted delivery can be attempted:

- Fetal position known, with cephalic presentation.
- Presenting part descended to the ischial spines or below with <1/5 palpable abdominally.
- Cervix fully dilated and membranes ruptured.
- Maternal bladder empty (to limit trauma).
- Adequate analgesia.
- Consent of the mother.

Lactation

Mammary development

During pregnancy the breast undergoes hormone-induced adaptations in preparation for lactation after birth. This section describes these changes together with the control and process of lactation. The development of the breast is described along with the other organs of reproduction in Chapter 11. The structure and disorders of the adult breast can be found in Chapter 12.

Changes during pregnancy

After puberty the female breast is composed of 15–20 lobes divided into secretory lobules, each with 10–100 acini. These acini are surrounded by fatty connective tissue; they drain into the lactiferous ducts. The breast remains in this state until pregnancy.

Development of the breasts during pregnancy is caused by the rising levels of four hormones:

- Estrogens—cause the ductal system to grow and branch and fat to be stored in the stroma; inhibit milk production.
- Progesterone—causes growth and an increased number of acini.
- hPL—causes development of the acini cells so that they are capable of milk secretion.
- Prolactin—causes development of the acini similar to hPL.

In the last few weeks of pregnancy, estrogen fails to inhibit breast secretion completely so that small quantities of a yellowish fluid called colostrum are secreted. Colostrum contains virtually no fat and has high concentrations of antibodies.

After birth the estrogen, progesterone, and hPL levels fall because the placenta is expelled. Prolactin secretion continues if the mother breastfeeds the baby; this maintains the breast changes brought about by the other hormones. The lack of estrogen allows prolactin to stimulate production of milk instead of colostrum, although it takes a few days for the change to occur.

The breast changes caused by estrogens and progesterone occur to a lesser degree toward the end of each menstrual cycle. The breasts often become swollen and tender.

Hormonal control

Lactation is caused by the effects of two hormones:

- Prolactin—causes milk secretion.
- Oxytocin—causes milk ejection.

Both hormones are secreted by the pituitary gland in response to nipple stimulation. Prolactin is secreted by the anterior pituitary gland and oxytocin is secreted by the hypothalamus and released from the posterior pituitary. The synthesis and secretion of these hormones are described in Chapter 2.

Prolactin

Prolactin secretion increases throughout pregnancy, causing the acinar cells of the breast to develop. During pregnancy, milk production is inhibited by high estrogen levels. After childbirth, estrogen levels

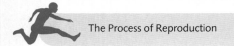
fall dramatically so that prolactin can stimulate the secretion of milk.

During breastfeeding, stimulation of the nipple causes prolactin secretion, resulting in milk secretion and maintenance of the breast. The milk accumulates within the breast, causing swelling unless oxytocin triggers the milk to be ejected. This neuroendocrine reflex is shown in Fig. 14.19. Once breastfeeding is stopped, nipple stimulation diminishes so that prolactin secretion and milk production cease.

The high levels of prolactin during lactation inhibit LH and FSH secretion, giving breastfeeding a contraceptive effect. This is only effective while the baby is suckling regularly. Once lactation ceases, the normal ovarian cycle and fertility return within 4–5 weeks.

The production of milk is a very good example of biological supply and demand. The more the baby suckles, the more prolactin is secreted and the more milk is produced. Women who are having difficulty producing "enough milk" should be encouraged to allow the baby to suckle more.

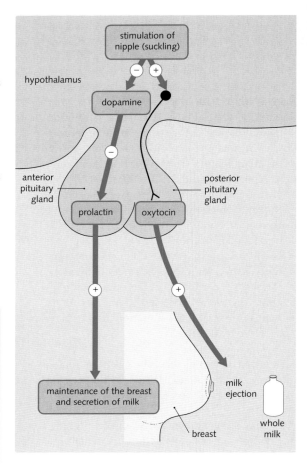

Fig. 14.19 Regulation of lactation by prolactin and oxytocin.

Oxytocin

Milk is ejected from the breast by the action of hormonal rather than neural signals on the smooth muscle in the breast. Oxytocin induces the smooth muscle cells surrounding the acini to contract so that milk is squeezed out of the nipple. Suckling stimulates this oxytocin release, causing milk ejection within about 30 seconds. The reflex is shown in Fig. 14.19. Even the sound of the baby crying can stimulate the release of oxytocin and the ejection of milk. On the other hand, stress can inhibit this reflex, and this can be a particular problem if the woman is worried about her ability to breastfeed.

Colostrum and milk

Colostrum is a pale-yellow fluid that lacks the fat content of milk. It is richer in antibodies so that it protects the neonate against early infection; this is called passive immunity.

Breast milk is a mixture of essential nutrients in water. The main constituents are:
- Lipids (fat).
- Casein (protein).
- Lactose (sugar).

It also contains vitamins, minerals, and antibodies. Milk produced by other mammals has a different composition, making it unsuitable for human babies. For example, cow's milk contains less lactose but more casein than human milk. Special formula milks are available for women who choose not to breastfeed.

It is important to consider whether a woman is breastfeeding when prescribing medications. A number of chemicals can enter breast milk and affect the baby, including estrogen (e.g., combined oral contraceptive pill) and alcohol. HIV-positive mothers are advised not to breastfeed, since there is a risk of the virus infecting the baby through the milk.

Lactation is a very energy-intensive process, even more so than pregnancy. The woman will require about 120% of her normal energy usage. This extra energy is derived from stored fat and the diet.

Disorders of pregnancy and the placenta

Ectopic pregnancies

It is important to consider the possibility of an ectopic pregnancy in any woman presenting with abdominal or pelvic pain. A pregnancy is described as "ectopic" if the blastocyst implants in any location other than the endometrium of the uterus. Ninety-nine per cent of the time this means the fallopian tubes, but it can also occur on the ovary or the abdomen. The incidence is about 1 in 100 pregnancies in developed countries; the risk is increased by factors that slow the transport of the oocyte:

- Pelvic inflammatory disease.
- Previous pelvic surgery.
- Previous ectopic pregnancy.
- Pregnancy despite progesterone-only pill or IUD use.
- Pregnancy from assisted fertilization (e.g., IVF).

Once the blastocyst has implanted, the trophoblast attempts to form a placenta by invading the surrounding structures. Initially this allows the embryo to grow, but the pregnancy usually terminates after 6–10 weeks owing to a lack of space and nutrients. This is called tubal abortion.

There is a high risk of complications following ectopic pregnancy, the most serious of which is tubal rupture. The trophoblast erodes through the wall of the fallopian tube, causing intraperitoneal bleeding. In a minority of cases this can be severe and life-threatening.

Symptoms and signs
Subacute
The majority of patients with ectopic pregnancies present following tubal abortion or mild rupture. The most common symptoms are:

- Unilateral abdominal pain and tenderness.
- Recent amenorrhea.
- Vaginal bleeding.

On vaginal examination there may be a tender mass in a fallopian tube. The abdominal pain may be so mild that it is ignored until vaginal bleeding occurs.

Acute
In severe tubal rupture the patient presents with severe abdominal pain and sudden collapse. They will have hypovolemic shock and an acute abdomen (tender with guarding).

Investigations
Diagnosis of subacute ectopic pregnancies from the history and examination alone is very difficult owing to the nonspecific symptoms. Blood tests for hCG will be positive, indicating a pregnancy (if measured over a couple of days it may rise more slowly than expected). An ultrasound scan will show an empty uterus and may reveal the mass in the fallopian tube. If the embryo is not found, a laparoscopy is performed to examine the tubes directly.

Acute tubal rupture is a surgical emergency. It is investigated and treated by laparotomy to remove the entire affected fallopian tube as soon as possible.

Treatment
If ectopic pregnancies are diagnosed before abortion or rupture occur, they are treated surgically using laparoscopy ("keyhole" techniques) or laparotomy (opening the abdomen); there are three treatment options:

- Removal of the entire fallopian tube that contains the embryo.
- Removal of just the embryo through an incision in the tube.
- Injection of methotrexate (cytotoxic drug) into the embryo, inducing early abortion.

Since there is a high risk of recurrence or infertility following ectopic pregnancy, any further pregnancies need careful monitoring.

Miscarriage
Miscarriage (spontaneous abortion) is the expulsion of a fetus from the uterus before it is capable of independent survival; clinically, this is before 24 weeks or below 500 g. After 24 weeks, it is termed a premature delivery. Miscarriage is very common, affecting about 10% of pregnancies, usually between the 6th and 10th weeks, although more may occur before the mother realizes she is pregnant. It is caused by:

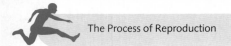

- Fetal abnormalities, often due to chromosomal disorders (60%).
- Abnormal implantation or placenta.
- Uterine abnormality.
- Maternal illness.
- Idiopathic (unknown).

Symptoms and investigations

Miscarriage is suspected if a pregnant woman experiences vaginal bleeding. Ultrasound is used to visualize the fetus and normally shows that the fetus is alive and well.

If the bleeding is associated with cervical dilatation and uterine contractions (which may be described as pelvic pain), miscarriage becomes inevitable. The woman must be admitted to hospital to ensure that the entire fetus and placenta are expelled. This is done by inspecting the expelled material and performing a further ultrasound scan of the uterus. Any retained material must be extracted surgically through the cervix.

Placenta previa

If the placenta is located over the lower uterine segment (sometimes including the cervix), the condition is called placenta previa; the incidence is about 1 in 200 pregnancies. It is important not to perform a vaginal examination if placenta previa is suspected. The severity of placenta previa is graded 1–4, according the distance from the cervix (1 being the farthest). The placenta is prone to bleeding as the uterus grows or when the cervix dilates in labor. The bleeding is usually painless, and the uterus remains soft and nontender; it may also present with the fetus in an abnormal position owing to the location of the placenta. The risk of placenta previa is increased by multiple pregnancies and previous cesarean sections. It is diagnosed and monitored by ultrasound. Delivery is performed by cesarean section at 37 weeks (or earlier if bleeding is severe), except grade 1, which may allow normal vaginal delivery.

Placental abruption

Placental abruption occurs when the placenta separates from the uterine wall before the fetus has been delivered, resulting in bleeding. Vaginal bleeding is usually obvious; however, the blood is concealed within the uterus in about 20% of cases. The bleeding ranges from mild to severe and life-threatening. It is a common disorder (about 1 in 80 pregnancies) that is predisposed by hypertension, smoking, multiple pregnancies, and polyhydramnios (excess amniotic fluid). It presents with:

- Vaginal bleeding.
- Abdominal pain and tenderness.
- Rigid uterus.
- Evidence of fetal compromise.

Placental abruption can be diagnosed using ultrasound to visualize concealed blood clots and to distinguish it from placenta previa. The extent of bleeding is determined using signs of shock and blood tests to measure hemoglobin and platelet concentration. Fetal compromise is recorded using fetal heart monitoring. The mother should be resuscitated and stabilized; induced delivery or emergency cesarean section may be indicated.

Preeclampsia and eclampsia

Eclampsia is a disease that presents in the second half of pregnancy with convulsions caused by hypertension. It is preceded by an increase in blood pressure called preeclampsia.

Preeclampsia

Preeclampsia (also called pregnancy-induced hypertension [PIH]) affects about 5% of women during pregnancy to varying degrees. Treatment is needed if the blood pressure rises above 140/100 mmHg or if urine protein is consistently greater than 300 mg/L.

Preeclampsia is largely asymptomatic, although generalized edema can occur at any stage. If the following symptoms and signs develop, an eclamptic convulsion is likely:

- Severe headache.
- Irritability.
- Blurred vision.
- Epigastric pain.
- Vomiting.
- Brisk reflexes.

Eclampsia

Careful blood pressure and urine monitoring aims to prevent the progression of preeclampsia to eclampsia; in developed countries eclampsia affects only 0.0005% of pregnancies (i.e., it is very rare). The woman experiences a brief period of disorientation followed by a tonic–clonic seizure. The initial seizure can be followed by further seizures, coma, or hemorrhagic stroke. There is a risk of death for both the mother and fetus, but this is usually prevented by early detection and treatment of preeclampsia.

Etiology

The underlying cause of preeclampsia and eclampsia occurs early in pregnancy during implantation. The trophoblast fails to invade the endometrial spiral arteries sufficiently, resulting in poor placental perfusion. This deficient invasion may be due to a maternal immunological response against the embryo.

Both the placenta and fetus become ischemic, leading to poor development; thus fetal growth retardation is often associated with preeclampsia. Cells from the ischemic placenta can be carried (embolize) into the maternal circulation, where they trigger the release of thromboplastins. The thromboplastins cause vasoconstriction and poor renal perfusion, resulting in:

- Hypertension.
- Proteinuria.
- Edema.

These signs characterize preeclampsia. If the condition continues, cerebral hypoxia and edema can result, causing the convulsions of eclampsia. There is also a high risk of blood clots forming in the blood vessels (disseminated intravascular coagulation [DIC]) that can produce tissue infarctions. The etiology of preeclampsia is shown in Fig. 14.20.

Death can occur from:

- Cerebral hemorrhage (stroke) or edema.
- Cardiac failure.
- Cardiorespiratory arrest.
- Organ failure following DIC.

Treatment

Even mild preeclampsia requires frequent blood pressure checks. If the blood pressure exceeds 140/100 mmHg or there is significant proteinuria, the woman needs to be admitted and treated.

The only cure for preeclampsia and eclampsia is delivery of the baby, often by cesarean section, although eclamptic fits can still occur up to 48 hours later. Several medications may slow the rise in blood pressure so that the baby has more time to mature. Diuretics cannot be used because they lower the blood volume, making the placental ischemia worse.

Magnesium sulphate is used in severe PIH or eclampsia. It causes the arteries to relax, restoring

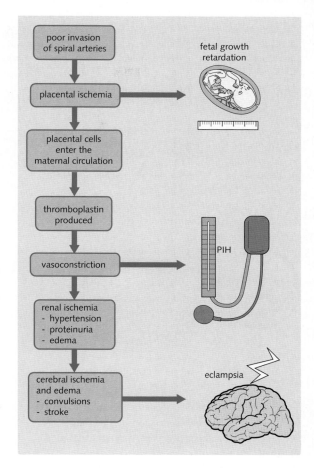

Fig. 14.20 The etiology of pregnancy-induced hypertension (PIH; preeclampsia).

blood flow to the brain, and also inhibits coagulation. Treatment must be monitored because it can depress breathing.

Neoplasia of trophoblastic origin

During implantation the trophoblast normally invades the endometrium. If this process is disrupted, there is a high chance of the trophoblast forming an invasive tumor.

Hydatidiform mole

Hydatidiform moles are benign tumors of the chorion that forms the placenta. Chorionic villi enlarge to form grapelike vesicles that secrete hCG and progesterone. It is usually caused by major abnormalities of fertilization. There are two types: partial and complete (Fig. 14.21).

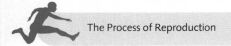
Comparison of partial and complete hydatidiform mole		
Feature	**Partial mole**	**Complete mole**
Extent of placental involvement	Only a section	Entire placenta
Fetal tissue	Present but fetus is normally nonviable	Not present
Usual cause	Two sperms fertilizing the oocyte (polyspermy)	Sperm entering an oocyte that has lost its nucleus (haploid zygote)
Risk of developing malignancy	Low	High

Fig. 14.21 Comparison of partial and complete hydatidiform mole.

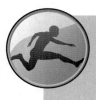

Hydatidiform moles are named from the Greek word *hydratid*, meaning water droplet. This is due to the appearance of the vesicles that make up the mole.

Hydatidiform moles occur in about 1 in 2000 of U.S. pregnancies. The secretion of hCG and progesterone causes exaggerated symptoms of pregnancy:
- Severe morning sickness.
- Early preeclampsia.
- Abnormally large and doughy uterus.
- Vaginal bleeding.

Moles produce the following results on investigation:
- Absence of fetal heart sounds.
- "Snowstorm-like" appearance on ultrasound scans.
- Extremely high hCG levels.

They are treated by suction evacuation of the uterus, followed by hCG level monitoring to detect the recurrence seen in 10% of cases, often in a malignant form called choriocarcinoma.

Invasive mole
This represents the middle ground between a hydatidiform mole and choriocarcinoma. The tumor invades the myometrium, but it does not spread outside of the uterus. There is a higher risk of recurrence and further invasion.

Choriocarcinoma
This is a highly malignant tumor of the trophoblast without recognizable chorionic villi. It is usually preceded by the recurrence of a hydatidiform mole. It can also occur following pregnancies (1 in 50,000) or miscarriages (1 in 5000). The cancer contains many areas of hemorrhage and necrosis; while villi are not formed, it does secrete high levels of hCG.

It presents in the same manner as a hydatidiform mole or with symptoms and signs of metastasis. Histological examination is used to determine the degree of malignancy.

The prognosis is excellent despite the early blood-borne metastasis to the brain, liver, and lungs. It responds to chemotherapy very well, and hCG levels can be monitored to guide treatment. Fertility is often not affected.

- Describe the two components of sexual arousal and the physical changes that they cause.
- Describe the physiological changes that accompany sexual intercourse and orgasm.
- Describe the physical changes that occur during male and female orgasm.
- What are the common causes of male and female sexual dysfunction?
- Describe the mature sperm and mature oocyte and where they meet.
- Describe the process of fertilization. What prevents polyspermy?
- Describe the early development of the zygote and implantation.
- Discuss methods of contraception.
- List the advantages and disadvantages of different types of hormonal contraception.
- Make a table showing the common causes of infertility and their treatments.
- Describe the development of the placenta including the three phases of the chorionic villi.
- Describe the functions of the placenta.
- List the hormonal changes and their source throughout pregnancy.
- Describe the actions of estrogen, progesterone, and hCG during pregnancy.
- Describe four maternal adaptations to pregnancy.
- Describe the three stages of birth and list the factors that stimulate labor.
- Describe the changes of the breast through pregnancy and the stimulation of lactation along with the hormones responsible.
- Describe the presentation, etiology, and treatment of ectopic pregnancies.
- Describe the presentation, etiology, and treatment of preeclampsia and eclampsia.
- Describe the presentation, etiology, and treatment of hydatidiform moles and choriocarcinoma.

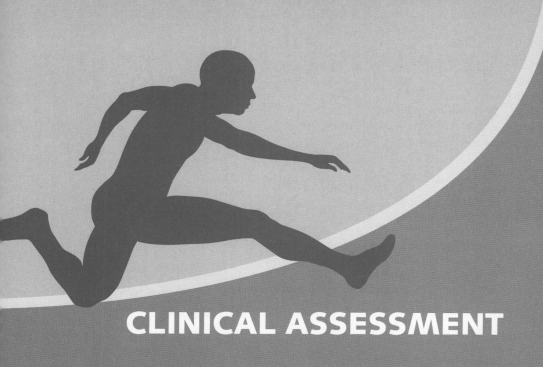

CLINICAL ASSESSMENT

15. Common Presentations of Endocrine and Reproductive Disease

This section gives examples of presenting complaints that are commonly associated with endocrine and reproductive disorders. It does not include the many presentations in which these systems are uncommon causes. Since the disorders of these two systems have a substantial overlap, the disorders are presented together in alphabetical order. The important questions in the history are outlined along with a guide to differential diagnosis. The following disorders are included:

- Amenorrhea.
- Breast lumps.
- Galactorrhea.
- Gynecomastia (male).
- Hirsutism (female).
- Loss of consciousness and coma.
- Menorrhagia and intermenstrual bleeding (female).
- Polyuria.
- Scrotal lumps.
- Sexual dysfunction (male and female).
- Thyroid lumps and goiters.
- Weight gain and obesity.
- Weight loss.

Amenorrhea

This is a complete failure in menstruation lasting longer than 70 days; there are two types:

- Primary—failure to start menstruating by 16 years of age.
- Secondary—absent menstruation after starting during puberty.

Important questions in history taking are shown in Fig. 15.1. Primary amenorrhea is usually just late puberty, while secondary amenorrhea is most commonly caused by low body weight. A number of endocrine disorders can also be responsible, including hyperprolactinemia.

Breast lumps

Breast lumps are a common presentation, especially since breast self-examination has recently been encouraged. While breast cancer is very common and can occur at any age, the majority of breast lumps are benign. Despite this, every lump needs careful examination and further investigation (Fig. 15.2).

Galactorrhea

Galactorrhea (Fig. 15.3) is the inappropriate production of milk from the breasts (i.e., without a recent birth). It usually affects women, but in rare cases it can affect men.

Hyperprolactinemia is the most common cause, but the reason for this excess is often not found.

Gynecomastia

Gynecomastia is growth of the breasts in men caused by an abnormal balance between testosterone and estrogen. It is not the same as simple fat deposition caused by obesity or old age. It is a normal finding during puberty, but otherwise medications or drugs are the most common cause (Fig. 15.4).

Hirsutism

Hirsutism occurs when a woman develops a male pattern of facial and body hair (Fig. 15.5). It should not be confused with excessive hair growth (hypertrichosis) or development of male secondary sexual characteristics (virilism). Polycystic ovarian disease is the most common cause, but in many cases a cause is never found (idiopathic hirsutism).

Loss of consciousness and coma

Loss of consciousness can be caused by many disorders; endocrine and reproductive disturbance are not the most common. Other causes are excluded from Fig. 15.6.

Menorrhagia and intermenstrual bleeding

Menorrhagia is excessive bleeding during menstruation (>80 mL per period). Intermenstrual bleeding is blood discharged from the vagina between periods. The most common cause of both conditions

Fig. 15.1 Important questions and causes of amenorrhea.

Important questions and causes of amenorrhea		
Find out	**Findings**	**Differential diagnosis**
Age	>50 years	Menopause, can also be premature
Weight	Low	Low weight is a very common cause
Growth and sexual development	No secondary sexual characteristics, short stature	Turner syndrome
	Minimal pubic hair	Testicular feminization
Sexual history and contraception	Recent intercourse, no contraception	Pregnancy
	Recently started a progesterone-only form of contraception	May cause amenorrhea
	Recently came off the pill	Pituitary insensitivity
Systems review	Galactorrhea, previous sparse periods, weight gain	Hyperprolactinemia
	Weight gain, hirsutism, acne	Polycystic ovarian syndrome
	Weight loss, irritability, sweating	Hyperthyroidism
Social and medical history	Recent stress or illness	Pituitary insensitivity

Important questions and causes of breast lumps		
Find out	**Findings**	**Differential diagnosis**
Age	Young	Fibroadenoma
	Premenopause	Fibrocystic change, duct ectasia, or duct papilloma
	Elderly	Fibrocystic change, fat necrosis, breast cancer, or phyllodes tumor
Obstetric history	No pregnancies	Slightly higher risk of breast cancer
	Recent pregnancy	Breast abscess
Systems review	Bone pain or jaundice	Metastasis from breast cancer
	Creamy nipple discharge and nipple retraction	Duct ectasia
	Bloody nipple discharge and nipple retraction	Breast cancer
	Eczema round the nipple	Paget's disease (breast cancer)
Family history	Strong family history of breast or ovarian cancer	Breast cancer (*BRAC* genes)

Fig. 15.2 Important questions and causes of breast lumps.

Fig. 15.3 Important questions and causes of abnormal milk secretion (galactorrhea).

Important questions and causes of galactorrhea		
Find out	**Findings**	**Differential diagnosis**
Sexual history and contraception	Recent intercourse, no contraception	Pregnancy
Obstetric history	Recent miscarriage or termination	The hyperprolactinemia of pregnancy takes time to return to normal
Systems review	Female: amenorrhea, weight gain	Hyperprolactinemia
	Male: impotence, less facial hair, visual disturbance, gynecomastia	Hyperprolactinemia
	Visual disturbance, headache	Pituitary tumor loss of dopamine inhibition
	Weight gain and lethargy	Hypothyroidism is a rare cause
Medical history	Chronic renal failure	Can cause hyperprolactinemia
Drug history	Methyldopa, estrogens, tricyclic antidepressants, haloperidol	Drug-induced hyperprolactinemia

Important questions and causes of gynecomastia		
Find out	**Findings**	**Differential diagnosis**
Age	10–16 years	Puberty
Medical history	Testicular torsion, infection, or maldescent	Testosterone deficiency
	Chronic renal failure	Excess estrogen
System review	Small genitalia, tall stature, female fat distribution	Klinefelter syndrome
	Impotence, less facial hair, visual disturbance	Hyperprolactinemia
Drug history	Spironolactone, tricyclic antidepressants, estrogens, griseofulvin	Induce gynecomastia
Family history	Very strong history of breast or ovarian cancer	Male breast cancer (*BRAC* genes)
Social history	Frequent use of amphetamines or cannabis	Induce gynecomastia
	Chronic alcoholism	Liver disease, excess estrogen

Fig. 15.4 Important questions and causes of male breast enlargement (gynecomastia).

Important questions and cause of hirsutism		
Find out	**Findings**	**Differential diagnosis**
Age of onset	Childhood	Congenital adrenal hyperplasia
	>50	Menopause
Systems review	Associated virilism	Androgen-producing tumors or congenital adrenal hyperplasia
	Amenorrhea, weight gain, acne	Polycystic ovarian syndrome
	Weight gain, skin bruising, muscle weakness	Cushing's syndrome
Family history	Other relatives affected	Familial hirsutism
Drug history	Use of high dose steroids	Induces hirsutism in the same manner as Cushing's syndrome
	Danazol for endometriosis	Androgenic effects
Social history	Use of androgens to enhance sporting ability	Excess androgens

Fig. 15.5 Important questions and causes of male pattern body hair in females (hirsutism).

Important questions and endocrine/reproductive causes of loss of conciousness and coma		
Find out	**Findings**	**Differential diagnosis**
Age	Young	IDDM (diabetic ketoacidosis)
Obstetric history	Over 20 weeks pregnant	Eclampsia
Sexual history	Recent intercourse, no contraception	Ruptured ectopic pregnancy
	Current use of combined contraceptive pill	Thromboembolism
Systems review	Weight loss, sweating, palpitations, cardiac arrhythmia	Thyrotoxicosis (hyperthyroidism)
	Weight gain, hypothermia, lethargy, recent illness	Myxedema coma (hypothyroidism)
	Weight loss, polyuria, thirst for several months	NIDDM (HONK)
	Recent weight loss, polyuria, thirst, and sweet-smelling breath	IDDM (diabetic ketoacidosis)
	Pigmentation, weight loss, anorexia, nausea, and vomiting	Addison's disease
	Headache, visual disturbances, gynecomastia	Raised intracranial pressure following pituitary adenoma

Fig. 15.6 Important questions and endocrine/reproductive causes of loss of consciousness and coma. (IDDM, insulin-dependent diabetes mellitus; NIDDM, non-IDDM.)

Fig. 15.7 Important questions and causes of heavy periods (menorrhagia) and intermenstrual bleeding. (HRT, hormone replacement therapy; IUD, intrauterine device.)

Important questions and causes of menorrhagia and intermenstrual bleeding		
Find out	**Findings**	**Differential diagnosis**
Age	Young	Dysfunctional uterine bleeding
	Premenopause	Dysfunctional uterine bleeding, fibroids, uterine polyps, ovarian cysts, endometriosis
	Postmenopause	Endometrial or cervical carcinoma
Sexual history	Recently started using the pill	Breakthrough bleeding is common for a few months
	Use of copper IUD	Causes menorrhagia
	Risk of pregnancy	Ectopic pregnancy, miscarriage
	Pregnant	Miscarriage, placenta previa, placental abruption
Systems review	Pelvic pain, dyspareunia	Fibroids, polyps, endometriosis, and adenomyosis
	Fever, malaise, pelvic pain	Pelvic inflammatory disease
	Hirsutism, weight gain, acne	Polycystic ovarian syndrome
	Weight loss, irritability, sweating	Hyperthyroidism
	Weight gain and lethargy	Hypothyroidism
Drug history	Estrogen (e.g., HRT)	Endometrial hyperplasia

is dysfunctional uterine bleeding, especially at the extremes of reproductive age (Fig. 15.7).

Polyuria

A number of endocrine disorders can upset the kidneys to cause polyuria (Fig. 15.8). This is the excretion of an excess volume of dilute urine causing dehydration and thirst (polydipsia). It is not the same as frequency, in which only small amounts of urine are passed frequently so the total volume is not great.

Scrotal lumps

Lumps in the scrotum are common presenting complaints, and self-examination is being encouraged (Fig. 15.9). Scrotal lumps can arise from the testis, other structures in the scrotum, or the abdominal cavity. There is a wide variety of underlying causes including tumors, infections, and trauma. Testicular cancer is the most common malignancy in young adult males.

Sexual dysfunction
Female

In women the presenting complaints are:
- Lack of sexual desire (decreased libido).
- Failure to reach orgasm (anorgasmia).
- Pain on intercourse (dyspareunia).

Decreased libido and anorgasmia often stem from psychological causes or difficulties within the relationship. Dyspareunia tends to have more physical causes. (See Fig. 15.10.)

Male

In men the presenting complaints are decreased libido and impotence. Medications and alcohol are the most common causes (Fig. 15.11).

Thyroid lumps and goiter

A goiter is an enlarged thyroid gland. The enlargement may be caused by the entire gland or by a nodule; any lumps must be investigated to exclude malignancy. Thyroid lumps are often associated with disorders of the thyroid hormones

Fig. 15.8 Important questions and causes of polyuria.

Important questions and causes of polyuria		
Find out	**Findings**	**Differential diagnosis**
Age	Young	IDDM
	Middle-aged or elderly	NIDDM
Medical history	Renal disease	Nephrogenic diabetes insipidus
	Trauma or surgery to the head	Cranial diabetes insipidus
Fluid intake	Excess intravenous fluids	Iatrogenic diabetes
Systems review	Tiredness, thirst, weight loss	Diabetes mellitus
	Bone pain, muscle weakness, headaches, confusion	Hypercalcemia
Drug history	Any diuretic	Iatrogenic diabetes
	Opiates	Cranial diabetes insipidus
	Lithium, demeclocycline	Nephrogenic diabetes insipidus
	Anticholinergics	Cause a dry mouth and excessive fluid intake
Family history	Diabetes mellitus	Especially NIDDM
	Diabetes insipidus	X-linked inheritance (rarely)
Social history	Psychological problems, abuse	Psychogenic polydipsia

Important questions and causes of scrotal lumps		
Find out	**Findings**	**Differential diagnosis**
Age of onset	Congenital	Indirect hernia, hydrocele, varicocele
	Puberty	Testicular torsion, epididymo-orchitis
	Young	Teratomas are common
	Middle-aged	Epididymal cyst or may be a seminoma
	>50 years	Hydrocele, chronic epididymitis, or lymphoma
Medical history	Recent trauma	Hematoma, hematocele
	Recent vasectomy	Sperm granuloma, hematocele
	Tuberculosis or syphilis	Infectious granuloma
Systems review	Infertility	Varicocele
	Fever, malaise, scrotal pain, UTI	Epidiymo-orchitis
	Weight loss, scrotum feels heavy	Testicular tumor
Social history	Intensive exercise	Testicular torsion
	Recent lifting, e.g. moved house	Indirect hernia

Fig. 15.9 Important questions and causes of scrotal lumps. (UTI, urinary tract infection.)

Fig. 15.10 Important questions and causes of sexual dysfunction in females.

Important questions and causes of sexual dysfunction in females		
Find out	**Findings**	**Differential diagnosis**
Age	Postmenopause	Estrogen deficiency causing a lack of lubrication
Sexual history	Muscles of the vagina tense on attempted intercourse	Vaginismus causing dyspareunia
	Never achieved orgasm	Anorgasmia
Medical history	Previous surgery or trauma	Dyspareunia
Systems review	Fever, malaise, dyspareunia	Infections of the urethra, vulva, vagina, or pelvic inflammatory disease
	Menorrhagia, pelvic pain, deep dyspareunia	Ovarian cysts and tumors, endometriosis, fibroids
	Amenorrhea, galactorrhea, and decreased libido	Hyperprolactinemia
Social history	Lack of communication with partner	Decreased libido and anorgasmia
	Lack of sexual awareness	Anorgasmia

Important questions and causes of sexual dysfunction in males		
Find out	**Findings**	**Differential diagnosis**
Medical history	Diabetes mellitus	Impotence is a chronic complication of diabetes mellitus
	Multiple sclerosis	Inhibits sexual arousal
Systems review	Gynecomastia, visual disturbance	Hyperprolactinemia
	Small testes, deficient male pattern hair	Hypogonadism
Drug history	Antihypertensives and diuretics	Iatrogenic impotence
	Antidepressants, antipsychotics, estrogens	Decreased libido
Social history	Lack of communication with partner	Psychological impotence and decreased libido
	Excessive alcohol intake	Causes acute and chronic impotence

Fig. 15.11 Important questions and causes of sexual dysfunction in males.

and are especially common in women. (See Fig. 15.12.)

Weight gain and obesity

Obesity is defined as a body mass index (BMI; see box) greater than 30, while 25–30 is classified as overweight. The cause of obesity is unknown in the vast majority of patients, although current research into the regulation of eating may change this. Currently obesity alone does not warrant investigation, whereas unexplained weight gain does. The causes of weight gain can lead to obesity so the two are considered together (Fig. 15.13).

Important questions and causes of thyroid lumps and goiters

Find out	Findings	Differential diagnosis
Age	10–16	Temporary physiological goiter
	Young	Papillary carcinoma
	Middle-aged	Autoimmune causes, medullary or follicular carcinoma
	Elderly	Multinodular goiter, medullary, anaplastic carcinoma or lymphoma
Obstetric history	Pregnancy	Temporary physiological goiter
Systems review	Weight loss, sweating, palpitations, irritability, heat intolerance	Graves' disease, multinodular goiter, toxic adenoma
	Weight gain, cold intolerance, tiredness, lethargy, dry skin and hair	Hashimoto's thyroiditis, de Quervain's thyroiditis
	Fever, malaise, and painful neck	Infectious goiter (e.g., de Quervain's thyroiditis)
	Bone pain	Metastases from thyroid cancer
Family history	Thyroid disease	Autoimmune thyroid disease
	Medullary carcinoma	MEN IIa and IIb syndromes
Social history	Unusual diet or immigration from inland developing country	Iodine deficiency

Fig. 15.12 Important questions and causes of thyroid lumps and goiters. (MEN, multiple endocrine neoplasia.)

Important questions and causes of weight gain and obesity

Find out	Findings	Differential diagnosis
Systems review	Abnormal fat distribution, easy bruising, muscle weakness, hirsutism	Cushing's syndrome
	Lethargy, depression, cold intolerance	Hypothyroidism
	Amenorrhea, acne, hirsutism	Polycystic ovarian syndrome
Drug history	Steroids, antidepressants	Stimulate eating
Family history	Other obese members	Genetic or environmental causes
Social history	Stress or history of binge eating	Psychological cause
	Recently gave up smoking	Often slight weight gain

Fig. 15.13 Important questions and causes of weight gain and obesity.

Fig. 15.14 Important questions and causes of weight loss.

Important questions and causes of weight loss		
Find out	**Findings**	**Differential diagnosis**
Age	Elderly	Malignancy or organ failure are most likely
Systems review	Increased appetite, sweating, palpitations, heat intolerance	Hyperthyroidism
	Reduced appetite, malaise, vomiting	Addison's disease, malignancy, or organ failure
	Polyuria, thirst, tiredness	Diabetes mellitus
	Light-colored, chronic diarrhea, large appetite	Malabsorption
Social history	Perception of weight	Eating disorders (e.g., anorexia nervosa)
	Unprotected sexual intercourse or intravenous drug use	HIV infection

BMI is calculated from the weight in kg and height in m. The weight is divided by the height squared. For example, a man weighing 85 kg with a height of 1.65 m has a BMI of $85/(1.65 \times 1.65) = 31.2$.

Weight loss

Weight loss is often a sign of fairly severe disease, so it must be taken seriously. It can be caused by the failure of the heart, kidneys, or liver, but also by several endocrine disorders (Fig. 15.14).

16. History and Examination

The processes of taking a history and examining a patient form the core of a doctor's job. This chapter includes a description of these two tasks along with the major signs associated with common endocrine and reproductive disorders. Chapter 15 describes common presenting complaints along with useful questions to ask in the history. The diversity of the endocrine and reproductive systems makes both the history and examination difficult to describe in a general manner. Both tasks should be directed toward the presenting complaint.

After reading this chapter you should be able to:
- Take and present a history (or at least try).
- Examine a patient.
- List the common findings of endocrine and reproductive disease on examination.

History

Taking a history seems simple in practice, but the presence of a patient induces amnesia and stuttering in most students. It takes a lot of practice to develop a smooth technique and even longer to learn what questions are important and which answers are relevant. This process is neither quick nor easy, but that is why medical training takes so many years.

A proper history involves many components, each of which is described below. These sections are very important for the correct diagnosis to be made; however, they are derived from a doctor-centered approach. To understand the problem from the patient's point of view, the following questions should also be asked:
- Why has the patient sought medical help? Why now?
- What does the patient believe could be causing the problem?
- What does the patient want (e.g., reassurance or treatment)?

In many ways you act as an interpreter for the patient between English and medical jargon; in the same way you should speak to the patient only in plain English.

Preparations

Before taking a history it is important for you, the patient, and the surroundings to be suitably prepared. Several factors can help:
- Check that the patient is available and comfortable.
- Find a quiet and private location. This is often difficult in practice but should always be attempted.
- Be dressed appropriately.
- Have a visible ID badge.
- Think about a possible differential diagnosis from the presenting complaint.
- Write out the components of a history if you need to do so.

Structure of a history

Apart from introducing yourself and asking permission, there is no prescribed structure to taking a history. However, the standard structure used is required for presenting the history in the notes and to medical staff. It also serves as a mental framework that will, in the future, help you to remember a patient's history without having to write everything down! That said, it is a good idea to let the patient tell you about the problem at first in the order with which the patient is comfortable and then use specific questions to fill in the gaps. Possible answers to some of these questions are included in Chapter 15.

Introduction and permission

Always introduce yourself, including your status (e.g., medical student). Explain to the patient what you would like to do (i.e., take a history) and ask the patient's permission.

Example: "My name is Stephen, and I'm a medical student. May I have a chat with you about your illness?"

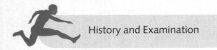

Note that patients usually respond well to the use of first names. If you really *must* introduce yourself as "Dr Huntington-Smythe," all well and good, but remember that "Call me Stephen" is more likely to put the patient at ease.

1) Patient details

It is good practice to obtain basic details about the patient before starting the history. These details are often written above the history in the notes. They should include:

- Patient's name; check that you are with the right patient.
- Age.
- Sex.
- Occupation.

Example: Mr D. Vader is a 34-year-old man who works in the military.

2) Presenting complaint (PC)

The history should begin with an open question along the lines of:

- What brought you into hospital?
- Tell me about your problem.
- What led you to go to your doctor?

The presenting complaint is the main symptom(s) that led the patient to seek medical help. It should be written in the patient's words, not medical jargon.

The presenting complaint should be presented as:

- How the patient came to see you.
- The symptom, in the patient's words.
- The duration.

Example: The patient was referred by his PCP because of "strange breathing noises" over the past three days.

> When a patient answers, "An ambulance" to the question, "What brought you to the hospital?," the patient believes this to be an original and funny joke, deserving at least a smile in recognition.

3) History of presenting complaint (HPC)

This section forms the bulk of the history and includes all details relevant to the presenting complaint. Ideally, the patient will tell you the complete history with only minor prompting, although in practice many patients will need to be led through it. The HPC should include any previous episodes of a similar nature and the systems review questions relevant to the presenting complaint.

The presenting complaint of pain prompts a series of questions to describe it fully. These can be remembered by the mnemonic **SOCRATES**:

- **S** = **S**ite—where the pain is.
- **O** = **O**nset—sudden or gradual.
- **C** = **C**haracter—sharp/crushing/burning.
- **R** = **R**adiation—is it felt anywhere else?
- **A** = **A**lleviating features—what makes it better?
- **T** = **T**iming—when did it start; does it come and go?
- **E** = **E**xacerbating features—what makes it worse?
- **S** = **S**everity—compare with other types of pain.

When presenting this section of the history, you should begin with the time when the patient last felt completely well and continue in order until the present. If any aspect of other sections of the history is relevant (e.g., family history), it should be placed appropriately within this section.

Example: Mr Vader felt completely well until 1 week ago when he began to wake at night with a cough. This coincided with his working at the dusty construction site of a new battleship. Three days ago he developed a wheeze on expiration that has become progressively worse.

He remembers going to the doctor with a similar wheeze when he was young but cannot recall any further details. His aunt and uncle on his mother's side both suffer from asthma, and his daughter has mild eczema. He has no history of smoking.

4) Past medical history (PMH)

This section includes any previous hospital admissions, chronic illness, acute illness, or operations, along with when they occurred. The patient should be asked to describe any previous illness he or she has suffered and then asked specifically about diabetes, tuberculosis (TB), asthma, jaundice, rheumatic fever, hypertension, heart attacks, strokes, and epilepsy.

Extra sections can be added depending on the patient (e.g., obstetric history in women, immunization history in children).

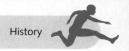

Relevant medical history or negative responses should be included in the HPC, whereas the details and any unrelated illnesses are included here. Unrelated negative responses are not presented but should be written in the notes, often abbreviated (e.g., ^{0}DM/TB).

Example: The patient suffered severe trauma during his late teenage years following a natural disaster that still causes him recurrent back pain. He has no history of surgery or other significant illness.

5) Drug history (DH)

This section is about any medications that the patient takes regularly, not the use of recreational drugs. Accordingly, it is better to ask, "Do you take any medications?" rather than "Do you take any drugs?" The DH includes medications of any form that the patient gets by prescription or over the counter (OTC). Two other questions are important:

- In women of reproductive age: Are you on the pill?
- Everyone: Do you have any allergies? What about penicillin?

The medication should be presented along with the reason for taking it. It is vital to write down the dose and frequency for each drug—don't forget that you will have to write out the drug chart!

Example: He takes 200 mg of ibuprofen 4 times/day for back pain. He has no known allergies.

6) Family history (FH)

Ask the patient if anyone else in his or her family has had similar or related problems and ask specifically about asthma, epilepsy, diabetes, and heart disease. Record the relationship between the patient and affected relatives along with the age, health/cause of death of parents, siblings, and children. It is good practice to sketch the family tree.

Example: Alongside a history of asthma and eczema detailed in the HPC, his grandfather suffered from epilepsy. His father was killed in an accident soon after Mr. Vader was born, and he has lost touch with his mother. He has no siblings. He has two children (twins) aged 6 years, both of whom are well.

7) Social history (SH)

The social history can be very important to diagnosis and appropriate treatment but must be approached in a sensitive and nonjudgmental manner. It is often useful to know about:

- Who the patient lives with and their relationship (e.g., children, wife/partner).
- Leisure activities, exercise, smoking, alcohol, illicit drugs.
- Living status, type of house, financial problems, community help.
- Travel abroad.

Example: Mr. Vader lives alone in military accommodation following separation from his partner. He does not visit his children and is unaware of their whereabouts. He does not smoke and consumes about 20 units of alcohol a week. He has traveled extensively with his occupation.

8) Review of systems

This is essentially a quick checklist of the other systems in the body to prevent missing important symptoms or other problems. The extent to which each system is investigated depends on the presenting complaint. Learning which questions are necessary takes experience and practice. Examples of these questions are shown in Fig. 16.1.

Only the questions with positive answers should be presented, although all answers can be written in the notes.

Example: He has slight constipation and had a headache 1 day ago.

9) Summary

Having taken the perfect history, you should present it back to the patient in simple language, covering all the important points. This can be very difficult; again, experience and practice are essential. It may be easier to summarize parts of the history as you go along.

When presenting the history, a summary is also required before describing the examination. This allows anyone who was not paying attention to catch up and look knowledgeable. It should include:

- The patient's name and age.
- The presenting complaint along with the duration and means of referral.
- A brief summary of the history of the presenting complaint.
- The differential diagnosis.

Example: Mr. D. Vader is a 34-year-old man who was referred by his PCP because of "strange breathing noises" over the past three days. He has had a cough for the last week and developed a

Review of systems	
General health • Weight loss, appetite, night sweats, fevers, any lumps, itch, fatigue, apathy **Cardiovascular system** • Chest pain • Palpitations (awareness of the heart beating) • Exertional dyspnea (quantify exercise tolerance, e.g., number of flights of stairs that can be managed) • Orthopnea (breathlessness on lying flat—symptom of left ventricular failure) • Paroxysmal nocturnal dyspnea (repeated bouts of breathlessness at night) • Claudication (calf pain on walking) • Ankle edema (sign of right-sided heart failure) • Skin sores/ulcers **Respiratory system** • Cough • Sputum (amount, color) • Hemoptysis (coughing up blood) • Shortness of breath • Wheeze **Gastrointestinal system** • Appetite, weight, diet, taste • Nausea, vomiting • Difficulty swallowing • Hematemesis (vomiting blood) • Heartburn • Indigestion • Abdominal pain (site, severity, character, relationship to eating, previous episodes, etc.) • Bowel habit (frequency, change, difficulties) • Rectal bleeding **Urinary system** ("How are the waterworks?") • Frequency • Nocturia (needing to pass urine in the night) • Urine stream (hesitancy, dribbling) • Dysuria (pain on passing urine) • Hematuria (blood in the urine) • Incontinence	**Nervous system** • Headaches, fits, faints, loss of consciousness • Changes in vision, hearing, speech, memory • Anxiety, depression, sleep disturbances • Paresthesia (pins and needles) • Sensory disturbances (numbness) • Weakness **Reproductive system (female)** • Periods (length, cycle, menarche, menopause) • First day of last menstrual period (LMP) • Contraception • Postmenstrual/intermenstrual bleeding • Vaginal discharge • Dyspareunia (pain on intercourse) • Pregnancies, terminations, births • Problems in pregnancy • Breast symptoms **Reproductive system (male)** • Impotence/loss of libido • Scrotal swelling **Musculoskeletal system** • Aches or pains in muscles, bones, or joints • Swelling of joints • Limitation of joint movements • Weakness of muscles **Skin** • Rashes **Risk factors** • Smoking, alcohol consumption, drug abuse • Allergies, foreign travel

Fig. 16.1 Symptoms to ask about in the review of systems.

wheeze three days ago that has progressed since. This is consistent with an episode of asthma or a viral infection.

Communication skills

Many medical schools now place great emphasis on teaching communication skills—partly as a response to public criticism of the medical profession over the past few decades. As a student, it is easy to dismiss this teaching as less important than the more factual elements of the course and even as an insult to a group of people who are surely perfectly capable of talking to patients.

However, when it comes to clinical assessment, most clerkships now feature some form of structured clinical skills examination. In preparation for these types of exams, you should remember these important points:

- None of us is as good at communicating as we like to think we are.
- A lot of this material seems to be stating the obvious—but the obvious can be easy to forget under pressure, and reminding ourselves of the basics is a useful exercise.
- Communication skills account for nearly half the marks in the clinical exams—even in the systems examination stations there are marks for your approach to the patient.
- Practicing a few communication scenarios with friends before the exam is an easy way to pick up a lot of extra marks.
- If you get on the right side of the patient or actor in a clinical exam, he or she is likely to divulge information much more easily.

Obstacles to communication

Many factors can make it difficult to talk with patients and colleagues. It is important to be aware of these and address those you can do something about, while making allowances for those you cannot.

- Noisy environment and lack of privacy—try to find a quiet room or cubicle to see your patient if possible.
- Nervousness—both yours and the patient's. You can help yourself with practice. The patient can be put more at ease by a sensitive approach (more on this later).
- Pain—does the patient need analgesia now rather than after the history?
- Other medical factors—breathlessness, hearing impairment, and confusion (acute or chronic) can make communication difficult. Patience and persistence are required in these situations.
- Language and cultural barriers—try to take the history with a member of the family who can interpret. If this is not possible, an interpreter may be provided. In an acute situation you will have to make do with smiles and gestures to establish the important points, such as the presence and site of pain.
- Hostility—some people may feel (rightly or wrongly) aggrieved by some aspect of the treatment they have already received. It is vital that you do not take this personally or be drawn into a confrontation. Try to remain calm and civil; empathize with the patient and apologize if appropriate. If all else fails, politely explain that

you don't feel anything is being achieved and come back later.

Nonverbal communication skills

A large proportion of our communication "bandwidth" is nonverbal. Examples include body posture, facial expression, eye movements, and gestures. We are conscious of some of these things, but most are subconscious. Nonverbal cues are very important in a clinical setting, both in achieving a rapport with the patient and in gaining insight into the patient's condition.

The following points may be helpful during a consultation:

- Sit with the patient so that your eyes are on roughly the same level; avoid looking down at the patient. Maintain a comfortable distance between you and try to face the patient while you are talking. It is also useful to make sure that you have a comfortable position to write when you are taking a history—kneeling by the bedside is sometimes the best option!
- Maintain good eye contact, even if the patient does not.
- Use nonverbal cues to show that you are listening, and encourage the patient. Nodding, smiling, and even appropriate laughter can help to put the patient at ease. Smiling is particularly important!
- It is worth having practice sessions with friends before you go into an exam. Friends can point out any nervous habits of which you might be unaware.

Verbal communication skills

The things we say and how we say them. It is important to put the patient at ease during a consultation, although this is often easier said than done since people are often understandably concerned in the clinical situation. The following are important skills:

- Empathize with the patient: this means understanding the patient's point of view and is not the same as sympathy. It is perfectly good practice to use such phrases as "I understand" or "That must have been very frightening" when a patient is relating the details of the history.
- Use open questions at first, such as "What made you come to see a doctor today?" or "Have you any other problems that have been worrying you?" It is a good idea to let the patient talk freely for the first minute or so, before you focus the history

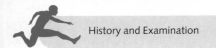

with closed questions such as "Does the pain catch you when you breathe in?"

- Use verbal cues such as "I see" or "I understand" to help the flow of conversation.
- Check that you have understood what the patient has told you by repeating a summary to the patient.
- Use plain English rather than medical jargon. Having said that, try to assess the educational level of your patient and pitch your vocabulary appropriately.

Objectives in the consultation

It is important to have a mental checklist of objectives when you go into a consultation with a patient—especially when this is part of an exam. Once again, the key to this is practice: preferably on the wards, but you can also run through mock scenarios in a study group if you are short of time. You may also need to produce the following kind of list in a short-answer exam paper or viva:

- Introduce yourself and establish a rapport with the patient.
- Find out why the patient has presented to you.
- Find out what the patient understands about the problem and whether the patient has his or her own theory about the cause.
- What are the patient's expectations of this consultation—what does the patient want from you?
- Explore the problem with history and examination and formulate a plan for further management—investigations, treatment, etc.
- Explain your findings and plan to the patient clearly.
- Check that the patient understands what you have said.
- Ask the patient if there is anything he or she is not happy with.
- Literature—provide leaflets or write things down for the patient to take away.
- Follow-up—make sure the patient knows what the next point of contact will be (e.g., an outpatient appointment).

Examination

The diversity of the endocrine system makes examination especially difficult. There is no specific "endocrine examination" comparable to the

examination of the cardiovascular system; instead the examination must include aspects of six major examination sequences:

- Cardiovascular.
- Respiratory.
- Abdominal.
- Cranial nerves.
- Peripheral nerves.
- Examination of a lump.

The extent to which these systems are examined depends on the presenting complaint and differential diagnosis. It takes experience to know which systems to examine, although the history should guide this decision.

The situation is slightly better for the reproductive system, although there are still three sequences that must be examined:

- Female reproductive system.
- Breast.
- Male reproductive system.

This section includes a general examination sequence that covers the major systems, followed by a description of the three reproductive examinations. Common findings together with the potential disorders are shown throughout.

General examination
Introduction and permission
Before examining a patient, you must introduce yourself, unless you have already done so for the history. You must always explain what you intend to do and ask the patient's permission.

General inspection
When meeting a patient and taking a history, it is important to be aware of signs that give information about the patient's condition. These can include their surroundings (e.g., walking sticks), speech, and mental state. Some physical signs can also be seen while taking the history, in particular:

- Facial features and obvious eye signs (Fig. 16.2).
- Skin complexion (Fig. 16.3).
- Body physique and posture (Fig. 16.4).

The area to be examined should also be inspected specifically from the end of the bed before any active examination. The area must be exposed before inspection and the patient should be reassured that you are not just staring.

Inspection of the face	
Findings	**Diagnostic inference**
Harsh facial features, large nose, protruding jaw, and large hands	Acromegaly
Infant with a broad flat face, widely spaced eyes, and a protruding tongue	Cretinism (resulting from hypothyroidism)
Eyes that appear to be bulging out of their sockets, i.e., exophthalmos	Graves' disease (not in other forms of hyperthyroidism)

Fig. 16.2 Common findings on inspection of the face.

Inspection of the skin	
Findings	**Diagnostic inference**
Generalized pigmentation of the skin	Addison's disease, Cushing's disease (not in Cushing's syndrome)
Flushed, red skin with excessive sweating	Thyrotoxicosis, pheochromocytoma
Boils/skin infections	Undiagnosed or poorly controlled diabetes mellitus

Fig. 16.3 Common findings on inspection of the skin.

Common findings on inspection of the body		
Findings		**Diagnostic inference**
Short stature	Failure to grow	Dwarfism
	Infant with flat face	Hypothyroidism (cretinism)
	Bone deformities	Rickets (vitamin D deficiency)
	Female with masculine body shape and webbing of the neck	Turner syndrome (45 chromosomes, XO)
Tall stature	Male with female fat distribution (breasts and hips)	Kleinfelter syndrome (47 chromosomes, XXY)
	Child with excess growth	Gigantism
Overweight	Abnormal fat distribution, wasted arms and legs	Cushing's syndrome
	Purely abdominal	Pregnancy
	Lethargic	Hypothyroidism
Underweight	Young with recent weight loss and wasting	Diabetes mellitus (IDDM)

Fig. 16.4 Common findings on inspection of the body.

Examination of the hands, limbs, and feet

Examination always begins with the hands. This provides a lot of information and is a nonintrusive start that reassures the patient. The specific features to look for in the hands, nails, limbs, and feet are outlined in Figs. 16.5 to 16.8.

Examination sequence
1. Inspect the nails.
2. Test capillary refill.
3. Inspect the hand and skin creases.
4. Feel and count the pulse.
5. Take the blood pressure.
6. Inspect the limbs and feet.
7. Test tone and power of the limbs.
8. Test reflexes of the limbs.
9. Test sensation of the limbs.
10. Test coordination of the limbs.

Examination of the head and neck

Signs found in the head, eyes, and neck that suggest endocrine disorders are shown in Figs. 16.9 to 16.12.

Examination sequence
1. Inspect the face, eyes, and neck.
2. Test the visual acuity and visual fields.
3. Test the eye movements and look for lid lag.
4. Inspect the fundi.

219

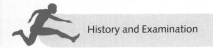

Fig. 16.5 Common findings on examination of the hands. (ACTH, adrenocorticotropic hormone.)

Examination of the hands	
Findings	**Diagnostic inference**
Hands are enlarged, greasy, spadelike, with thickened skin	Acromegaly
Palms are warm and moist ± tremor	Thyrotoxicosis
Palms are cold and dry	Hypothyroidism
Palmar creases are pigmented	Addison's disease, Cushing's disease, ectopic ACTH syndrome
Note the extent of the areas where the patient complains of "pins and needles" (paresthesia) or numbness (anesthesia) in the fingers and hands	Diabetes mellitus (complication), hypocalcemia
Trousseau's sign, showing neuromuscular irritability—test by occluding the blood flow to the hands, using an inflated blood pressure cuff around the upper arm, which causes a typical contraction of the hand (thumb adducts, fingers extend) within 2 minutes	Hypocalcemia
Tinel's sign, showing carpal tunnel syndrome—diagnosed by tapping over the flexor retinaculum and causing paresthesia in the medial fingers	Hypothyroidism, acromegaly
Decreased skin turgor, signifying dehydration—present if skin on the back of the hand does not return to normal immediately after being pinched	Uncontrolled diabetes mellitus, diabetes insipidus, hypercalcemia

Inspection of the nails	
Findings	**Diagnostic inference**
Separation of the nail from its bed (onycholysis) and nail tips appear white	Thyrotoxicosis
Clubbing of the fingertips, caused by swelling of the soft tissue at the base of the nail	Graves' disease (not in other forms of thyrotoxicosis)
Nails look broken and weak (fragile nails)	Hypocalcemia
Deformed nails with inflammation of the surrounding skin is a sign of infection (often caused by *Candida albicans*)	Uncontrolled diabetes mellitus

Fig. 16.6 Common findings on inspection of the nails.

Fig. 16.7 Common findings on examination of the limbs.

	Examination of the limbs	
Feature	**Findings**	**Diagnostic inference**
Pulse rate and rhythm	Rapid pulse rate of >100 beats per minute (tachycardia)	Thyrotoxicosis, pheochromocytoma
	Slow pulse rate of <60 beats per minute (bradycardia)	Hypothyroidism
	Irregular pulse rhythm (signifying cardiac arrhythmias)	Thyrotoxicosis and hypercalcemia
	Reduced or absent pulses in the feet and legs (caused by peripheral vascular disease)	Diabetes mellitus (complication)
Skin, muscle, and bone structure of the limbs	Infected or ulcerated skin (look especially on the lower leg and ankles)	Diabetes mellitus (complication), Cushing's syndrome (both cause poor wound healing)
	Multiple bruising over the skin, with no history of trauma	Cushing's syndrome
	Thickened skin over the tibia, with elevated dermal nodules and plaques (pretibial myxedema)	Graves' disease (not in other forms of thyrotoxicosis)
	Proximal muscle wasting (observe and feel the biceps and quadriceps muscles)	Cushing's syndrome, hypothyroidism, thyrotoxicosis
	Bone deformity, e.g., "bow-legs" or "knock-knees" (observe when the patient is standing)	Rickets (vitamin D deficiency: rare in US)
	Pitting edema at the ankles (caused by salt and water retention)	Cushing's syndrome (SIADH does not cause edema)
Blood pressure	High blood pressure (hypertension)	Cushing's syndrome, diabetes mellitus (complication), acromegaly
	Low blood pressure whilst moving from lying to standing position (postural hypotension)	Addison's disease, diabetic autonomic neuropathy

Examination of the feet	
Findings	**Diagnostic inference**
Feet are large and wide and patient's shoe size has recently increased	Acromegaly
Skin ulcers and/or gangrene	Diabetes mellitus
Dry, cold, hairless skin of the feet and weak or absent foot pulses may signify ischemia caused by peripheral vascular disease (check by testing capillary refill)	Diabetes mellitus (complication)
Note the extent of the areas where the patient complains of "pins and needles" (paresthesia) or numbness (anesthesia) in the feet and lower legs	Diabetes mellitus (complication), hypocalcemia

Fig. 16.8 Common findings on examination of the feet.

221

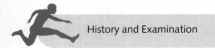

Examination of the head		
Feature	**Findings**	**Diagnostic inference**
Bone structure, facial features, and complexion	Increased head circumference, protruding jaw, coarse facial features, nose and jaw enlarged, malaligned teeth with spaces between them in the lower jaw, thickened facial skin folds	Acromegaly
	Protruding forehead	Rickets (vitamin D deficiency; rare in US)
	Pale, puffy face with coarse features	Hypothyroidism
	Round "moon-face"	Cushing's syndrome
	Acne on face, neck, and chest	Cushing's syndrome, acromegaly and polycystic ovarian syndrome
	Chvostek's sign, showing neuromuscular irritability—diagnosed by gently tapping the facial nerve where it passes through the parotid gland and causing the facial muscles to twitch briskly on the same side of the face	Hypocalcemia
Hair distribution	Lack of normal beard growth in postpubescent males	Delayed puberty, hypopituitarism causing gonadotropin deficiency
	Excessive facial hair (hirsutism) in females	Polycystic ovarian syndrome
Mouth	Hyperpigmented buccal mucosa	Addison's disease, Cushing's disease (not in Cushing's syndrome)
	Malaligned teeth, enlarged tongue (possibly causing dysarthria, i.e., difficulty in pronunciation)	Acromegaly
	Swollen tongue and a hoarse, croaky voice	Hypothyroidism

Fig. 16.9 Common findings on examination of the head.

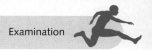

Fig. 16.10 Common findings on examination of the eyes.

Examination of the eyes	
Findings	**Diagnostic inference**
Lid lag—slow descent of the upper lid, lags behind the descent of the eyeball	Hyperthyroidism
Lid retraction—at rest, the superior limbus of the iris and possibly even some sclera above it (white of the eye) is visible (see Fig. 16.11)	Hyperthyroidism
Exophthalmos—the eye appears to bulge out of its socket and it is possible to see the whole of the iris and sometimes even sclera surrounding its circumference (see Fig. 16.11)	Graves' disease (not in other forms of thyrotoxicosis)
Anemia—the inner surface of the lower lid looks pale if anemia is present	Menorrhagia
Retinal disease—look for ischemic change and neovascularization using an ophthalmoscope (appearance of "dots" and "blots" signifies presence of microaneurysms and microhemorrhages, respectively)	Diabetes mellitus (complication)
Papilledema (caused by raised intracranial pressure)—both optic disks appear convex and their margins appear blurred	Pituitary tumor
Impaired visual acuity—test the visual acuity in both eyes separately using an eye chart	Diabetes mellitus (complication)
Bitemporal hemianopia visual field deficits—test the visual fields in each eye separately	Pituitary tumor

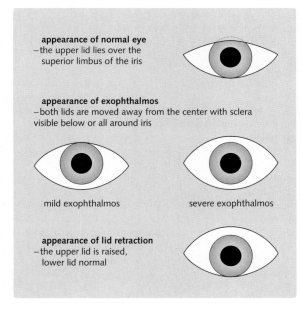

Fig. 16.11 Appearance of the eyes indicating hyperthyroidism.

Examination of the neck	
Findings	**Diagnostic inference**
Anterior neck swelling in the thyroid position which ascends during swallowing	Goiter
Swelling in the neck between the chin and the 2nd tracheal ring which rises when the tongue is stuck out	Congenital thyroglossal cyst

Fig. 16.12 Common findings on examination of the neck.

5. Test the sensation and power of the face.
6. Listen to their speech.
7. Feel for lymph nodes.
8. Examine any lumps present.
9. Look for the height of the jugular venous pressure (JVP).
10. Feel for tracheal deviation or tug.

Examination of the thorax
Signs found in the thorax suggestive of endocrine disorders are shown in Fig. 16.13. The patient should

223

be examined whilst he or she is reclined at an angle of 45°.

Examination sequence

1. Inspect the front, sides, and back of the chest.
2. Count the respiratory rate.
3. Locate the apex beat.
4. Feel for heaves or thrills.
5. Palpate the chest movement on the front and back.
6. Percuss the lungs on the front, sides, and back.
7. Auscultate the heart (four positions).
8. Listen at the apex with the bell while the patient lies on the left side (mitral stenosis).
9. Listen in the tricuspid area with the patient sitting forward and the breath held on

expiration using the diaphragm (aortic regurgitation).

10. Auscultate the lungs on the front, sides, and back.

Examination of the abdomen

Signs found in the abdomen which suggest endocrine and reproductive disorders are shown in Figs. 16.14 and 16.15. The patient should be examined while lying flat.

Examination of the thorax	
Findings	**Diagnostic inference**
A "pigeon chest" or "rickety rosary" (outward bowing and thickening of the costochondral junctions)	Rickets (vitamin D deficiency; rare in US)
Truncal obesity (abnormal fat distribution) and increased chest hair in men and women	Cushing's syndrome
Respiratory distress—deep, rapid hyperventilation ("air-hunger"), called Kussmaul's breathing	Diabetic ketoacidosis

Fig. 16.13 Common findings on examination of the thorax.

Inspection of the abdomen	
Findings	**Diagnostic inference**
Scars	Previous surgery possibly to treat an endocrine or reproductive system disorder
Wide purple striae (linear wrinkled "stretch" marks) in both sexes and increased abdominal hair (hirsutism) in women	Cushing's syndrome
Abdominal distension (can be caused by fat, fluid, fetus, flatus, feces, or large solid tumors)	Cushing's syndrome (fat), hypothyroidism (fat), pelvic mass (e.g., fibroids, ovarian disease, or pregnancy)
Excessive outward curvature of the spine (kyphosis) or excessive inward curvature of the spine (lordosis) can be caused by vertebral collapse	Osteoporosis secondary to menopausal hormone failure, Cushing's syndrome, or thyrotoxicosis

Fig. 16.14 Common findings on inspection of the abdomen.

Palpation and percussion of the abdomen	
Findings	**Diagnostic inference**
Enlarged liver, spleen, and kidneys (organomegaly)	Acromegaly
Mass with impalpable lower border	Pelvic mass (e.g., fibroids, pregnancy)
Body tenderness	Osteoporosis secondary to menopause, Cushing's syndrome, or thyrotoxicosis
	Bony metastases
Lower abdominal tenderness	Pelvic inflammatory disease, ectopic pregnancy
Shifting dullness	Ascites following malignancy

Fig. 16.15 Common findings on palpation and percussion of the abdomen.

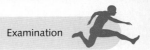

Examination sequence

1. Inspect the abdomen.
2. Lightly palpate the abdomen starting away from tender areas.
3. Palpate the abdomen more deeply.
4. Examine any lump present.
5. Palpate for the liver edge from the right iliac fossa.
6. Palpate for the spleen edge from the right iliac fossa.
7. Ballot the kidneys.
8. Percuss for the liver, spleen, and ascites.
9. Auscultate for bowel sounds or fetal heart sounds.
10. Rectal examination.

Fetal heart sounds can be heard over a pregnant uterus using Doppler ultrasound at 10 weeks gestation and with a stethoscope at 25 weeks.

Examination of a lump or mass

If a lump is detected, it must be assessed for the features shown in Fig. 16.16. This is a very common presentation, and assessment guidelines apply to lumps found in all locations.

Examination of the female reproductive system

It is essential to explain carefully the examination that you wish to perform when it involves intimate body parts. A member of staff of the same sex as the patient should be present at every examination for medicolegal reasons and to reassure the patient.

Examination of a lump	
Feature	**Findings**
Skin changes	Color, scarring, ulceration, edema
Temperature	Hot, cold
Tenderness	Is it painful when touched?
Location	Accurate anatomical description
Size and shape	Estimates of diameter
Surface	Irregular, lobular, smooth
Edge	Sharp, rounded, indistinct
Consistency	Firm, hard, soft
Translucency	Cysts allow light to pass through
Relations	What structures is it attached to?

Fig. 16.16 Examination and description of a lump.

Examination of the vulva (external genitalia)

The vulva should be examined with the patient lying on her back with the legs apart and knees bent. The common signs of vulval disease are shown in Fig. 16.17.

Examination sequence

1. Inspect the entire vulva.
2. Look for vaginal discharge.
3. Ask the patient to cough or push down.
4. Look for vaginal prolapse and urinary incontinence.

Internal examination with a speculum

This examination should not be performed on a virgin. A warmed vaginal speculum can be used to visualize the cervix and obtain swabs or a cervical smear. Three swabs are routinely taken if there is a risk of infection:

- High vaginal swab.
- Cervical swab.
- Cervical swab for *Chlamydia*.

If a smear is required, the speculum should be inserted without lubricant. A wooden spatula is used to sample the cells of the cervix; the sample is smeared onto a slide and fixed immediately, before being sent for analysis.

Bimanual examination of the vagina and uterus

This examination often follows examination with a speculum and, likewise, it should not be performed on a virgin. The signs of disease of the internal female reproductive system are shown in Fig. 16.18.

Examination sequence

1. Lubricate your index and middle finger.
2. Insert gently into the vagina.
3. Rotate upward.
4. Palpate the cervix.
5. Press above the pubis with the other hand to feel the uterus.
6. Palpate laterally; the ovaries should not be palpable.

Breast examination

Breast examination is usually aimed at finding and describing a lump (see Fig. 16.16). If a lump is found, further investigation is always required to exclude the possibility of malignancy. This cannot be determined from the history and examination alone.

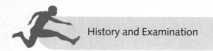

Fig. 16.17 Common findings on inspection of the vulva.

Inspection of the vulva	
Findings	**Diagnostic inference**
Rashes (redness, swelling, or white thickened areas called leukoplakia)	Often caused by infections, dermatological conditions (e.g., lichen sclerosus), chemical irritants, or allergies
Injury or scars	Can be due to trauma (e.g., childbirth, female circumcision, or sexual abuse)
Enlarged clitoris (clitoromegaly)	Congenital adrenal hyperplasia (excessive androgen secretion)
Red painful cystic lump beneath the posterior part of the labia majora	Bartholin's cyst or abscess
Bloody vaginal discharge	Menstruation, miscarriage, cancer, cervical polyp, or erosion
Purulent vaginal discharge	Infection, e.g., vaginitis, cervicitis, endometritis
Frothy, watery, pale, yellow-white, or purulent discharge and pruritus	Infection caused by *Trichomonas vaginalis*
Thick, white, cottage-cheese-like discharge and inflammation of the skin and mucous membranes	Infection caused by *Candida albicans*

Examination of the female internal genitalia	
Findings	**Diagnostic inference**
Difficult to insert a lubricated finger	Vaginismus
Impalpable uterus	Retroverted uterus
Palpable mass laterally	Mass in the ovary or fallopian tube
Enlarged, nodular uterus	Fibroids
Enlarged, smooth uterus	Pregnancy or cancer

Fig. 16.18 Common findings on examination of the female internal genitalia.

The potential findings of breast examination are shown in Figs. 16.19 and 16.20. Always examine both breasts. To avoid the patient wondering what you are doing, explain that you always "start with the good side so you can compare it with the affected side."

Examination sequence
1. Inspect sitting up.
2. Inspect sitting forward.
3. Inspect with arms lifted.
4. Inspect with hands pressed on hips.
5. Palpate both breasts and describe any lumps.
6. Examine axillary and supraclavicular lymph nodes.

Examination of the male genitalia
Examination of the external genitalia
The common abnormalities of the male external genitalia found on examination are shown in Figs. 16.21 and 16.22.

Examination sequence
1. Inspect skin color and texture.
2. Inspect the ventral and dorsal sides of the penis.
3. Locate the urethral meatus (hole).

Examination of a scrotal mass
The possible causes of lumps and swellings in the scrotum are illustrated in Fig. 16.23. The exact location of a lump relative to the testes and abdomen is especially important.

Examination sequence
1. Inspect the scrotum.
2. Palpate the testes, epididymis, and spermatic cords.
3. Describe any abnormal lumps present.

Fig. 16.19 Common findings on inspection of the breast.

Inspection of the breast	
Findings	**Diagnostic inference**
Scar due to mastectomy (removal of breast)	Previous breast carcinoma
Breast size decreased bilaterally in women	Hypopituitarism
Enlargement of the female breast (unilateral or bilateral)	Benign hyperplasia of the breast, breast infection/inflammation, breast neoplasia
Enlargement of the male breast (unilateral or bilateral)	Gynecomastia (see Fig. 15.4), breast carcinoma
Skin appears pulled in and puckered	Underlying breast carcinoma
Skin has an "orange peel" appearance (peau d'orange) because of edema-induced widening of the orifices of sweat glands and hair follicles	Breast carcinoma that is blocking the lymphatic drainage and causing edema
Skin nodules, abnormal skin texture and color	Skin infiltrated with tumor cells from a breast carcinoma
Skin is erythematous (reddened) + hot	Infection of the breast or the overlying skin
Skin ulceration (determine its position, size, shape, color, edge, and base)	Advanced breast carcinoma
Nipple and surrounding skin is thickened, red, encrusted, and oozy, with an underlying breast lump	Paget's disease of the nipple (breast carcinoma)
Recent nipple pigmentation increased	Addison's disease or pregnancy
Nipple asymmetry and/or retraction	Underlying breast carcinoma
Nipple discharge	Infection, benign or malignant breast tumors, lactation
Nipple duplication—can occur anywhere along the line from the axilla to the groin	Supernumerary nipples
Redness and swelling of the axilla and arm (caused by lymphadenopathy and edema)	Metastases in the axillary lymph nodes from a breast carcinoma

Examination of the breast	
Findings	**Diagnostic inference**
A solitary, stony-hard, painless lump with an irregular surface and an indistinct edge, which may involve the skin, underlying muscle, and regional lymph nodes	Breast carcinoma
A young patient with a solitary, firm, painless lump with a spherical (or knobbly) surface, which tends to be highly mobile and no lymphadenopathy	Fibroadenoma—but further investigations must be performed
In a pregnant woman with a lump or diffuse swelling that is tender, soft/solid, and spherical with hot overlying skin and lymphadenopathy	Breast abscess
Palpable regional lymph nodes	Breast infection, breast carcinoma

Fig. 16.20 Common findings on examination of the breast.

Inspection of the male external genitalia	
Findings	**Diagnostic inference**
Skin/mucosal rashes or ulceration	Infection, inflammation, connective tissue disease, squamous cell carcinoma
Decreased pubic hair	Hypogonadism, hypopituitarism
Small penis	Hypogonadism
Abnormal position of the external urethral meatus ± hooded foreskin	Hypospadias

Fig. 16.21 Common findings on inspection of the male external genitalia.

Examination of the male external genitalia	
Findings	**Diagnostic inference**
Urethral discharge	Infection or inflammation
Empty scrotum (unilateral or bilateral)	Undescended or retractile testis, previous excision
Small firm testes (bilateral)	Hypogonadism, testicular atrophy due to alcohol or drugs
Small firm testis (other testis normal)	Mumps orchitis
Exquisitely tender testis with edematous swelling of the entire scrotal contents	Torsion of the testis (epididymo-orchitis)

Fig. 16.22 Common findings on examination of the male external genitalia.

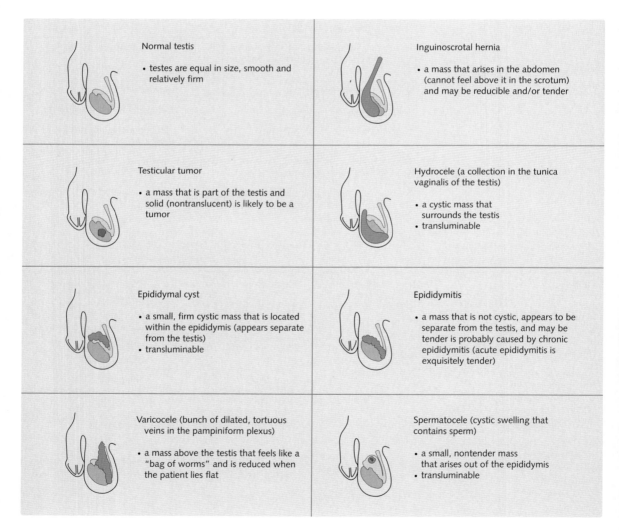

Normal testis

- testes are equal in size, smooth and relatively firm

Inguinoscrotal hernia

- a mass that arises in the abdomen (cannot feel above it in the scrotum) and may be reducible and/or tender

Testicular tumor

- a mass that is part of the testis and solid (nontranslucent) is likely to be a tumor

Hydrocele (a collection in the tunica vaginalis of the testis)

- a cystic mass that surrounds the testis
- transluminable

Epididymal cyst

- a small, firm cystic mass that is located within the epididymis (appears separate from the testis)
- transluminable

Epididymitis

- a mass that is not cystic, appears to be separate from the testis, and may be tender is probably caused by chronic epididymitis (acute epididymitis is exquisitely tender)

Varicocele (bunch of dilated, tortuous veins in the pampiniform plexus)

- a mass above the testis that feels like a "bag of worms" and is reduced when the patient lies flat

Spermatocele (cystic swelling that contains sperm)

- a small, nontender mass that arises out of the epididymis
- transluminable

Fig. 16.23 Common findings on examination of a lump in the scrotum.

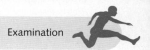

4. Determine the location of any lumps.
5. Try to transluminate any lumps.

Examination of the prostate gland

The prostate gland and seminal vesicles can be examined by rectal palpation. The common findings are shown in Fig. 16.24.

Common findings on examination of the prostate	
Findings	**Diagnostic inference**
Smooth, firm gland, 2–3 cm across, with two lobes separated by narrow sulcus	Normal prostate
Enlarged and mobile gland with lobules	Benign hypertrophy
Large, irregular, and hard gland fixed to the rectal mucosa with a distorted central sulcus	Prostatic carcinoma

Fig. 16.24 Common findings on examination of the prostate.

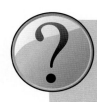

- Write out the nine components of a history in the order they are presented.
- Take a history from a friend who pretends to have a suitable condition.
- Present the history.
- Summarize the most important points of the history.
- Perform a cardiovascular examination and present the findings.
- Perform a respiratory examination and present the findings.
- Perform an abdominal examination and present the findings.
- Perform a neurological examination and present the findings.
- Examine a lump and present the findings.
- Describe how the male and female reproductive systems are examined.

17. Investigations and Imaging

Following the history and examination, an endocrine or reproductive disorder may be suspected. Many tests can be used to investigate endocrine function; however, the results can be misleading unless the appropriate test is used.

Proper investigation of a suspected endocrine disorder follows the following steps:
- Measure the level of hormone in the blood/urine or its biological effects.
- If a deficiency is suspected, use a stimulation test.
- If an excess is suspected, use a suppression test.
- If an abnormality is confirmed, image the suspected gland.

After reading this chapter you should be able to:
- List the types of tests available.
- Outline the tests relevant to the hormone under investigation.
- Describe other tests that may contribute to diagnosis.
- Discuss the imaging techniques available.

Investigating hormones

Measuring methods
This section outlines the tests used to measure hormone levels and how they change upon stimulation or suppression. These tests are performed if a hormone excess or deficiency is suspected from the history and examination; they aim to confirm the diagnosis and investigate its cause. The four main methods of investigating hormones are described below.

Direct measurement
The levels of hormones in the plasma and urine can be measured using enzyme-linked immunosorbent assays (ELISAs). The sample is mixed with a known concentration of hormone bound to fluorescent markers. Monoclonal antibodies specific to the hormone are added and the hormone–antibody complexes formed are separated from the solution. The degree of fluorescence is inversely proportional to the original hormone concentration because the native hormone competes with the labeled hormone for antibodies to bind to (Fig. 17.1). In the past radioimmunoassay (RIA) was used, but this test is less sensitive. The normal concentrations of commonly measured hormones are shown in Fig. 17.2.

Indirect measurement
Some hormones produce metabolic changes that are easier to measure than the hormone itself. There are two main examples:
- Blood glucose is used to determine insulin levels.
- Urine vs. blood osmolality is used to determine antidiuretic hormone (ADH) levels.

Stimulation tests
If a hormone deficiency is suspected, secretion is stimulated to record the response. Blood levels are measured before and after stimulation.

Suppression tests
If a hormone excess is suspected, the hormone secretion is suppressed to record the response. Blood levels are measured before and after suppression.

Hypothalamic function
The quantities of hormones secreted by the hypothalamus are generally too low to be measured clinically. Hypothalamic dysfunction is investigated by measuring the relevant pituitary hormones and their response to stimulation or suppression.

Anterior pituitary function
Hormone assays
Pituitary adenomas can affect the secretion of all anterior pituitary hormones. For this reason a suspected abnormality in one anterior pituitary hormone prompts investigation of all the others.

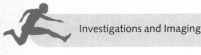

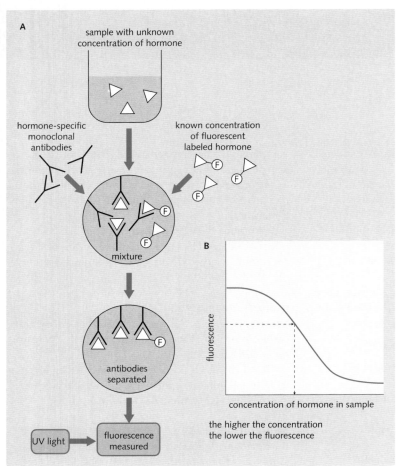

Fig. 17.1 (A) Measuring hormone levels by enzyme-linked immunosorbent assay (ELISA). (B) Interpretation of the results.

Hormones secreted by the anterior pituitary gland are measured along with the hormones that they stimulate. The tests for the following hormones are usually available:

- Thyroid-stimulating hormone (TSH), along with triiodothyronine (T_3) and thyroxine (T_4).
- Luteinizing hormone (LH) and follicle-stimulating hormone (FSH), along with estrogen or testosterone.
- Growth hormone (GH), along with insulin-like growth factor 1 (IGF-1) and glucose; circadian variation must be considered.
- Prolactin.

Triple stimulation test

The combined pituitary test (CPT) stimulates the anterior pituitary gland to secrete the six major hormones. It is used to investigate hypopituitarism,

usually caused by a pituitary adenoma. Three stimulatory substances are injected intravenously:

- Insulin—causes hypoglycemia which stimulates ACTH, GH, and prolactin secretion (Fig. 17.3).
- Thyrotropin-releasing hormone (TRH)— stimulates TSH and prolactin secretion.
- Gonadotropin-releasing hormone (GnRH)— stimulates LH and FSH secretion.

The levels of all six hormones and the hormones that they stimulate are measured before and several times after the stimulation.

Individual tests for secretion

Stimulation and suppression tests are especially important for measuring GH and ACTH because of their circadian variation. Hypothalamic function can be assessed only by these tests. The tests for TSH,

LH, FSH, and ACTH are described under the relevant endocrine organ. There is no further test for prolactin, and the tests for GH are described below.

Normal ranges of commonly measured hormones	
Hormone	Normal levels
Prolactin	Men: <450μL (2–15ng/mL) Women: <600μL (2–20ng/mL)
Adrenocorticotropic hormone (ACTH)	<80ng/L (80pg/mL)
Growth hormone (GH)	<20mU/L (<5ng/mL)
Thyroid-stimulating hormone (TSH)	0.5–5.7μU/mL
Thyroxine (T$_4$)	70–140nmol/L (5–12μg/dL)
Triiodothyronine (T$_3$)	1.2–3nmol/L (70–190ng/dL)
Calcitonin	<0.1μg/L (3–26pg/mL)
Cortisol (morning)	200–700nmol/L (6–23μg/dL)
Aldosterone	80–250pmol/L (<2–9ng/dL)
Renin (standing)	2.8–4.5pmol/mL/hr
Testosterone	Men: 10–35nmol/L (3–10ng/mL) Women: <3.5nmol/L (<1ng/mL)

Fig. 17.2 The normal ranges of commonly measured hormones.

Stimulation test

Used for GH deficiency; GH can be stimulated by:
- Insulin-induced hypoglycemia (Fig. 17.3).
- Oral clonidine.

Blood samples are measured for glucose and GH before the test and several times over the following 2 hours. To create a suitable stimulus, blood glucose must fall below 2.2mmol/L (40mg/dL), causing symptoms of hypoglycemia. Sugar may need to be given if blood glucose falls too low. GH deficiency is confirmed if secretion does not rise by >20mU/L.

Suppression test

Used for GH excess; GH is measured every 30 minutes for 2 hours following administration of glucose, i.e., an oral glucose tolerance test (see p. 235). Increased blood glucose normally suppresses GH secretion, but in acromegaly or gigantism GH levels fail to decrease.

Posterior pituitary function
Hormone assays
Antidiuretic hormone

Plasma levels of antidiuretic hormone (ADH) can be measured by ELISA, but they are of little value unless combined with stimulation tests. The comparison between urine and blood osmolality is a more useful clinical measure:
- Dilute urine, concentrated blood: ADH excess (diabetes insipidus).

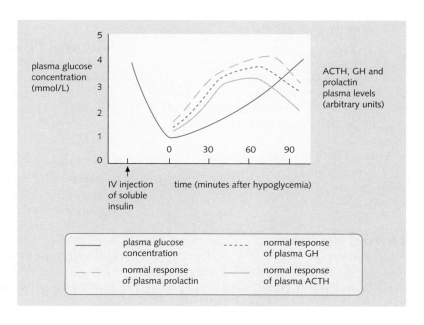

Fig. 17.3 Normal response of adrenocorticotropic hormone (ACTH), growth hormone (GH), and prolactin to insulin-induced hypoglycemia. (Adapted from Jeffcoate WJ: Lecture Notes on Endocrinology, 5th ed. London, Blackwell Science, 1993.)

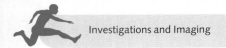

- Concentrated urine, dilute blood: ADH deficiency (syndrome of inappropriate ADH secretion; SIADH).

Oxytocin
Since abnormal plasma levels do not cause any recognized pathology, secretion is not tested.

Water deprivation test
This is a stimulation test used for suspected ADH deficiency (i.e., diabetes insipidus). ADH release is stimulated by high plasma osmolality caused by water deprivation.

After a night's sleep and fasting the patient is deprived of food and water for 8 hours, during which plasma osmolality and urine osmolality are measured repeatedly. The patient is also weighed, and the test is abandoned if the patient loses >3% body weight. At the end of the test desmopressin (an ADH analog) is given, and urine and plasma osmolality continue to be measured. This section of the test is described below under the desmopressin test.

Diabetes insipidus is diagnosed if urine osmolality is <400 mosmol/kg; the normal range is >600 mosmol/kg. The plasma osmolality should have risen to >295 mosmol/kg to induce this fall.

Desmopressin test
This is a suppression test that identifies the cause of diabetes insipidus (DI) once it has been confirmed by a water deprivation test. It can be caused by:
- Cranial DI—deficient pituitary secretion of ADH.
- Nephrogenic DI—failure of the kidney to respond to ADH.

The ADH analog desmopressin is injected intramuscularly, and the patient is allowed to drink water. Plasma and urine osmolality are measured 1 and 2 hours later. If DI is caused by ADH deficiency (i.e., cranial DI), this should return urine osmolality to normal:
- Cranial DI—urine osmolality increases to >750 mosmol/kg.
- Nephrogenic DI—urine osmolality remains <400 mosmol/kg.

Thyroid function
Hormone assays
If abnormalities of thyroid function are suspected, then plasma levels of TSH, T_4, and T_3 should be measured. Both thyroid hormones are measured because variations in thyroxine-binding globulin (TBG) levels can give inaccurate results. Further investigation is often not needed:
- Low levels of T_4 and T_3—hypothyroidism.
- High levels of T_4 and T_3—hyperthyroidism.

TSH is measured with T_3 and T_4 to locate the lesion. In hypothyroidism a low TSH suggests a pituitary/hypothalamic lesion, while a high TSH suggests a thyroid gland problem. In hyperthyroidism TSH will almost always be low.

TSH is also measured to guide thyroxine treatment of thyroid disorders. The correct dose of thyroxine or carbimazole is being administered when TSH levels return to normal.

Thyrotropin-releasing hormone stimulation test
This stimulation test is used if TSH deficiency is suspected. However, TSH measurement is now so sensitive that it is rarely used. Hypothalamic TRH is administered intravenously, and plasma TSH levels are measured before and after.

Thyroid autoantibody assays
ELISA can also be used to detect thyroid autoantibodies caused by the common autoimmune thyroid diseases:
- Thyroid-stimulating antibodies (TsAb) suggest Graves' disease.
- Antithyroid-peroxidase (anti-TPO) and antithyroglobulin (anti-TgAb) antibodies suggest Hashimoto's thyroiditis.

Adrenal function
Cortisol assays
24-hour urinary free cortisol
Urine is collected over a 24-hour period, and the quantity of cortisol is measured. It is normally <280 nmol/24 hr. This gives an accurate guide to plasma levels.

Basal plasma cortisol and adrenocorticotropic hormone
These are measured at 09:00 and 22:00 because of circadian variation. This test is not as reliable as 24-hour urinary free cortisol.

Aldosterone assays
Plasma levels of aldosterone are measured, along with renin and potassium, to assess the appropriateness of aldosterone secretion.

Aldosterone is normally secreted in response to high renin or high potassium. Conn's syndrome is suggested by high aldosterone in the presence of low renin and potassium.

Catecholamine assays

Catecholamine levels can be measured directly or, more commonly, by measuring their metabolites such as vanillylmandelic acid (VMA). Both tests are performed on 24-hour urine samples. Pheochromocytoma causes VMA levels to rise above 48 mol/24 hr.

Dexamethasone suppression test

This test is used if excess cortisol (Cushing's syndrome) is suspected. Dexamethasone is a synthetic corticosteroid that normally suppresses hypothalamic CRH and pituitary ACTH secretion, causing cortisol secretion to drop. High or low doses of dexamethasone may be used, as described below.

Low-dose

This is used to investigate excess cortisol (i.e., Cushing's syndrome). Plasma cortisol is measured in the morning; then 0.5 mg/6 hr dexamethasone is given orally for 48 hours. Plasma cortisol is measured again in the morning after the last dose. A 24-hour urinary cortisol is also collected on the second day of stimulation. Cushing's syndrome is diagnosed if the test fails to suppress plasma cortisol.

High-dose

This is used if the patient has clear signs of Cushing's syndrome or has had a positive low-dose test. 2 mg/6 hr dexamethasone is given orally for 48 hours, and the same measurements are collected as in the low-dose test.

- **Slight cortisol depression**—Cushing's disease; ACTH-secreting pituitary tumor.
- **No cortisol depression**—ectopic ACTH-secreting or adrenal tumor.

Synacthen® stimulation test

This test is used to investigate cortisol deficiency (e.g., Addison's disease). Synacthen® (also called tetracosactrin) is a synthetic analog of ACTH that normally stimulates cortisol secretion. There are two versions of the test (see below).

Short Synacthen® test

This test is used to exclude Addison's disease. 0.25 mg Synacthen® is given intramuscularly, and plasma cortisol levels are measured before and 30 minutes later. Addison's is excluded if:

- First plasma cortisol level is >140 nmol/L.
- Second plasma cortisol is >500 nmol/L.
- Second plasma cortisol is >200 nmol/L higher than the first.

Prolonged Synacthen® test

This test is used if the short test fails to exclude Addison's disease. 1.0 mg Synacthen® is given intramuscularly on three successive days, and plasma cortisol levels are measured before and 6 hours after each injection. The diagnosis can be made from the plasma cortisol 6 hours after the third injection:

- <690 nmol/L—Addison's disease.
- >690 nmol/L—pituitary ACTH deficiency.

The name Synacthen® is made by combining *syn*thetic with ACTH.

Pancreatic function

Random and fasting blood glucose assays

Endocrine investigation of the pancreas is aimed at diagnosing suspected diabetes mellitus. Insulin deficiency causes abnormally high plasma glucose levels (hyperglycemia) and sometimes glycosuria. Insulin levels are never measured directly because blood glucose gives a more consistent measure of insulin action, especially if insulin resistance is present.

Diabetes mellitus is diagnosed using blood glucose measurements after an overnight fast on two occasions. Fasting blood glucose levels are normally 3.5–5.5 mmol/L (60–100 mg/dL). The results are interpreted as follows:

- >7.8 mmol/L (>140 mg/dL)—diabetes mellitus confirmed.
- 6–7.8 mmol/L (108–140 mg/dL—impaired glucose tolerance.
- <6 mmol/L (<108 mg/dL)—not diabetic.

Oral glucose tolerance test

If the fasting blood glucose measurements show impaired glucose tolerance, an oral glucose tolerance test (OGTT) is indicated. This is a stimulation test to check for insulin deficiency; however, glucose is measured, not insulin. The patient fasts overnight

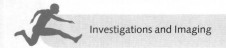

Interpretation of oral glucose tolerance test results			
Blood glucose level (mg/dL)	Normal	IGT	Diabetes mellitus
After an overnight fast	<108	108–140	>140
2 hours after glucose intake	<140	140–200	>200

Fig. 17.4 Interpretation of blood glucose measurements during an oral glucose tolerance test. (IGT, impaired glucose tolerance.)

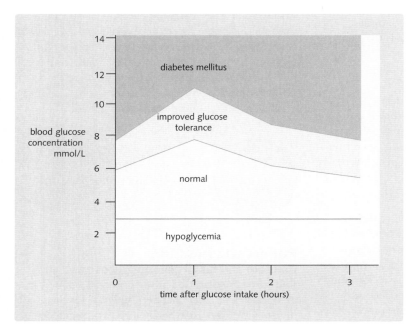

Fig. 17.5 Changes in blood glucose following an oral glucose tolerance test and interpretation of the results.

and then drinks 75 g glucose in water. Plasma glucose is measured before and 2 hours after the drink. The results are shown in Figs. 17.4 and 17.5. In patients with normal glucose tolerance the blood glucose should return to the fasting level within 2 hours.

Gonadal function and pregnancy testing
Hormone assays
Male
The male reproductive hormones are measured to exclude gonadal failure causing infertility following two abnormal sperm counts. Plasma levels of the following hormones are measured:

- FSH and LH.
- Testosterone.
- Prolactin.

Testosterone requires three blood samples to be taken in the morning at 20-minute intervals because it is secreted in a pulsatile manner with a circadian rhythm.

Female
A similar set of hormones are investigated in a woman with amenorrhea or infertility to exclude gonadal failure. Estradiol-17β and progesterone are measured instead of testosterone. The stage of the menstrual cycle must be calculated because normal levels of FSH, LH, estradiol-17β, and progesterone vary throughout the cycle.

Primary gonadal failure
Low levels of gonadal steroids along with high levels of LH and FSH indicate primary gonadal failure.

Hypothalamic–pituitary dysfunction
Low levels of gonadal steroids with low or normal levels of LH and FSH indicate hypothalamic–pituitary dysfunction. Raised prolactin levels can cause this pattern.

Gonadotropin-releasing hormone stimulation test

This test is used to investigate gonadal steroid deficiency (i.e., gonadal failure in both men and women). GnRH normally raises secretion of LH and FSH.

100 μg GnRH is injected intravenously and the plasma levels of the reproductive hormones are measured before and four times in the hour after the test. The levels of all the reproductive hormones should be increased following this test. Failure of LH and FSH levels to rise confirms pituitary dysfunction, while an excessive rise suggests hypothalamic dysfunction.

Pregnancy test

Pregnancy can be diagnosed by detecting human chorionic gonadotropin (hCG) in the urine. The test will be positive approximately 10 days after conception.

Other investigations

Information about endocrine and reproductive disorders can be gathered from tests not specifically designed to investigate hormone levels or organs.

Clinical chemistry

The clinical chemistry laboratory measures the concentrations of ionic and organic components in the blood and urine (e.g., U + Es). Figure 17.6 shows endocrine causes of disordered chemical levels. These results must be viewed alongside the history,

Component and its normal range	Endocrine causes of abnormally high concentration	Endocrine causes of abnormally low concentration
Plasma sodium: 135–145 mmol/L	Diabetes insipidus, Cushing's syndrome, Conn's syndrome	Syndrome of inappropriate antidiuretic hormone secretion (SIADH), Addison's disease, diabetes mellitus
Plasma potassium: 3.5–5.0 mmol/L	Addison's disease, diabetes insipidus, diabetes mellitus	Cushing's syndrome, hyperaldosteronism, SIADH, hyperthyroidism
Plasma urea: 2.5–7.5 mmol/L; plasma creatinine: <120 mmol/L	Diabetes insipidus, diabetes mellitus, Addison's disease	SIADH
Plasma osmolality: 270–300 mosmol/kg	Diabetes insipidus, diabetes mellitus (N.B. abnormal aldosterone levels do not affect osmolality)	SIADH
pH: 7.35–7.45; bicarbonate: 24–30 mmol/L	Cushing's syndrome, Conn's syndrome	Addison's syndrome, diabetic ketoacidosis, hyperparathyroidism (mild)
Plasma calcium: 2.25–2.55 mmol/L	Hyperparathyroidism, vitamin D toxicity, hyperthyroidism, acromegaly, Addison's disease (N.B. abnormal calcitonin levels do not affect plasma calcium levels)	Hypoparathyroidism, vitamin D deficiency, Cushing's syndrome
Plasma phosphate: 0.8–1.5 mmol/L	Hypoparathyroidism, hyperthyroidism, acromegaly	Hyperparathyroidism, vitamin D deficiency, diabetes mellitus
Fasting blood glucose: 3.5–6.0 mmol/L	Diabetes mellitus, Cushing's syndrome, acromegaly, hyperthyroidism, pheochromocytoma	Exogenous insulin overdose, Addison's disease, pituitary insufficiency
Fasting plasma triglycerides: 0.55–1.90 mmol/L	Diabetes mellitus	
Plasma ketone bodies: not normally present in the blood	Diabetes mellitus	

Fig. 17.6 Normal concentration ranges for ionic and organic components of the blood and endocrine causes of abnormally high or low concentrations.

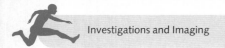

examination, and other tests, since endocrine diseases are rarely the most common cause.

Hematology

Investigations of the components that make up blood can suggest specific disorders:

- Low hemoglobin—chronic blood loss.
- Raised hematocrit—dehydration.
- Increased percentage of HBA_{1C}—diabetes mellitus.
- Raised erythrocyte sedimentation rate (ESR)—inflammation or infection.

Microbiology and virology

If an infection is suspected, an appropriate specimen can be tested for microorganisms. Specimens can be collected by swabbing, scraping, or aspirating the infected region. Infections of endocrine organs are uncommon, but the reproductive system is prone to sexually transmitted diseases.

The following endocrine disorders can predispose to infection elsewhere in the body:

- Diabetes mellitus.
- Cushing's syndrome.
- Hypothyroidism.

Histopathology and cytology

Histopathological examination requires an intact sample of the tissue called a biopsy. Biopsies can be taken from many organs in the endocrine and reproductive systems if an abnormality or tumor is suspected. The specimens are examined for abnormal cells and tissue structure:

- Inflammatory cells—show the presence of inflammation or infection.
- Tissue structure changes (e.g., necrosis, hyperplasia).

Cytology requires only a cell sample (e.g., cervical smear). A full biopsy is not needed, but it can be used. The cells are examined for cancerous changes called dysplasia.

Imaging of the endocrine and reproductive systems

Plain x-ray radiography

Plain x-rays demonstrate bony structures and calcified areas within organs because these tissues are radiopaque (white), while soft tissues are radiolucent (gray to black). They are used to investigate endocrine and reproductive disorders that cause bone abnormalities:

- Acromegaly—thickened skull, enlarged jaw and hands (Fig. 17.7).
- Hyperparathyroidism and rickets—osteomalacia.
- Cushing's syndrome and thyrotoxicosis—osteoporosis.
- Prostate bony metastases—osteosclerotic lesions.
- Other bony metastases—osteolytic lesions.
- Size of the pituitary fossa—enlarged with large adenomas.
- Organ calcification—following disease in the adrenal glands.

Contrast media

Contrast media and dyes can be used to image soft tissues. Contrast media are used with x-rays; they must be radiopaque and inert to prevent damage to the organ. The contrast medium or dye can be ingested or injected into a specific body compartment to allow visualization with x-rays.

Angiography

A contrast medium is injected into the arteries (intraarterially) or veins (intravenously), allowing these blood vessels and the organs they supply to be visualized (Fig. 17.8).

Fluorescein angiography

This is a form of angiography used to visualize the retinal vessels. A fluorescein contrast medium is injected intravenously and the retina is photographed using ultraviolet light that causes the fluorescein to fluoresce. This technique is especially useful in the investigation of diabetic retinopathy.

Hysterosalpingography

A contrast medium is injected into the uterus and fallopian tubes via the cervix. Its progression along the fallopian tubes is imaged using real-time x-ray screening (Fig. 17.9).

Mammography

Mammography is one method of investigating and screening for breast lesions. Early detection of breast cancer by mammography may improve the prognosis. An example of a normal breast and one affected by cancer are shown in Fig. 17.10.

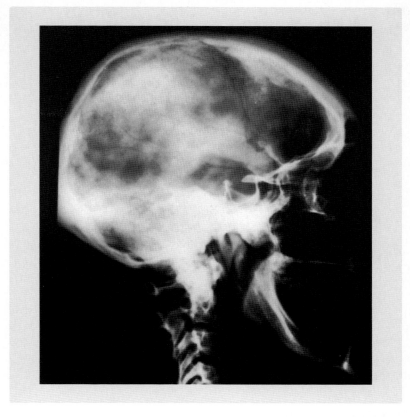

Fig. 17.7 Plain x-ray of the skull of a patient with acromegaly. It shows a large, protruding jaw, a large pituitary fossa, and a thick skull. (From Grainger R, Allison D, eds.: Diagnostic Radiology: A Textbook of Medical Imaging, 4th ed. London, Churchill Livingstone, 1996.)

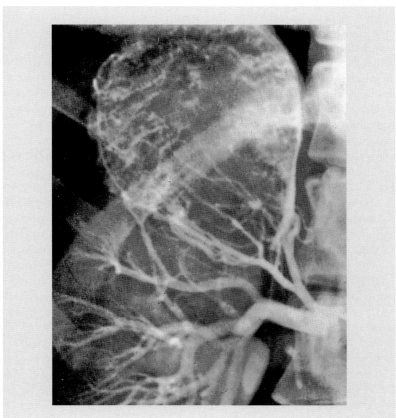

Fig. 17.8 Selective arteriogram of a pheochromocytoma. (From Sutton D: Textbook of Radiology and Imaging, 6th ed. London, Churchill Livingstone, 1995.)

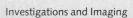
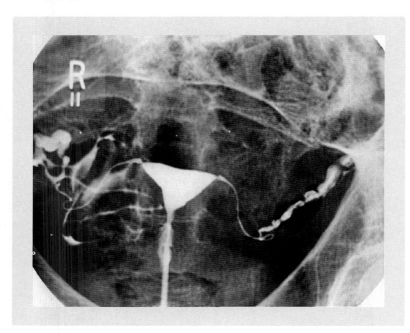

Fig. 17.9 Hysterosalpingogram of a normal uterus and fallopian tubes. (From Grainger R, Allison D, eds.: Diagnostic Radiology: A Textbook of Medical Imaging, 4th ed. London, Churchill Livingstone, 1996.)

Ultrasonography

Ultrasonography uses the reflection of harmless, high-frequency sound waves to determine the composition of various tissues throughout the body. The reflected sound waves are processed to produce an image in which fluid appears black and denser structures appear white.

Ultrasonography may be used to evaluate the size and composition of masses, determining if they are cystic or solid. Masses are commonly examined by ultrasound in the breast, ovaries, testes, thyroid gland, and adrenal glands. An example is shown in Fig. 17.11.

Ultrasound imaging is routinely used to examine the developing fetus and to investigate any abnormalities that may be suspected clinically. An example is shown in Fig. 17.12.

Computed tomography

Computed tomography (CT) produces cross-sectional images using x-rays, typically in the axial or horizontal plane. The x-ray emitter rotates about the patient, and the computer reconstructs an image by combining views from the multiple x-ray detectors. The computer can differentiate over 2000 densities; this is significantly more than conventional x-ray films. Bone appears white, and other soft tissues are gray to black. An example is shown in Fig. 17.13.

CT scanning has applications in almost all disease processes, particularly oncology and neurology. It can also be used for planning accurate biopsy and interventions.

In a similar manner to conventional radiography, contrast media are routinely used in CT to enhance imaging of tissues and vasculature. The same contrast media can be used as for conventional radiography.

Magnetic resonance imaging

Magnetic resonance imaging (MRI) produces cross-sectional images without using ionizing radiation. MRI uses strong external magnetic fields formed by magnetic coils around the patient to manipulate the protons that form the nucleus of hydrogen atoms. The protons behave like miniature magnets that line up to the strong magnetic field and gain energy in the process. Once the magnetic field is turned off, the protons release the energy they gained by inducing a current in the magnetic coils that produced the magnetic field. This current is detected and processed into a computerized image.

The hydrogen atoms detected are generally in water (H_2O). There are two main methods of processing the image:

- T1-weighted images: good anatomical detail; water is black.

Fig. 17.10 (A) Mammogram of a normal breast. (B) Mammogram of a breast containing a carcinoma. (From Sutton D: Textbook of Radiology and Imaging, 6th ed. London, Churchill Livingstone, 1995.)

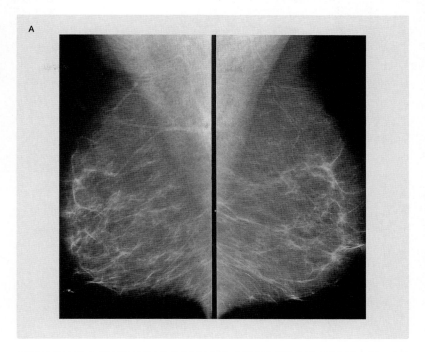

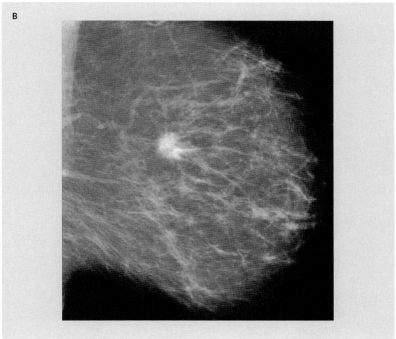

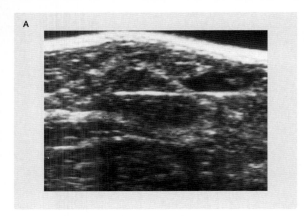

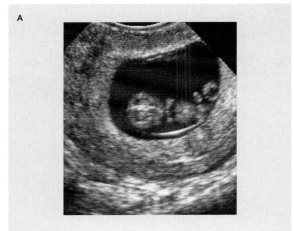

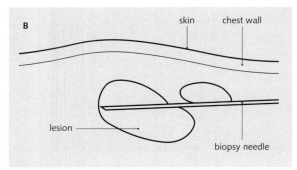

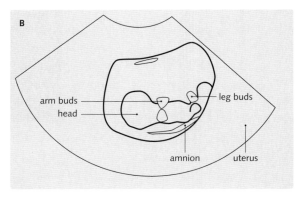

Fig. 17.11 (A) Ultrasound-guided needle biopsy of a breast mass. (B) Line drawing of A. Note that the needle is introduced parallel to the chest wall. (A, from Sutton D: Textbook of Radiology and Imaging, 6th ed. London, Churchill Livingstone, 1995.)

Fig. 17.12 (A) Transvaginal ultrasound scan of a normal 8–9-week fetus. (B) Line drawing of A. (A from Grainger R, Allison D, eds.: Diagnostic Radiology: A Textbook of Medical Imaging, 4th ed. London, Churchill Livingstone, 1996.)

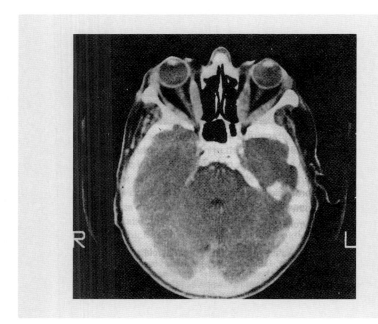

Fig. 17.13 CT scan showing exophthalmos in a patient with Graves' disease. (From Edwards CRW et al., eds.: Davidson's Principles and Practice of Medicine, 17th ed. London, Churchill Livingstone, 1997.)

Fig. 17.14 MRI scan (T2-weighted spin echo image) of large uterine leiomyomas, showing areas of high signal (curved arrow) and low signal (straight arrow). b, bladder; r, rectum. (From Sutton D: Textbook of Radiology and Imaging, 6th ed. London, Churchill Livingstone, 1995.)

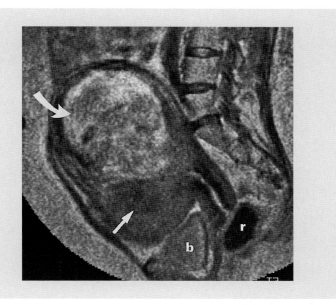

- T2-weighted images: good detail for pathological changes; water is white.

An example is shown in Fig. 17.14.

Radioisotope scans
Certain chemicals are absorbed more rapidly by different tissues. For example, iodine is actively absorbed by the thyroid gland. By tagging a chemical with a radioactive element (i.e., a radioisotope), uptake in the target tissue can be monitored using a gamma camera (this is called scintigraphy). This pattern of isotope uptake within the gland can expose abnormal areas.

This method is especially suitable for the thyroid gland because of the highly selective uptake of iodine. By administering an oral dose of ^{123}I (a radioactive isotope of iodine), the activity of different areas within the gland can be detected between 5 and 24 hours later. It allows measurement of:
- Hyperactivity.
- Abnormal anatomy.
- Tumors or nodules, including size and location.

Most tumors show up as inactive "cold" spots; however, hypersecretory tumors show up as active "hot" spots.

A better resolution can be achieved using intravenous technetium-99m pertechnetate. This substance is also less toxic and allows scanning just 20 minutes after injection. Examples are shown in Fig. 17.15.

Different substances can be used to scan the parathyroid and adrenal glands:
- Parathyroid glands—technetium-99m Sestamibi.
- Adrenal cortex—^{131}I-iodonorcholesterol (NP-59) or ^{75}Se-selenomethylnorcholesterol.
- Adrenal medulla—^{131}I-metaiodobenzylguanidine (mIBG).

Radioactive iodine is potentially harmful to the thyroid gland. Lugol's solution, which contains nonradioactive iodine, is given both the day before and on the test day to reduce the uptake of radioactive iodine by the thyroid gland.

243

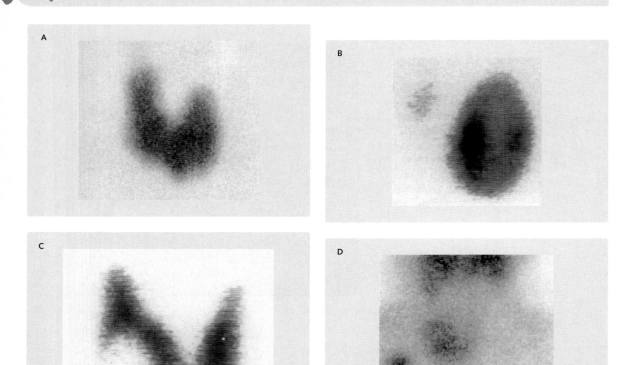

Fig. 17.15 Radioisotope thyroid images using technetium-99m pertechnetate. (A) Scan showing increased uptake throughout the gland in a patient with Graves' disease. (B) A patient with a single toxic nodule; the remainder of the gland is suppressed. (C) Increased uptake in a patient with Graves' disease but decreased uptake in a nontoxic (cold) lump (arrowed) consistent with a thyroid cancer or cyst. (D) ^{99m}Tc MIBI scan of recurrent papillary thyroid carcinoma not seen on ^{131}I scanning. (A, from Grainger R, Allison D, eds.: Diagnostic Radiology: A Textbook of Medical Imaging, 4th ed. London, Churchill Livingstone, 1996; B–D, from Murray IPC, Ell PJ, eds.: Nuclear Medicine, 2nd ed. London, Churchill Livingstone, 1996.)

- Describe the ELISA technique and its use in endocrinology.
- Which hormones are measured indirectly? Why?
- With an example, describe the situations in which a suppression test is used.
- With an example, describe the situations in which a stimulation test is used.
- Describe the triple stimulation test of pituitary function. Why are all these hormones tested together?
- With examples, describe how laboratory-based investigations other than for hormone levels can aid diagnosis.
- Describe the use of plain and contrast-enhanced radiography in diagnosis of endocrine and reproductive disorders.
- Describe the use of ultrasound in diagnosis of endocrine and reproductive disorders.
- Describe the use of CT and MRI scans in diagnosis of endocrine and reproductive disorders.
- Describe the use of radioisotope scans in diagnosis of endocrine and reproductive disorders.

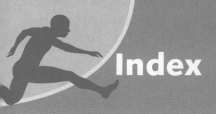

Index

Page numbers in *italics* refer to figures and tables

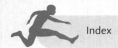

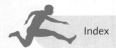

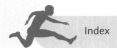

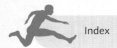

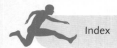

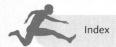

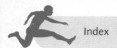

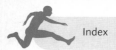

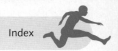